Nurses' Handbook of Health Assessment

fifth edition

Janet R. Weber, RN, EdD
Professor
Department of Nursing
Southeast Missouri State University
Cape Girardeau, Missouri

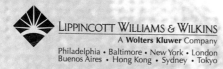

LIPPINCOTT WILLIAMS & WILKINS
A **Wolters Kluwer** Company
Philadelphia • Baltimore • New York • London
Buenos Aires • Hong Kong • Sydney • Tokyo

Senior Acquisitions Editor: Elizabeth Nieginski
Developmental Editor: Deedie McMahon
Editorial Assistant: Josh Levandoski
Director of Nursing Production: Helen Ewan
Managing Editor / Production: Erika Kors
Art Director: Carolyn O'Brien
Design Coordinator: Brett MacNaughton
Interior Designer: Joan Wendt
Cover Designer: Melissa Walter
Senior Manufacturing Manager: William Alberti
Indexer: Gaye Tarallo
Compositor: Circle Graphics
Printer: R.R. Donnelley, Crawfordsville

5th Edition

9 8 7 6 5 4 3 2

Library of Congress Cataloging-in-Publication Data

Weber, Janet.
  Nurses' handbook of health assessment / Janet R. Weber.— 5th ed.
      p. ; cm.
  Includes bibliographical references and index.
  ISBN 0-7817-5340-6 (alk. paper)
  1. Nursing assessment—Handbooks, manuals, etc. I. Title.
  [DNLM: 1. Nursing assessment—methods—Handbooks. 2. Medical History Taking—methods—Handbooks. 3. Physical Examination—methods—Handbooks. WY 49 W374n 2005]
RT48.N863 2005
616.07'5—dc22   2004008378

LWW.com

To my loving husband, Bill, for all
your wise encouragement, patience
and confidence

To my son, Joe, for teaching me to
live more fully by relaxing and
taking risks

To my son, Wesley, for your
endless, energizing humor and wise
insights

To my mom for photocopying and
tending to details

To my colleagues, Jane and Ann,
for all your contributions that hold
this guide together

To all my students who teach me
how to teach

To all the nurses who inspire me to
continue to write

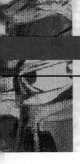

Contributors

Jill Cash, RN-CS, MSN, FNP
Family Nurse Practitioner
Carbondale Family Medicine
Carbondale, Illinois
Instructor, Graduate Family Nurse Practitioner Program
Southern Illinois University
Edwardsville, Illinois

Jane Kelley, RN, PhD
Professor of Nursing
School of Nursing University of Mississippi
    Medical Center
Jackson, Mississippi

Rosie Danker, RN, BSN, CDE
Diabetes Clinician
St. Francis Medical Center
Cape Girardeau, Missouri

Ann Sprengel, RN, EdD
Professor of Nursing
Southeast Missouri State University
Cape Girardeau, Missouri

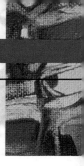

Preface

PURPOSE

The fifth edition of the *Nurses' Handbook of Health Assessment* continues to provide students and practicing nurses with an up-to-date reference and guide to assist with interviewing clients and performing a physical assessment.

This guide will remind the student or nurse of questions to ask, examinations to make, and procedures to carry out when assessing the client. In addition, it clearly identifies normal versus abnormal findings and supplies examples of precise descriptive language that will make documentation easy and accurate.

COLORFUL NEW LOOK

New to the fifth edition are full-color anatomy and physiology images, illustrations of normal and abnormal physiologic findings, and highlighted risk factors. A feature carried over from the fourth edition is the three-column format of assessment procedures and the spiral binding that allows the handbook to stay open on any flat surface.

STREAMLINED ORGANIZATION

The handbook has 20 chapters. The first three provide an overview of the nursing assessment process and its rationale.

Chapter 1 explains the purpose of a nursing health history. *Chapter 2* contains guidelines needed to elicit subjective data for a complete nursing health history, and begins with questions for a client profile and developmental history followed by health history questions organized according to Gordon's 11 functional health patterns (Gordon, 1994). The reader is referred to specific physical assessment chapters for related objective data as appropriate. A list of associated nursing diagnoses that may be identified by client response follows each section. The nursing diagnoses are based on the currently accepted North American Nursing Diagnosis Association (NANDA) taxonomy of diagnostic categories. The functional health patterns format focuses the health history within the independent domain of professional nursing. *Chapter 3* consists of guidelines for performing the physical assessment.

Chapters 4 through *20* present assessment procedures in an easy to understand format. Each chapter contains the following:

- Focus questions specific to the body system being assessed
- Illustration of relevant anatomy or physiologic processes
- Equipment needed for the examination
- Physical assessment procedure
- Pediatric variations
- Geriatric variations
- Cultural variations
- Selected and related collaborative problems
- Teaching tips

Chapters 18, 19, and *20* are a guide to special assessments:

- Nutritional assessment
- Maternal assessment
- Newborn assessment

COLLECTION OF STANDARD ASSESSMENT TOOLS

Twelve appendices bring together in one convenient place the many reference tools needed for health assessment. These include nursing assessment forms, developmental norms, growth charts, immunization schedules, sample of an adult health history and physical assessment, a family assessment, breast and skin self-examination guides, blood pressure classification and management guide, nursing diagnoses, and collaborative problems.

Janet R. Weber, RN, EdD

Acknowledgments

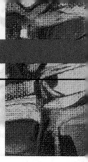

I would like to thank the instructors who offered insight and suggestions for this revision

Paula Herberg, RN, PhD
Associate Professor of Nursing
California State University, Fullerton
Fullerton, California

Catherine T. Horat, RN, MSN, CS, C-FNP
Assistant Professor
Georgia Baptist College of Nursing of Mercer University
Atlanta, Georgia

Sharon Jensen, RN, MN
Instructor, Nursing
Seattle University
Seattle, Washington

Joshua Nelson Roberts, RN, NS
Student Nurse (RN)
South Puget Sound Community College
Olympia, Washington

Eric G. Stennes
Student
South Puget Sound Community College
Olympia, Washington

Delores Williams, RN, MS
Professor, Department of Nursing
Central Texas College
Killeen, Texas

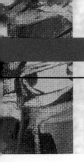

Contents

1 The Nursing Health History   1

2 Components of the Nursing Health History   13

3 Physical Assessment   35

4 General Physical Survey   45

5 Skin, Hair, and Nail Assessment   62

6 Head, Neck, and Cervical Lymph Node Assessment   82

7 Mouth, Oropharynx, Nose, and Sinus Assessment   96

8 Eye Assessment   122

9 Ear Assessment   151

10 Thoracic and Lung Assessment   170

11 Cardiac Assessment   198

12 Peripheral Vascular Assessment   223

13 Breast Assessment   252

14 Abdominal Assessment   269

15 Genitourinary-Reproductive Assessment   296
   Assessment of Female Genitalia/296
   Assessment of Male Genitalia/308
   Assessment of Inguinal Area/313
   Assessment of Rectum/316

16 Musculoskeletal Assessment   338

17 Neurologic Assessment   372
   Mental Status Assessment/378
   Cranial Nerve Assessment/395
   Sensory Nerve Assessment/402
   Motor Assessment/406
   Cerebellar Assessment/406
   Reflex Assessment/412

18 Nutritional Assessment 424
19 Maternal Physical Assessment 444
20 Initial Newborn Physical Assessment 482

APPENDICES

Appendix 1: Nursing Assessment Form Based on Functional Health Patterns 512
Appendix 2: Developmental Information—Age 1 Month to 18 Years 522
Appendix 3: Recommended Childhood and Adolescent Immunization Schedule—United States, 2003 529
Appendix 4: Psychosocial Development 535
Appendix 5: Height–Weight–Head Circumference Charts for Children 537
Appendix 6: How to Examine Your Own Skin 546
Appendix 7: Breast Self-Examination (BSE) 550
Appendix 8: Classification and Management of Blood Pressure for Adults 553
Appendix 9: Sample Adult Nursing Health History and Physical Assessment 555
Appendix 10: Assessment of Family Functional Health Patterns 569
Appendix 11: Nursing Diagnoses (Wellness, Risk, and Actual) Grouped According to Functional Health Patterns 577
Appendix 12: Collaborative Problems 583

References 585

Index 591

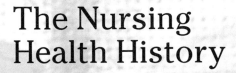
The Nursing Health History

DEFINITION AND PURPOSE

A nursing health history can be defined as the systematic collection of subjective data (stated by the client) and objective data (observed by the nurse) used to determine a client's functional health pattern status (Table 1–1). The nurse collects physiologic, psychological, sociocultural, developmental, and spiritual client data. These data assist the nurse in identifying nursing diagnoses and/or collaborative problems.

The North American Nursing Diagnoses Association (NANDA, 2003–2004) defines a nursing diagnosis as a clinical judgment about individual, family, or community responses to actual and potential health problems and life processes. A nursing diagnosis provides the basis for selection of nursing interventions to achieve outcomes for which the nurse is accountable. Nursing diagnoses fall into three categories: (1) wellness diagnoses (opportunity to enhance health status), (2) risk diagnoses, and/or (3) actual nursing diagnoses.

Wellness diagnoses may be described as opportunities for enhancement of a healthy state (Kelley, Avant, & Frisch, 1995). There are occasions when clients are ready to improve an already healthy level of function. When such an opportunity exists, the nurse can support the client's movement toward greater health and wellness by identifying "opportunities for enhancement." If a client does not have a diagnosis but data reveal a risk for its development, the nurse can focus on reducing factors for a *risk diagnosis* (Table 1–2). Actual diagnoses present a current client problem.

Carpenito (2004) defines collaborative problems as certain "physiological complications that nurses monitor to detect their onset or changes in status. Nurses manage collaborative problems using both physician-prescribed and nursing-prescribed interventions to minimize the complications of the events." The definitive treatment for a

TABLE 1–1	COMPARING SUBJECTIVE AND OBJECTIVE DATA	
	Subjective	**Objective**
Description	Data elicited and verified by the client	Data directly or indirectly observed through measurement
Sources	Client Family and significant others Client record Other health care professionals	Observations and physical assessment findings of the nurse or other health care professionals Documentation of assessments made in client record Observations made by the client's family or significant others
Methods used to obtain data	Client interview	Observation and physical examination
Skills needed to obtain data	Interview and therapeutic communication skills Caring ability and empathy Listening skills	Inspection Palpation Percussion Auscultation
Examples	"I have a headache." "It frightens me." "I am not hungry."	Respirations 16 per minute BP 180/100, apical pulse 80 and irregular X-ray film reveals fractured pelvis

nursing diagnosis is developed by the nurse; the definitive treatment for a collaborative problem is developed by both the nurse and the physician. Not all physiologic complications are collaborative problems. If the nurse can prevent the complication or provide the primary treatment, then the problem may very well be a nursing diagnosis. For example, nurses can prevent and treat pressure ulcers. The NANDA nursing diagnosis to use, therefore, is Risk for Impaired Skin Integrity.

TABLE 1–2 COMPARISON OF WELLNESS, RISK, AND ACTUAL NURSING DIAGNOSES

	Wellness Diagnoses	Risk Diagnoses	Actual Nursing Diagnoses
Client status	Human responses to levels of wellness that have a readiness for enhancement (NANDA, 2003–2004)	Human responses that may develop in a vulnerable individual, family, or community (NANDA, 2003–2004)	Human responses to health conditions/life processes that exist (NANDA, 2003–2004)
Format for stating	Readiness for Enhanced . . .	"Risk for . . ."	"Nursing diagnoses and related to clause"
Examples	Readiness for Enhanced Body Image Readiness for Enhanced Family Processes Readiness for Enhanced Effective Breast-feeding Readiness for Enhanced Skin Integrity	Risk for Disturbed Body Image Risk for Interrupted Family Processes Risk for Ineffective Breast-feeding Risk for Impaired Skin Integrity	Disturbed Body Image related to wound on hand that is not healing Dysfunctional Family Processes: Alcoholism Ineffective Breast-feeding related to poor mother–infant attachment Impaired Skin Integrity related to immobility

Nursing diagnoses, risk nursing diagnoses, wellness nursing diagnoses, and collaborative problems are listed in Appendices 11 and 12.

Collaborative problems are equivalent in importance to nursing diagnoses but represent the interdependent or collaborative role of nursing, whereas nursing diagnoses represent the independent role of the nurse (Carpenito 2004). Figure 1–1 illustrates the decision-making process involved in distinguishing a nursing diagnosis from a collaborative health problem. The nurse can use this model to decide whether the identified problem can be treated independently as a nursing diagnosis, or whether the nurse will monitor and use both medical and nursing interventions to treat or prevent the problem. If collaborative medical and nursing interventions are not needed, the problem is discharged from nursing care and referred to medicine and/or dentistry. The difference between a medical diagnosis, collaborative problem, and nursing diagnosis is explained in Table 1–3. Guidelines for formulating nursing diagnoses and collaborative problems can be found in Table 1–4.

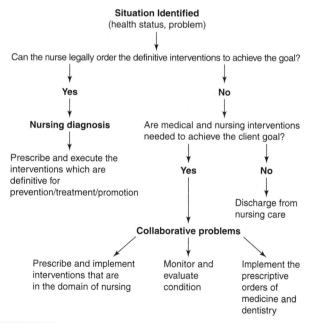

FIGURE 1–1 Differentiation of nursing diagnoses from collaborative problems. (Carpenito, L. J. [2004]. *Nursing Diagnoses: Application to Clinical Practice,* 10th ed. Philadelphia: Lippincott Williams & Wilkins, p. 22.)

TABLE 1–3 EXAMPLES OF MEDICAL DIAGNOSES, COLLABORATIVE PROBLEMS, AND NURSING DIAGNOSES

Medical Diagnoses	Collaborative Problems	Nursing Diagnoses
Fractured jaw	Potential complication: aspiration	Impaired Oral Mucous Membrane related to difficulty with hygiene secondary to fixation devices
		Chronic Pain related to tissue trauma
Diabetes mellitus	Potential complication: hyperglycemia	Impaired Skin Integrity related to poor circulation to lower extremities
		Deficient Knowledge related to the effects of exercise on need for insulin
Pneumonia	Potential complication: hypoglycemia	Ineffective Airway Clearance related to presence of excessive mucus
	Potential complication: hypoxemia	Deficient Fluid Volume related to poor fluid intake

TABLE 1–4   COMPARISON OF NURSING DIAGNOSES AND COLLABORATIVE PROBLEMS

Identifying Criteria of a Nursing Diagnosis	Identifying Criteria of a Collaborative Problem
1. The client problem is physiological, psychosocial, or spiritual.	1. The client problem is a physiologic complication.
2. The nurse monitors and treats.	2. The nurse monitors for signs and symptoms of the complication and notifies the physician if a change occurs. (In some cases the nurse may initiate interventions.)
3. The nurse independently orders and implements the primary nursing interventions.	3. The physician orders the primary treatment, and the nurse collaborates to implement additional treatments that are licensed to be implemented, and monitors for responses to and effectiveness of treatments.
Format for Stating Nursing Diagnoses	**Format for Stating Collaborative Problems**
1. Use problem + "related to" + etiology.	1. Use "Potential complication: _____."
2. Write specific client goals.	2. Write nursing goals.
3. Write specific nursing orders (interventions), including assessments, teaching, counseling, referrals, and direct client care.	3. Write which parameters the nurse must monitor, including how often. Indicate when the physician should be notified. Identify nursing interventions to prevent the complication and those to be initiated if a change occurs.

A nursing health history usually precedes the physical assessment and guides the nurse as to which body systems must be assessed. It also assists the nurse in establishing a nurse–client relationship, and allows client participation in identifying problems and goals. The primary source of data is the client; valuable information may also be obtained from the family, other health team members, and the client record.

NURSING MODEL VERSUS MEDICAL MODEL

Several models of nursing may be used to guide the nurse in data collection. Marjory Gordon's Functional Health Pattern assessment framework (1994) is particularly useful, however, in collecting health data to formulate nursing diagnoses. Gordon has defined 11 functional health patterns that provide for a holistic client database. A pattern is a sequence of related behaviors that assists the nurse in collecting and categorizing data. These 11 functional health patterns can be used for nursing assessment in any practice areas for clients of all ages and in the assessment of families and communities. For the purpose of this handbook, assessment is focused on the individual. However, guideline questions for families organized according to functional health patterns are included in Appendix 10. The NANDA list of accepted nursing diagnoses has been grouped according to the appropriate functional health patterns. These diagnoses are listed at the end of each functional health pattern section in Chapter 2. Box 1–1 presents a brief overview of the subjective and objective assessment focus data needed for each functional health pattern.*

Using a functional health pattern framework assists the nurse with collecting data necessary to identify and validate nursing diagnoses. This approach eliminates repetition of medical data already obtained by physicians and other members of the health care team. The medical systems model (biographical data, chief complaint, present health history, past medical history, family history, psychosocial history, and review of systems) is more useful for the physician in making medical diagnoses. Clients often complain that the same information is requested by both nurses and physicians. A nursing history based on functional health patterns, however, will help eliminate this problem by assisting the nurse to assess client responses associated with nursing diagnoses and collaborative problems.

It is important for the nurse to assess each functional health pattern with clients because alterations in health can affect functioning in any of these areas, and alterations in functional health patterns can, in turn, affect health. See Appendix 1 for a sample nursing assessment form based on functional health patterns.

*Adapted from Gordon, M. (1994). *Nursing Diagnosis: Process and Application,* (3rd ed). St. Louis: Mosby—Year Book.

BOX 1–1. Subjective and Objective Assessment Focus for Functional Health Patterns

1. Health Perception–Health Management Pattern
   Subjective data: Perception of health status and health practices used by client to maintain health
   Objective data: Appearance, grooming, posture, expression, vital signs, height, weight

2. Nutritional–Metabolic Pattern
   Subjective data: Dietary habits, including food and fluid intake
   Objective data: General physical survey, including examination of skin, mouth, abdomen, and cranial nerves (CN) V, IX, X, and XII

3. Elimination Pattern
   Subjective data: Regularity and control of bowel and bladder habits
   Objective data: Skin examination, rectal examination

4. Activity–Exercise Pattern
   Subjective data: Activities of daily living that require energy expenditure
   Objective data: Examination of musculoskeletal system, including gait, posture, range of motion (ROM) of joints, muscle tone, and strength; cardiovascular examination; peripheral vascular examination; thoracic examination

5. Sexuality–Reproduction Pattern
   Subjective data: Sexual identity, activities, and relationships; expression of sexuality and level of satisfaction with sexual patterns; reproduction patterns
   Objective data: Genitalia examination, breast examination

6. Sleep–Rest Pattern
   Subjective data: Perception of effectiveness of sleep and rest habits
   Objective data: Appearance and attention span

7. Cognitive–Perceptual Pattern
   For the purposes of this handbook, the cognitive–perceptual pattern has been divided into two parts: (1) the sensory–perceptual pattern, to include the senses of hearing, vision, smell, taste, and touch, and (2) the cognitive pattern, to include knowledge, thought perception, and language.
   a. Sensory–Perceptual Pattern
      Subjective data: Perception of ability to hear, see, smell, taste, and feel (including light touch, pain, and vibratory sensation)

> **BOX 1–1.** (*continued*)
>
> > **Objective data:** Visual and hearing examinations, pain perception, cranial nerve examination; testing for taste, smell, and touch
> >
> > b. Cognitive Pattern
> >
> > **Subjective data:** Perception of messages, decision making, thought processes
> >
> > **Objective data:** Mental status examination
>
> 8. Role–Relationship Pattern
>
>   **Subjective data:** Perception of and level of satisfaction with family, work, and social roles
>
>   **Objective data:** Communication with significant others, visits from significant others and family, family genogram
>
> 9. Self-perception–Self-concept Pattern
>
>   **Subjective data:** Perception of self-worth, personal identity, feelings
>
>   **Objective data:** Body posture, movement, eye contact, voice and speech pattern, emotions, moods, and thought content
>
> 10. Coping–Stress Tolerance Pattern
>
>   **Subjective data:** Perception of stressful life events and ability to cope
>
>   **Objective data:** Behavior, thought processes
>
> 11. Value–Belief Pattern
>
>   **Subjective data:** Perception of what is good, correct, proper, and meaningful; philosophical beliefs; values and beliefs that guide choices
>
>   **Objective data:** Presence of religious articles, religious actions and routines, and visits from clergy

GUIDELINES FOR OBTAINING A NURSING HEALTH HISTORY

Phases of the Nursing Interview

Professional interpersonal and interviewing skills are necessary to obtain a valid nursing health history. The nursing interview is a communication process that focuses on the client's developmental, psychological, physiologic, sociocultural, and spiritual responses that can be treated with nursing and collaborative interventions. The nursing interview has three basic phases, explained below by describing the roles of the nurse and the client during each phase.

Introductory Phase

Introduce yourself and describe your role (ie, RN, student, etc). Address the client with surname. Next, explain the purpose of the interview to the client (ie, to collect data, to understand the client's needs, and to plan nursing care). Explain the purpose of note taking, confidentiality, and the type of questions to be asked. Provide comfort, privacy, and confidentiality.

Working Phase
Facilitate the client's comments about major biographical data, reason for seeking health care, and functional health pattern responses. Use critical thinking skills to listen for and observe cues, and to interpret and validate information received from the client. Collaborate with the client to identify problems and goals. The approach used for facilitation may be either free flowing or more structured with specific questions, depending on available time and type of data needed.

Summary and Closure Phase
Summarize information obtained during the working phase and validate problems and goals with the client. You may begin to discuss possible plans to resolve the problems (nursing diagnoses and collaborative problems). Allow the client time to express feelings, concerns, and questions.

Specific Communication Techniques

Specific communication techniques are used to facilitate the interview. Following are specific guidelines for phrasing statements and questions to promote an effective and productive interview.

Types of Questions to Use
- Use open-ended questions to elicit the client's feelings and perceptions. These questions begin with "What," "How," or "Which," and require more than a one-word response.
- Use closed-ended questions to obtain facts and zero in on specific information. The client can respond with one or two words. These questions begin with "Is," "Are," "Will," "When," or "Did," and help avoid rambling by the client.
- Use a laundry list (scrambled words) approach to obtain specific answers. For example, "Is the pain severe, dull, sharp, mild, cutting, piercing?" "Does the pain occur once every year, day, month, hour?" This reduces the likelihood of the client's perceiving and providing an expected answer.
- Explore all data that deviate from normal with the following questions: "What alleviates or aggravates the problem?" "How long has it occurred?" "How severe is it?" "Does it radiate?" "When does it occur?" "Is its onset gradual or sudden?"

Types of Statements to Use
- Rephrase or repeat your perception of the client's response to reflect or clarify information shared. For example, "You feel you have a serious illness?"
- Encourage verbalization of client by saying "Um hum," "Yes," or "I agree," or nodding.
- Describe what you observe in the client. For example, "It seems you have difficulty on the right side."

Additional Helpful Hints

● Accept the client; display a nonjudgmental attitude.
● Use silence to help the client and yourself reflect and reorganize thoughts.
● Provide the client with information during the interview as questions and concerns arise.

Communication Styles to Avoid

● Excessive or insufficient eye contact (varies with cultures).
● Doing other things while taking the history, and being mentally distant or physically far away from client (more than 2–3 feet).
● Biased or leading questions—for example, "You don't feel bad, do you?"
● Relying on memory to recall all the information or recording all the details.
● Rushing the client.
● Reading questions from the history form, distracting attention from the client.

Specific Age Variations

When interviewing the pediatric client from birth to early adolescence (through age 14 years), information from the history should be validated for reliability with the responsible significant other (eg, parent, grandparent).

Use the following guidelines when interviewing the geriatric patient:

● Use a gentle, genuine approach.
● Use simple, straightforward questions in lay terms. Let the client set the pace of the conversation. Be patient and listen well. Allow ample time.
● Introduce yourself, but remember that an older client may soon forget your name—you may have to write it for the client later in the interview.
● Use direct eye contact and sit at client's eye level. Establish and maintain privacy (especially important).
● Assess hearing acuity; with loss, speak slowly, face the client, and speak on the side on which hearing is more adequate. Speak louder only if you confirm client has a hearing deficit. Turn off any background noises.
● *Remember:* Age affects and often slows all body systems within an individual to varying degrees.
● Wear a name tag and provide written notes for the client to refer to in the future.

Emotional Variations

● *Angry client:* Approach in a calm, reassuring, in-control manner. Allow ventilation of client's feelings. Avoid arguing and provide personal space.
● *Anxious client:* Approach with simple, organized information. Explain your role and purpose.
● *Manipulative client:* Provide structure and set limits.

- *Depressed client:* Express interest and understanding in a neutral manner.
- *Sensitive issues* (eg, sexuality, dying, spirituality): Be aware of your own thoughts and feelings. These factors may affect the client's health and need to be discussed with someone. Such personal, sensitive topics may be referred when you do not feel comfortable discussing these topics.

Cultural Variations

Ethnic variations in communication and self-disclosure styles may seriously affect the information obtained. Be aware of possible variations in the communication styles of yourself and patient. If misunderstanding or difficulty in communicating is evident, seek help from a "culture broker" who is skilled at cross-cultural communication. Frequently noted ethnic variations include:

- Reluctance to reveal personal information to strangers for various culturally based reasons.
- Variation in willingness to express emotional distress or pain openly.
- Variation in ability to receive information and/or listen.
- Variation in meaning conveyed by use of language (eg, by non-native speakers, by use of slang).
- Variation in use and meaning of nonverbal communication: eye contact, stance, gestures, demeanor (eg, eye contact may be perceived as rude, aggressive, or immodest by some cultures, but lack of eye contact may be perceived as evasive, insecure, or inattentive by other cultures; slightly bowed stance may indicate respect in some groups; size of personal space affects one's comfortable interpersonal distance; touch may be perceived as comforting or threatening).
- Variation in disease/illness perception; culture-specific syndromes or disorders are accepted by some groups (eg, *susto* in Latin America). *Susto* (fright or emotional shock) is perceived to cause general malaise, insomnia, irritability, depression, nightmares, and wasting away (dePaula, Laganá, & Gonzalez–Ramirez, 1996, p. 217).
- Variation in past, present, or future time orientation (eg, United States dominant culture is future-oriented; other cultures vary).
- Variation in family decision-making process: person other than client or client's parent may be the major decision maker re: appointments, treatments, or follow-up care for client.

Assessing Non-English-Speaking Clients

- Use a bilingual interpreter familiar with the client's culture and with health care, when possible (eg, a nurse culture broker).
- Consider the relationship of the interpreter to the client. If the interpreter is a child or of a different sex, age, or social status, interpretation may be impaired.
- Not all clients can read. Basic care terms can be communicated best by pictures.

Components of the Nursing Health History

HEALTH HISTORY BY FUNCTIONAL HEALTH PATTERN

Following are the components of a nursing health history incorporating a functional health pattern approach (Gordon, 1994). Prior to data collection for each functional health pattern, a client profile and developmental history are obtained.

1. Client Profile
2. Developmental History
3. Health Perception–Health Management Pattern
4. Nutritional–Metabolic Pattern
5. Elimination Pattern
6. Activity–Exercise Pattern
7. Sexuality–Reproduction Pattern
8. Sleep–Rest Pattern
9. Sensory–Perceptual Pattern
10. Cognitive Pattern
11. Role–Relationship Pattern
12. Self-Perception–Self-Concept Pattern
13. Coping–Stress Tolerance Pattern
14. Value–Belief Pattern

The purpose of each nursing health history component will be explained, followed by guideline statements and questions to elicit subjective data from the client. Guideline questions should be preceded by open-ended statements to encourage the client to verbalize freely. Then specific questions are asked to obtain specific information. It is important to remember that not every question will apply to every client. Common sense and professional judgment must be used to determine which questions are a priority and appropriate for each individual client.

Certain factors such as comfort level, anxiety level, age, and current health status must be considered as they influence the client's ability to participate fully in the interview. When appropriate, an objective data outline follows the subjective data questions and refers the examiner to the section where the specific examination technique, normal findings, and deviations from normal are located. At the end of each section is a list of corresponding nursing diagnostic categories for that specific nursing health history component. This list is divided into wellness nursing diagnoses, risk nursing diagnoses, and actual (problem) nursing diagnoses. Although clients can be at risk for most problem diagnoses, only NANDA-approved and a few selected other risk diagnoses are listed. Appendix 1 provides a documentation form for collection of subjective and objective data for each of the functional health patterns.

CLIENT PROFILE

Purpose

The purpose of the client profile is to determine biographical client data and to obtain an overview of past and present medical diagnoses and treatment that may alter a client's response. This section also helps the interviewer elicit collaborative health problems.

Subjective Data: Guideline Questions

Biographical Data

What is your name?
Tell me about your background.
When were you born?
What is your ethnic origin?
How old are you?
What level of education have you completed?
Have you ever served in the military?
Do you have a religious preference? Specify.
Where do you live?
What form of transportation do you use to come here or go other places?
Where is the closest health care facility to you that you would go to if ill or in an emergency?

Reason for Seeking Health Care and Current Understanding of Health

Explain your major reason for seeking health care.
What has the doctor told you regarding your health?
Do you understand your medical diagnosis? Explain.

Treatments/Medications

Describe the treatments and medications you have received.
How has your illness been treated in the past?

What is being planned for your treatment now?
Do you understand the purpose of your treatment?
Have you been satisfied with past treatments? Explain.
What prescribed medications are you taking?
What over-the-counter medications are you taking?
Do you have any difficulties with these medications?
How do they make you feel?
What is the purpose of these medications?

Past Illnesses/Hospitalizations

Tell me about any past illnesses/surgeries you have had.
Have you had other illnesses in the past? Specify.
How were the past illnesses treated?
Have you ever been in the hospital before? Where? For what purpose?
How did you feel about your past hospital stays?
How can we help to improve this hospital stay for you?
Have you received any home health care? Explain.
How satisfied were you with this care?

Allergies

Are you allergic to any drugs, foods, or other environmental substances (eg, dust, molds, pollens, latex)?
Describe the reaction you have when exposed to the allergen.
What do you do for your allergies?

DEVELOPMENTAL HISTORY

Purpose

The purpose of the developmental history is to determine the physical, cognitive, and psychosocial development of the client to assess any developmental delays. Subjective data obtained from assessment of the functional health patterns (Role–Relationship, Cognitive, Value–Belief, and Coping–Stress Tolerance) will assist you in determining cognitive and psychosocial development. Appendix 2 provides a comparison developmental table for the child. Psychosocial development of the adult and aging adult is provided in Appendix 4. Objective data obtained from the physical examination regarding height, weight, and musculoskeletal function provide a basis for determining physical development (see Developmental Information, Appendix 2, and growth charts, Appendix 5).

Subjective Data: Guideline Questions

Describe any physical handicaps you have.
Tell me about your health and growth as a child.
Tell me about your accomplishments in life.
What are your lifelong goals?
Has your illness interfered with these goals?

Objective Data

Appendices 2, 4, and 5 provide normal information and developmental norms based on age to provide a baseline by which to compare your client's physical, psychosocial, and cognitive development.

Does this client have obvious developmental lags that need further assessment?

Does this client's illness interfere with the ability to accomplish the necessary developmental, physical, psychosocial, and cognitive tasks required at each age level for normal development?

Does this client have any physical, psychosocial, or cognitive developmental lags that aggravate his or her illness or inhibit self-care?

HEALTH PERCEPTION–HEALTH MANAGEMENT PATTERN

Purpose

The purpose of assessing the client's health perception–health maintenance pattern is to determine how the client perceives and manages his or her health. Compliance with current and past nursing and medical recommendations is assessed. The client's ability to perceive the relationship between activities of daily living and health is also determined.

Subjective Data: Guideline Questions

Client's Perception of Health

Describe your health

How would you rate your health on a scale of 1 to 10 (10 is excellent) now, 5 years ago, and 5 years ahead?

Client's Perception of Illness

Describe your illness or current health problem.

How has this affected your normal daily activities?

How do you feel your current daily activities have affected your health?

What do you believe caused your illness?

What course do you predict your illness will take?

How do you believe your illness should be treated?

Do you have or anticipate any difficulties in caring for yourself or others at home? If yes, explain.

Health Management and Habits

Tell me what you do when you have a health problem.

When do you seek nursing or medical advice?

How often do you go for professional exams (dental, Pap smears, breast, blood pressure)?

What activities do you believe keep you healthy? Contribute to illness?

Do you perform self-exams (blood pressure, breast, testicular)?
When were your last immunizations? Are they up to date?
   (See immunization Schedule, Appendix 3.)
Do you use alcohol, tobacco, drugs, caffeine? Describe the
   amount and length of time used.
Are you exposed to pollutants or toxins? Describe.

Compliance with Prescribed Medications and Treatments

Have you been able to take your prescribed medications? If not,
   what caused your inability to do so?
Have you been able to follow through with your prescribed
   nursing and medical treatment (eg, diet, exercise)? If not, what
   caused your inability to do so?

Objective Data

Refer to Chapter 4, General Physical Survey.

Associated Nursing Diagnostic Categories to Consider

Wellness Diagnoses

Effective Therapeutic Regimen Management: Individual
Health–Seeking Behaviors

Risk Diagnoses

Risk for Delayed Development
Risk for Delayed Growth
Risk for Injury
Risk for Perioperative Positioning Injury
Risk for Poisoning
Risk for Suffocation
Risk for Trauma

Actual Diagnoses

Delayed Growth and Development
Ineffective Health Maintenance
Disturbed Energy Field
Ineffective Therapeutic Regimen Management: Community
Ineffective Therapeutic Regimen Management: Family
Ineffective Therapeutic Regimen Management: Individual
Noncompliance (Specify)

NUTRITIONAL–METABOLIC PATTERN

Purpose

The purpose of assessing the client's nutritional–metabolic pattern is
to determine the client's dietary habits and metabolic needs. The conditions of hair, skin, nails, teeth, and mucous membranes are assessed.

Subjective Data: Guideline Questions

Dietary and Fluid Intake

Describe the type and amount of food you eat at breakfast, lunch, and supper on an average day.

Do you attempt to follow any certain type of diet? Explain.

What time do you usually eat your meals?

Do you find it difficult to eat meals on time? Explain.

What types of snacks do you eat? How often?

Do you take any vitamin supplements? Describe.

Do you take herbal supplements? Describe.

Do you consider your diet high in fat? Sugar? Salt?

Do you find it difficult to tolerate certain foods? Specify.

What kind of fluids do you usually drink? How much per day?

Do you have difficulty chewing or swallowing food?

When was your last dental exam? What were the results?

Do you ever experience a sore throat, sore tongue, or sore gums? Describe.

Do you ever experience nausea and vomiting? Describe.

Do you ever experience abdominal pains? Describe.

Do you use antacids? How often? What kind?

Condition of Skin

Describe the condition of your skin.

Describe your bathing routine.

Do you use sunscreens, lotions, oils? Describe.

How well and how quickly does your skin heal?

Do you have any skin lesions? Describe.

Do you have excessively oily or dry skin?

Do you have any itching? What do you do for relief?

Condition of Hair and Nails

Describe the condition of your hair and nails.

Do you use artificial nails? How often? How long? Have you ever had problems with these nails?

Do you have excessively oily or dry hair?

Have you had difficulty with scalp itching or sores?

Do you use any special hair or scalp care products (ie, permanents, coloring, straighteners)?

Have you noticed any changes in your nails? Color? Cracking? Shape? Lines?

Metabolism

What would you consider to be your ideal weight?

Have you had any recent weight gains or losses? Describe.

Have you used any measures to gain or lose weight? Describe.

Do you have any intolerances to heat or cold?

Have you noted any changes in your eating or drinking habits? Explain.

Have you noticed any voice changes?

Have you had difficulty with nervousness?

Objective Data

Assess the client's temperature, pulse, respirations, and height and weight. Refer to Chapter 5, Skin, Hair, and Nail Assessment; Chapter 6, Head, Neck, and Throat Assessment; and Chapter 7, Mouth, Nose, and Sinuses Assessment

Associated Nursing Diagnostic Categories to Consider

Wellness Diagnoses

Readiness for Enhanced Effective Breast-feeding
Readiness for Enhanced Nutritional Metabolic Pattern
Readiness for Enhanced Skin Integrity

Risk Diagnoses

Imbalanced Nutrition: Risk for Less Than Body Requirements
Imbalanced Nutrition: Risk for More Than Body Requirements
Risk for Delayed Surgical Recovery
Risk for Imbalanced Body Temperature
   Hypothermia
   Hyperthermia
Risk for Aspiration
Risk for Constipation
Risk for Imbalanced Fluid Volume
Risk for Impaired Skin Integrity
Risk for Infection

Actual Diagnoses

Impaired Dentition
Imbalanced Nutrition: Less Than Body Requirements
Imbalanced Nutrition: More Than Body Requirements
Impaired Oral Mucous Membrane
Ineffective Protection
Decreased Intracranial Adaptive Capacity
Deficient Fluid Volume
Excess Fluid Volume
Impaired Skin Integrity
Impaired Swallowing
Impaired Tissue Integrity
Ineffective Breast-feeding
Ineffective Infant Feeding Pattern
Ineffective Thermoregulation
Interrupted Breast-feeding

ELIMINATION PATTERN

Purpose

The purpose of assessing the client's elimination pattern is to determine the adequacy of function of the client's bowel and bladder for elimination. The client's bowel and urinary routines and habits are assessed. In addition, any bowel or urinary problems and use of urinary or bowel elimination devices are examined.

Subjective Data: Guideline Questions

Bowel Habits

Describe your bowel pattern. Have there been any recent changes?
How frequent are your bowel movements?
What is the color and consistency of your stools?
Do you use laxatives? What kind and how often do you use them?
Do you use enemas? How often and what kind?
Do you use suppositories? How often and what kind?
Do you have any discomfort with your bowel movements? Describe.
Have you ever had bowel surgery? What type? Ileostomy? Colostomy?

Bladder Habits

Describe your urinary habits.
How frequently do you urinate? (when and number of times)?
What is the amount and color of your urine?
Do you have any of the following problems with urinating:
   Pain?
   Blood in urine?
   Difficulty starting a stream?
   Incontinence?
   Voiding frequently at night?
   Voiding frequently during day?
   Bladder infections?
Have you ever had bladder surgery? Describe.
Have you ever had a urinary catheter? Describe. When? How long?

Objective Data

Refer to Chapter 14, Abdominal Assessment, and the External Rectal Area Assessment section in Chapter 15.

Associated Nursing Diagnostic Categories to Consider

Wellness Diagnoses

Readiness for Enhanced Bowel Elimination
Readiness for Enhanced Urinary Elimination

Risk Diagnoses

Risk for Impaired Urinary Elimination
Risk for Constipation

Actual Diagnoses

Bowel Incontinence
Diarrhea
Perceived Constipation
Risk for Constipation
Impaired Urinary Elimination
   Functional Urinary Incontinence
   Reflex Urinary Incontinence
   Stress Incontinence

Total Incontinence
Urge Incontinence
Urinary Retention

ACTIVITY–EXERCISE PATTERN

Purpose

The purpose of assessing the client's activity–exercise pattern is to determine the client's activities of daily living, including routines of exercise, leisure, and recreation. This includes activities necessary for personal hygiene, cooking, shopping, eating, maintaining the home, and working. An assessment is made of any factors that affect or interfere with the client's routine activities of daily living. Activities are evaluated in reference to the client's perception of their significance in his or her life.

Subjective Data: Guideline Questions

Activities of Daily Living

Describe your activities on a normal day (including hygiene activities, cooking activities, shopping activities, eating activities, house and yard activities, other self-care activities).
How satisfied are you with these activities?
Do you have difficulty with any of these self-care activities? Explain.
Does anyone help you with these activities? How?
Do you use any special devices to help you with your activities?
Does your current physical health affect any of these activities (eg, dyspnea, shortness of breath, palpitations, chest pain, pain, stiffness, weakness)? Explain.

Leisure Activities

Describe the leisure activities you enjoy.
Has your health affected your ability to enjoy your leisure? Explain.
Do you have time for leisure activities?
Describe any hobbies you have.

Exercise Routine

Describe those activities that you believe give you exercise.
How often are you able to do this type of exercise?
Has your health interfered with your exercise routine?

Occupational Activities

Describe what you do to make a living.
How satisfied are you with this job?
Do you believe it has affected your health? If yes, how?
How has your health affected your ability to work?

Objective Data

Refer to Chapter 10, Thoracic and Lung Assessment; Chapter 11, Cardiac Assessment; Chapter 12, Peripheral Vascular Assessment; and Chapter 16, Musculoskeletal Assessment.

Associated Nursing Diagnostic Categories to Consider

Wellness Diagnoses
Readiness for Enhanced Tissue Perfusion
Readiness for Enhanced Activity–Exercise Pattern
Readiness for Enhanced Breathing Pattern
Readiness for Enhanced Cardiac Output
Readiness for Enhanced Effective Diversional Activity Pattern
Readiness for Enhanced Home Maintenance Management
Readiness for Enhanced Self-Care Activities
Readiness for Enhanced Organized Infant Behavior

Risk Diagnoses
Risk for Impaired Respiratory Function
Risk for Disorganized Infant Behavior
Risk for Disuse Syndrome
Risk for Perioperative Positioning Injury
Risk for Peripheral Neurovascular Dysfunction

Actual Diagnoses
Activity Intolerance
Ineffective Tissue Perfusion (specify type: Cerebral,
    Cardiopulmonary, Renal, Gastrointestinal, Peripheral)
Decreased Intracranial Adaptive Capacity
Decreased Cardiac Output
Disorganized Infant Behavior
Deficient Diversional Activity
Dysfunctional Ventilatory Weaning Response
Impaired Bed Mobility
Impaired Gas Exchange
Impaired Home Maintenance
Impaired Physical Mobility
Impaired Walking
Impaired Wheelchair Mobility
Impaired Transfer Ability
Inability to Sustain Spontaneous Ventilation
Self-Care Deficit (specify type: Feeding, Bathing/Hygiene,
    Dressing/Grooming, Toileting)
Ineffective Airway Clearance
Ineffective Breathing Pattern

SEXUALITY–REPRODUCTION PATTERN

Purpose

The purpose of assessing the client's sexuality–reproduction pattern is to determine the client's fulfillment of sexual needs and perceived level of satisfaction. The reproductive pattern and developmental level of the client are determined, and perceived problems related to sexual activities, relationships, or self-concept are elicited. The physical and psychological effects of the client's current health status on his or her sexuality or sexual expression are examined.

Subjective Data: Guideline Questions

Female

● Menstrual history

How old were you when you began menstruating?

On what date did your last cycle begin?

How many days does your cycle normally last?

How many days elapse from the beginning of one cycle until the beginning of another?

Have you noticed any change in your menstrual cycle?

Have you noticed any bleeding between your menstrual cycles?

Do you experience episodes of flushing, chillings, or intolerance to temperature changes?

Describe any mood changes or discomfort before, during, or after your cycle.

What was the date of your last Pap smear? Results?

● Obstetric history

How many times have you been pregnant?

Describe the outcome of each of your pregnancies.

If you have children, what are the ages and sex of each?

Describe your feelings with each pregnancy.

Explain any health problems or concerns you had with each pregnancy.

If pregnant now:

Was this a planned or unexpected pregnancy?

Describe your feelings about this pregnancy.

What changes in your lifestyle do you anticipate with this pregnancy?

Describe any difficulties or discomfort you have had with this pregnancy.

How can I help you meet your needs during this pregnancy?

Male or Female

● Contraception

What do you or your partner do to prevent pregnancy?

How acceptable is this method to both of you?

Does this means of birth control affect your enjoyment of sexual relations?

Describe any discomfort or undesirable effects this method produces.

Have you had any difficulty with fertility? Explain.

Has infertility affected your relationship with your partner? Explain.

● Perception of sexual activities

Describe your sexual feelings. How comfortable are you with your feelings of femininity/masculinity?

Describe your level of satisfaction from your sexual relationship(s) on scale of 1 to 10 (with 10 being very satisfying).

Explain any changes in your sexual relationship(s) that your would like to make.

Describe any pain or discomfort you have during intercourse.

Have you (has your partner) experienced any difficulty achieving an orgasm or maintaining an erection? If so, how has this affected your relationship?

● Concerns related to illness

How has your illness affected your sexual relationship(s)?

How comfortable are you discussing sexual problems with your partner?

From whom would you seek help for sexual concerns?

● Special problems

Do you have or have you ever had a sexually transmitted disease? Describe.

What method do you use to prevent contracting a sexually transmitted disease?

Describe any pain, burning, or discomfort you have while voiding.

Describe any discharge or unusual odor you have from your penis/vagina.

● History of sexual abuse

Describe the time and place the incident occurred.

Explain the type of sexual contact that occurred.

Describe the person who assaulted you.

Identify any witnesses present.

Describe your feelings about this incident.

Have you had any difficulty sleeping, eating, or working since the incident occurred?

Objective Data

Refer to Chapter 13, Breast Assessment; Chapter 14, Abdominal Assessment; and Chapter 15, Genitourinary–Reproductive Assessment.

Associated Nursing Diagnostic Categories to Consider

Wellness Diagnosis
Readiness for Enhanced Sexuality Patterns

Risk Diagnosis
Risk for Ineffective Sexuality Pattern

Actual Diagnoses
Ineffective Sexuality Pattern
Sexual Dysfunction

SLEEP–REST PATTERN

Purpose

The purpose of assessing the client's sleep–rest pattern is to determine the client's perception of the quality of his or her sleep, relaxation, and energy levels. Methods used to promote relaxation and sleep are also assessed.

Subjective Data: Guideline Questions

Sleep Habits

Describe your usual sleeping time and habits (ie, reading, warm milk, medications, etc.) at home.

How long does it take you to fall asleep?

If you awaken, how long does it take you to fall asleep again?

Do you use anything to help you fall asleep (ie, medication, reading, eating)?

How would you rate the quality of your sleep?

Special Problems

Do you ever experience difficulty with falling asleep?

Remaining asleep?

Do you ever feel fatigued after a sleep period?

Has your current health altered your normal sleep habits? Explain.

Do you feel your sleep habits have contributed to your current illness? Explain.

Sleep Aids

What helps you fall asleep?

Medications?

Reading?

Relaxation technique?

Watching TV?

Listening to music?

Objective Data

Observe Appearance

Pale

Puffy eyes with dark circles

Observe Behavior

Yawning

Dozing during day

Irritability

Short attention span

Associated Nursing Diagnostic Categories to Consider

Wellness Diagnosis

Readiness for Enhanced Sleep

Risk Diagnoses

Risk for Sleep Deprivation

Risk for Disturbed Sleep Pattern

Actual Diagnoses

Disturbed Sleep Pattern

Sleep Deprivation

SENSORY–PERCEPTUAL PATTERN

Purpose

The purpose of assessing the client's sensory–perceptual pattern is to determine the functioning status of the five senses: vision, hearing, touch (including pain perception), taste, and smell. Devices and methods used to assist the client with deficits in any of these five senses are assessed.

Subjective Data: Guideline Questions

Perception of Senses

Describe your ability to see, hear, feel, taste, and smell.
Describe any difficulty you have with your vision, hearing, ability to feel (eg, touch, pain, heat, cold), taste (salty, sweet, bitter, sour), or smell.

Pain Assessment

Describe any pain you have now.
What brings it on? What relieves it?
When does it occur? How often? How long does it last?
What else do you feel when you have this pain?
Show me on this drawing (of a figure) where you have pain.
Rate your pain on a scale of 1 to 10, with 10 being the most severe pain. (Have a child use the Oucher Scale, with faces ranging from frowning to crying.)
How has your pain affected your activities of daily living?

Special Aids

What devices (eg, glasses, contact lenses, hearing aids) or methods do you use to help you with any of these problems?
Describe any medications you take to help you with these problems.

Objective Data

Refer to the section on Nose and Sinus Assessment in Chapter 7; Chapter 8, Eye Assessment; Chapter 9, Ear Assessment; and the section on Cranial Nerve Assessment in Chapter 17.

Associated Nursing Diagnostic Categories to Consider

Wellness Diagnosis

Readiness for Enhanced Physical Comfort

Risk Diagnoses

Risk for Aspiration
Risk for Acute Pain

Actual Diagnoses

Chronic Pain
Dysreflexia
Acute Pain

Disturbed Sensory Perception (specify: Visual, Auditory, Kinesthetic, Gustatory, Tactile, Olfactory)
Unilateral Neglect

COGNITIVE PATTERN

Purpose

The purpose of assessing the client's cognitive pattern is to determine the client's ability to understand, communicate, remember, and make decisions.

Subjective Data: Guideline Questions

Ability to Understand

Explain what your doctor has told you about your health.
Are you satisfied with your understanding of your illness and prescribed care? Explain.
What is the best way for you to learn something new (read, watch television, etc)?

Ability to Communicate

Can you tell me how you feel about your current state of health?
Are you able to ask questions about your treatments, medications, and so forth?
Do you ever have difficulty expressing yourself or explaining things to others? Explain.

Ability to Remember

Are you able to remember recent events and events of long ago? Explain.

Ability to Make Decisions

Describe how you feel when faced with a decision.
What assists you in making decisions?
Do you find decision making difficult, fairly easy, or variable? Describe.

Objective Data

Refer to the Mental Status Assessment section of Chapter 17.

Associated Nursing Diagnostic Categories to Consider

Wellness Diagnosis

Readiness for Enhanced Cognition

Risk Diagnosis

Risk for Disturbed Thought Processes

Actual Diagnoses

Acute Confusion
Disturbed Thought Processes

Chronic Confusion
Decisional Conflict (specify)
Impaired Environmental Interpretation Syndrome
Impaired Memory
Deficient Knowledge (specify)

ROLE–RELATIONSHIP PATTERN

Purpose

The purpose of assessing the client's role–relationship pattern is to determine the client's perceptions of responsibilities and roles in the family, at work, and in social life. The client's level of satisfaction with these is assessed. In addition, any difficulties in the client's relationships and interactions with others are examined.

Subjective Data: Guideline Questions

Perception of Major Roles and Responsibilities in Family

Describe your family.
Do you live with your family? Alone?
How does your family get along?
Who makes the major decisions in your family?
Who is the main financial supporter of your family?
How do you feel about your family?
What is your role in your family? Is this an important role?
What is your major responsibility in your family? How do you feel about this responsibility?
How does your family deal with problems?
Are there any major problems now?
Who is the person you feel closest to in your family? Explain.
How is your family coping with your current state of health?

Perception of Major Roles and Responsibilities at Work

Describe your occupation.
What is your major responsibility at work?
How do you feel about the people you work with?
If you could, what would you change about your work?
Are there any major problems you have at work? If yes, explain.

Perception of Major Social Roles and Responsibilities

Who is the most important person in your life? Explain.
Describe your neighborhood and the community in which you live.
How do you feel about the people in your community?
Do you participate in any social groups or neighborhood activities? If yes, describe.
What do you see as your contribution to society?
What would you change about your community if you could?

Objective Data

1. Outline a family genogram for your client. See Figure 2–1 for an example.
2. Observe your client's family members.
   a. How do they communicate with each other?
   b. How do they respond to the client?
   c. Do they visit, and how long do they stay with the client?

Associated Nursing Diagnostic Categories to Consider

Wellness Diagnoses

Readiness for Enhanced Caregiver Role
Readiness for Enhanced Communication
Readiness for Enhanced Grieving
Readiness for Enhanced Parenting
Readiness for Enhanced Relationships
Readiness for Enhanced Role Performance
Readiness for Enhanced Social Interaction

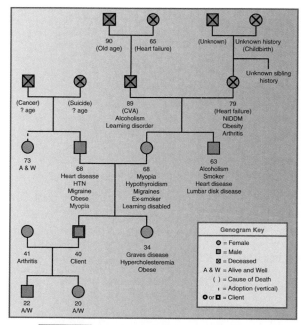

FIGURE 2–1 Genogram of a 40-year-old male client.

Risk Diagnoses
Risk for Impaired Parent/Infant/Child Attachment
Risk for Dysfunctional Grieving
Risk for Loneliness

Actual Diagnoses
Interrupted Family Processes
Dysfunctional Family Processes: Alcoholism
Impaired Parenting
Ineffective Role Performance
Anticipatory Grieving
Caregiver Role Strain
Dysfunctional Grieving
Impaired Social Interaction
Impaired Verbal Communication
Parental Role Conflict
Social Isolation

SELF-PERCEPTION–SELF-CONCEPT PATTERN

Purpose

The purpose of assessing the client's self-perception–self-concept pattern is to determine the client's perception of his or her identity, abilities, body image, and self-worth. The client's behavior, attitude, and emotional patterns are also assessed.

Subjective Data: Guideline Questions

Perception of Identity
Describe yourself.
Has your illness affected how you describe yourself?

Perception of Abilities and Self-Worth
What do you consider to be your strengths? Weaknesses?
How do you feel about yourself?
How does your family feel about you and your illness?

Body Image
How do you feel about your appearance?
Has this changed since your illness? Explain.
How would you change your appearance if you could?
How do you feel about other people with disabilities?

Objective Data

Refer to the procedures for observing appearance, behavior and mood in the Mental Status Assessment section of Chapter 17.

Associated Nursing Diagnostic Categories to Consider

Wellness Diagnoses
Readiness for Enhanced Self-Concept

Risk Diagnoses
Risk for Disturbed Body Image
Risk for Hopelessness
Risk for Chronic Low Self-Esteem

Actual Diagnoses
Anxiety
Disturbed Body Image
Chronic Low Self-Esteem
Death Anxiety
Fatigue
Fear
Hopelessness
Disturbed Personal Identity
Powerlessness
Disturbed Self-Esteem
Situational Low Self-Esteem

COPING–STRESS TOLERANCE PATTERN

Purpose

The purpose of assessing the client's coping–stress tolerance pattern is to determine the areas and amount of stress in a client's life and the effectiveness of coping methods used to deal with it. Availability and use of support systems such as family, friends, and religious beliefs are assessed.

Subjective Data: Guideline Questions

Perception of Stress and Problems in Life
Describe what you believe to be the most stressful situation in your life.
How has your illness affected the stress you feel? *or* How do you feel stress has affected your illness?
Has there been a personal loss or major change in your life over the last year? Explain.
What has helped you to cope with this change or loss?

Coping Methods and Support Systems
What do you usually do first when faced with a problem?
What helps you to relieve stress and tension?
To whom do you usually turn when you have a problem or feel under pressure?
How do you usually deal with problems?
Do you use medication, drugs, or alcohol to help relieve stress? Explain.

Objective Data

Refer to the Mental Status Assessment section of Chapter 17.

Associated Nursing Diagnostic Categories to Consider

Wellness Diagnoses
Readiness for Enhanced Individual Coping
Readiness for Enhanced Family Coping
Readiness for Enhanced Community Coping
Readiness for Enhanced Spiritual Well-Being

Risk Diagnoses
Risk for Ineffective Coping (Individual, Family, or Community)
Risk for Post-Trauma Syndrome
Risk for Self-Mutilation
Risk for Spiritual Distress
Risk for Suicide
Risk for Violence (specify: Self-Directed, Other-Directed)

Actual Diagnoses
Caregiver Role Strain
Chronic Sorrow
Impaired Adjustment
Ineffective Community Coping
Compromised Family Coping
Disabled Family Coping
Ineffective Individual Coping:
  Defensive Coping
  Ineffective Denial
Post-Trauma Syndrome
Rape–Trauma Syndrome
Relocation Stress Syndrome

VALUE–BELIEF PATTERN

Purpose

The purpose of assessing the client's value–belief pattern is to determine the client's life values and goals, philosophical beliefs, religious
beliefs, and spiritual beliefs that influence his or her choices and decisions. Conflicts between these values, goals, beliefs, and expectations that are related to health are assessed.

Subjective Data: Guideline Questions

Values, Goals, and Philosophical Beliefs
What is most important to you in life?
What do you hope to accomplish in your life?
What is the major influencing factor that helps you make
  decisions?
What is your major source of hope and strength in life?

Religious and Spiritual Beliefs
Do you have a religious affiliation?
Is this important to you?

r

Are there certain health practices or restrictions that are important for you to follow while you are ill or hospitalized? Explain.

Is there a significant person (eg, minister, priest) from your religious denomination whom you want to be contacted?

Would you like the hospital chaplain to visit?

Are there certain practices (eg, prayer, reading scripture) that are important to you?

Is a relationship with God an important part of your life? Explain.

Describe any other sources of strength that are important to you.

How can I help you continue with this source of spiritual strength while you are ill in the hospital?

Objective Data

Observe religious practices

Presence of religious articles in room (eg, Bible, cards, medals, statues)

Visits from clergy

Religious actions of client: prayer, visit to chapel, request for clergy, watching of religious TV programs or listening to religious radio stations

Observe client's behavior for signs of spiritual distress

Anxiety

Anger

Depression

Doubt

Hopelessness

Powerlessness

Associated Nursing Diagnostic Categories to Consider

Wellness Diagnosis

Readiness for Enhanced Spiritual Well-being

Risk Diagnosis

Risk for Spiritual Distress

Actual Diagnoses

Death Anxiety

Spiritual Distress

C H A P T E R
3

Physical
Assessment

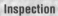

PHYSICAL ASSESSMENT SKILLS

Four basic techniques are used in performing a physical assessment: *inspection, palpation, percussion,* and *auscultation.* The definition and proper technique for each of these are described below. Always use Standard Precautions as recommended by the Hospital Injection Control Practices Advisory Committee (HICPAC) and the Communicable Disease Center (COC).

Inspection
Definition
Inspection is using the senses of vision, smell, and hearing to observe the condition of various body parts, including any deviations from normal.

Technique
- Expose body parts being observed while keeping the rest of the client properly draped.
- *Always* look before touching.
- Use good lighting. Tangential sunlight is best. Be alert for the effect of bluish red-tinted or fluorescent lighting that interferes with observing bruises, cyanosis, and erythema.
- Provide a warm room for examination of the client. (Too cold or hot an environment may alter skin color and appearance.)
- Observe for color, size, location, texture, symmetry, odors, and sounds.

Palpation

Definition

Palpation is touching and feeling body parts with your hands to determine the following characteristics:

- Texture (roughness/smoothness)
- Temperature (warm/hot/cold)
- Moisture (dry/wet/moist)
- Motion (stillness/vibration)
- Consistency of structures (solid/fluid filled)

Technique

- Examiner's fingernails should be short.
- The most sensitive part of the hand should be used to detect various sensations. See Table 3–1.
- Light palpation precedes deep palpation.
- Tender areas are palpated last.
- Three different types of palpation may be used depending on the purpose of the exam. The purpose and technique for each are described in Table 3–2.

Percussion

Definition

Percussion is tapping a portion of the body to elicit tenderness or sounds that vary with the density of underlying structures.

Technique

Two types of percussion may be used depending on purpose. These are explained in Table 3–3. Percussion notes elicited through indirect percussion vary with density of underlying structures. Five percussion notes are described in Table 3–4.

Auscultation

Definition

Auscultation is listening for various breath, heart, vasculature, and bowel sounds using a stethoscope.

TABLE 3–1	SENSITIVITY OF PARTS OF THE HAND
Hand Part Used	**Type of Sensation Felt**
Fingertips	Fine discriminations, pulsations
Palmar/ulnar surface	Vibratory sensations (eg, thrills, fremitus)
Dorsal surface (back of hand)	Temperature

TABLE 3–2 TYPES OF PALPATION

Type	Purpose	Technique
Light palpation	To determine surface variations (eg, texture, tenderness, temperature, moisture, elasticity, pulsations, superficial organs, masses)	Depress skin ½″ to ¾″ with finger pads.
Deep palpation	To feel internal organs and masses for size, shape, tenderness, symmetry, mobility	Depress skin 1½″ to 2″ with firm, deep pressure. May use one hand on top of the other to exert firmer pressure.

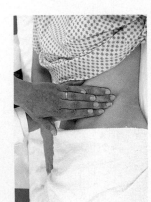

Deep palpation. (© B. Proud.)

(continued)

TABLE 3–2   TYPES OF PALPATION (*Continued*)

Type	Purpose	Technique
Bimanual palpation (use with caution as it may provoke internal injury)	To palpate breasts and deep abdominal organs	Use two hands, one on each side of body part or organs being felt. The upper hand is used to apply pressure while the lower hand is used to detect deep structures. Use one hand to push deeply on abdominal wall to move internal structure to the flank. Use the other hand to feel the structure.

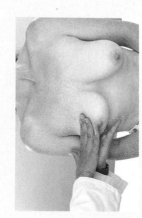

Bimanual palpation of the breast.
(© B. Proud.)

TABLE 3–3 TYPES OF PERCUSSION

Type	Purpose	Technique
Direct percussion	To elicit tenderness or pain	Directly tap body part with 1 or 2 fingertips.

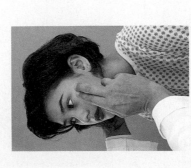

Direct percussion of sinuses.
(© B. Proud.)

(continued)

TABLE 3–3 TYPES OF PERCUSSION (*Continued*)

Type	Purpose	Technique
Indirect percussion	To elicit one of the following sounds over the chest or abdomen: tympany, resonance, hyperresonance, dullness, flatness (see Table 3–4)	Press middle finger of nondominant hand firmly on body part. Keep other fingers off body part. Strike the finger on the body part with the middle finger (with short fingernail) of the dominant hand. Flex dominant wrist (not forearm) quickly. Listen to sound. (Use quick wrist movement, as if giving an IM injection.)

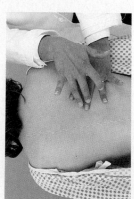

Indirect or mediate percussion of lungs.
(© B. Proud.)

TABLE 3–4 SOUNDS (TONES) ELICITED BY PERCUSSION

Sound	Intensity	Pitch	Length	Quality	Example of Origin
Resonance (heard over part air and part solid)	Loud	Low	Long	Hollow	Normal lung
Hyperresonance (heard over mostly air)	Very loud	Low	Long	Booming	Lung with emphysema
Tympany (heard over air)	Loud	High	Moderate	Drumlike	Puffed-out cheek, gastric bubble
Dullness (heard over more solid tissue)	Medium	Medium	Moderate	Thudlike	Diaphragm, pleural effusion, liver
Flatness (heard over very dense tissue)	Soft	High	Short	Flat	Muscle, bone, sternum, thigh

Technique

Use a good stethoscope that has the following:

- Snug-fitting ear plugs
- Tubing not longer than 15 inches and internal diameter not greater than 1 inch
- Diaphragm and bell

The diaphragm and bell are used differently to detect various sounds, as shown in Table 3–5.

BASIC GUIDELINES FOR PHYSICAL ASSESSMENT

Obtain a nursing history and survey the client's general physical status for an overall impression prior to physical assessment. This is done to determine which specific body systems should be examined (eg, if the client complains of chest pain, a thoracic and cardiac physical exam should be performed). A complete examination of all body systems may be done only on admission; otherwise, the physical assessment may only include one or a few body systems.

Maintain privacy and proper draping.

Explain the procedure and purpose of each part of the exam to the client.

Follow a planned examination order for each body system, using the four techniques described earlier. Specific history questions related to each body part being examined may be integrated with the physical exam. (For example, when examining vision, ask the date of the client's last eye exam, if he or she has a history of blurring or double vision.)

TABLE 3–5	USES FOR DIAPHRAGM AND BELL OF STETHOSCOPE	
	Purpose	**Technique**
Diaphragm	To detect high-pitched sounds (eg, breath sounds, normal heart sounds, bowel sounds)	Press firmly on body part.
Bell	To detect low-pitched sounds (eg, abnormal extra heart sounds, heart murmurs, carotid bruits)	Press lightly over body part.

First inspect, palpate, percuss, and then auscultate, except in the abdominal exam. To avoid alterations in bowel sounds: first auscultate and then percuss the abdomen *prior to* palpation.

Use each technique to compare symmetrical sides of the body and organs.

Assess both structure *and* function of each body part and organ (eg, the appearance and condition of the ear, as well as its hearing function).

When you identify an abnormality, assess for further data on the extent of the abnormality and the client's responses to the abnormality. Is there radiation of pain to other areas? Is there an effect on eating? Bowels? Activities of daily living? (For example, with left upper quadrant abdominal pain: Is there radiation of the pain?)

Integrate client education with the physical assessment (eg, breast self-exam, testicular self-exam, foot care for the client with diabetes).

Allow time for client questions.

Remember: The most important guideline for adequate physical assessment is conscious, continuous practice of physical assessment skills.

VARIATIONS IN PHYSICAL ASSESSMENT OF THE PEDIATRIC CLIENT

The physical assessment sequence is dependent upon the development level of the client. (For a detailed discussion, see Appendix 2, Developmental Information—Age 1 Month to 18 Years.)

Establishment of rapport with the child and significant others is the most essential step in obtaining meaningful physical assessment data.

Allowing time for interaction with the child prior to beginning the examination helps to reduce fears.

In certain age groups, portions of the assessment will require physical restraint of the client with the help of another adult.

Distraction and play should be intermingled throughout the examination to assist in maintaining rapport with the pediatric client.

Involving assistance from the child's significant caregiver may facilitate a more meaningful examination of the younger client.

Based on the child's responses, the examiner should be prepared to alter the order of the assessment and approach to the child.

Protest or an uncooperative attitude toward the examiner is a normal finding in children from birth to early adolescence, throughout parts or even all of the assessment process. Appendix 2 describes normal behavior at various developmental levels for the pediatric client.

If restraining is needed by another health team member, allow parent to comfort child *after* the procedure.

VARIATIONS IN PHYSICAL ASSESSMENT OF THE GERIATRIC CLIENT

Remember: Normal variations related to aging may be observed in all parts of the physical exam. To avoid fatiguing the older client, allow rest periods between parts of the physical assessment. Provide a room with a comfortable temperature setting and no drafts, close to the restroom.

Allow sufficient time for client to respond to directions and to change positions. Use silence to provide more time for the client to process thoughts and respond.

If possible, assess geriatric clients in a setting where they have an opportunity to perform normal activities of daily living to determine their optimum potential.

Conduct exam in an area with ample space to accommodate wheelchairs and other supportive devices.

General Physical Survey

Equipment Needed

- Balance beam scale
- Tape measure
- Thermometer
- Sphygmomanometer
- Stethoscope

Subjective Data: Focus Questions

Reason for seeking health care? Major concern about current health? Current age, height, and weight? Recent weight change? Change in pulse or heart rate? Problem with hypertension or hypotension? Difficulty with respirations? Explain.

Objective Data: Assessment Techniques

When you meet the client, observe the client from head to toe to note any gross abnormalities in appearance or behavior. Assess vital signs (temperature, pulse, respirations, and blood pressure) to detect any severe deviations and to acquire baseline data. Then weigh the client and measure height with shoes and heavy clothing removed.

GENERAL PHYSICAL SURVEY

PROCEDURE	NORMAL FINDINGS	DEVIATIONS FROM NORMAL
Observe the following:		
• Physical development	• Appears to be stated chronological age	• Appears older than age with hard manual labor, chronic illness, or alcoholism/smoking
• Behavior	• Cooperative attitude and behavior	• Uncooperative or bizarre, unpredictable behavior may be seen in angry, mentally ill, or violent client; apathy or crying seen in depression
• Mood	• Mild anxiety or tenseness	• Moderate to severe anxiety and tenseness, restlessness, or fidgeting seen in anxiety states
• Dress	• Dressed for occasion	• Dress bizarre and inappropriate for occasion seen in mentally ill, grieving, depressed, or poor clients
• Gait	• Erect posture, coordinated, smooth and steady gait	• Lordosis, scoliosis, or kyphosis; uncoordinated; shaky, unsteady, or stiff gait seen with Parkinson disease; stiff, rigid gait seen with arthritis
• Body build	• Bilateral, firm, developed muscles	• Lack of subcutaneous fat seen in the undernourished, abdominal ascites seen in starvation, abundant fatty tissue seen in obesity

GENERAL PHYSICAL SURVEY (continued)

PROCEDURE	NORMAL FINDINGS	DEVIATIONS FROM NORMAL
Monitor **temperature.** Electronic thermometers are quicker than glass thermometers. They may be used for oral, rectal, or axillary temperatures depending on the model and type of probe used.	Body temperature is usually lowest in early AM and highest in late PM. 96.0–99.9°F (35.6–37.7°C)	Hypothermia (less than 96.0°F or 35.6°C) may be seen in prolonged exposure to cold, sepsis, hypoglycemia, hypothyroidism, or starvation.
Oral. Place clean thermometer under tongue near vascular bed with lips closed for 5 minutes. Wait 15 minutes before taking temperature if client just drank hot/cold fluids.	Strenuous exercise, stress, and ovulation may elevate temperature to 101.0°F (38.3°C). Hot fluids, smoking, and gum chewing may elevate temperature, while cold fluids may lower it.	Hyperthermia (more than 100.0°F or 37.8°C) may be seen in viral or bacterial infections, malignancies, trauma, and various blood and immune disorders.
Rectal. Lubricate clean thermometer with water-soluble lubricant and insert 1–2 inches into rectum for 3 minutes. Use this method only when other routes are not practical.	0.7–1.0°F (0.4–0.5°C) higher than oral temperature. Strenuous exercise may elevate temperature to 104.0°F (40.0°C).	

GENERAL PHYSICAL SURVEY (continued)

PROCEDURE	NORMAL FINDINGS	DEVIATIONS FROM NORMAL
Axillary. Insert thermometer under axilla with arm down and across chest for 5–10 minutes.	1.0°F (0.5°C) lower than oral temperature. Environmental temperature may alter body temperature, and stress may raise body temperature.	
Tympanic. Use special electronic thermometer for tympanic membrane temperature. Place covered probe very gently at opening of ear canal for 2–3 seconds until temperature appears on digital screen. This is a safe, quick, non-invasive method that may be used with client of any age. (Fig. 4–1).	1.4°F (0.8°C) higher than the normal oral temperature.	
Monitor **pulse.**		
Radial. Use middle three fingers to palpate radial pulse for 30 seconds and multiply by two if pulse is regular (Fig. 4–2). If pulse is irregular, take for 1 full minute. Always start counting with zero so that second pulse felt is no. 1.		

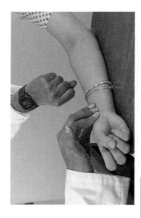

FIGURE 4–2 Timing the radial pulse rate. (© B. Proud.)

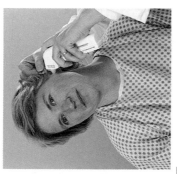

FIGURE 4–1 Taking a tympanic temperature. (© B. Proud.)

GENERAL PHYSICAL SURVEY (continued)

PROCEDURE	NORMAL FINDINGS	DEVIATIONS FROM NORMAL
Palpate for the following:		
• Rate	• 60–100 bpm (may be as low as 50 bpm in healthy athletes)	• More than 100 bpm equals tachycardia, seen in fever, stress, and with some medications; less than 60 bpm equals bradycardia, may be seen with prolonged sitting or standing; follow up with cardiac auscultation of apical pulse
• Rhythm (if irregular, feel for full minute)	• Regular	• Irregular (follow up with cardiac auscultation of apical pulse)
• Equality of strength	• Equal bilaterally in strength	• Asymmetrical in strength, bounding, weak, or thready; follow up with palpation of the carotid arteries (one at a time)
Apical. Auscultate heart sounds for 1 minute with stethoscope.		
• Rate	• 60–100 bpm	• More than 100 bpm equals tachycardia; less than 60 bpm equals bradycardia
• Rhythm	• Regular	• Irregular; pulse deficit (difference between apical and radial pulse) may indicate atrial fibrillation, atrial flutter, premature ventricular contractions, and various degrees of heart block

GENERAL PHYSICAL SURVEY (continued)

PROCEDURE	NORMAL FINDINGS	DEVIATIONS FROM NORMAL
Monitor **respirations** *1 full minute for the following:* • Rate • Rhythm • Depth See Table 4–1.	• 10–20 breaths/min • Regular and spontaneous • Equal bilateral chest expansion of 1–2 inches	• Less than 12/min, more than 20/min • Irregular • Unequal, shallow, or extremely deep chest expansion
Monitor **blood pressure** after client is seated or supine quietly for 10 minutes. Repeat after 2 minutes. Repeat with client standing. Verify blood pressure in the contralateral arm. Refer to Table 4–2.	Systolic: less than/equal to 139 mm Hg, diastolic: less than/equal to 89 mm Hg; varies with individuals	Higher or lower than normal systolic and diastolic readings (Tables 4–2 and 4–3)
Weigh client with light clothing and no shoes. Measure **height** of client.		

TABLE 4–1 TYPES OF RESPIRATIONS

	Description	Pattern
Normal	12–20/min and regular	∿∿∿
Apnea	Absence of respiration	——
Bradypnea	Slow, shallow respiration	∽
Tachypnea	More than 20/min and regular	∿∿∿∿∿∿
Hyperventilation	Increased rate and increased depth	∭∭∭
Hypoventilation	Decreased rate and decreased depth	⌒
Cheyne–Stokes	Periods of apnea and hyperventilation	∭___∭
Kussmaul	Very deep with normal rhythm	∿∿∿∿∿

TABLE 4–2 CLASSIFICATION AND MANAGEMENT OF BLOOD PRESSURE FOR ADULTS*

BP Classification	SBP* mmHg	DBP* mmHg	Lifestyle Modification	Initial Drug Therapy Without Compelling Indication	Initial Drug Therapy With Compelling Indications
Normal	<120	and <80	Encourage		
Prehypertension	120–139	or 80–89	Yes	No antihypertensive drug indicated	Drug(s) for compelling indications‡
Stage 1 hypertension	140–159	or 90–99	Yes	Thiazide-type diuretics for most; may consider ACEI, ARB, BB, CCB, or combination	Drug(s) for the compelling indications.‡ Other antihypertensive drugs (diuretics, ACEI, ARB, BB, CCB) as needed.
Stage 2 hypertension	≥160	or ≥100	Yes	Two-drug combination for most† (usually thiazide-type diuretic and ACEI or ARB or BB or CCB)	

DBP, diastolic blood pressure; SBP, systolic blood pressure.

Drug abbreviations: ACEI, angiotensin converting enzyme inhibitor; ARB, angiotensin receptor blocker; BB, beta-blocker; CCB, calcium channel blocker.

*Treatment determined by highest BP category.

†Initial combined therapy should be used cautiously in those at risk for orthostatic hypotension.

‡Treat patients with chronic kidney disease or diabetes to BP goal of <130/80 mm Hg.

Source: 7th Report of the Joint National Committee on Prevention, Detection, and Treatment of High Blood Pressure (2003).

Compelling Indication*	Recommended Drugs						Clinical Trial Basis†
	Diuretic	BB	ACEI	ARB	CCB	Aldo ANT	
Heart failure	•	•	•	•		•	ACC/AHA Heart Failure Guideline, MERIT-HF, COPERNICUS, CIBIS, SOLVD, AIRE, TRACE, ValHEFT, RALES
Postmyocardial infarction		•	•			•	ACC/AHA Post-MI Guideline, BHAT, SAVE, Capricorn, EPHESUS
High coronary disease risk	•	•	•		•		ALLHAT, HOPE, ANBP₂, LIFE, CONVINCE
Diabetes	•	•	•	•	•		NKF-ADA Guideline, UKPDS, ALLHAT
Chronic kidney disease			•	•			NKF Guideline, Captopril Trial, RENAAL, IDNT, REIN, AASK
Recurrent stroke prevention	•		•				PROGRESS

Drug abbreviations: ACEI, angiotensin converting enzyme inhibitor; Aldo ANT, aldosterone antagonist; ARB, angiotensin receptor blocker; BB, beta-blocker; CCB, calcium channel blocker.

*Compelling indications for antihypertensive drugs are based on benefits from outcome studies or existing clinical guidelines. The compelling indication is managed in parallel with the BP.

†Conditions for which clinical trials demonstrate benefit of specific classes of antihypertensive drugs.

Source: 7th Report of the Joint National Committee on Prevention, Detection, and Treatment of High Blood Pressure (2003).

PEDIATRIC VARIATIONS

Equipment Needed

- Tape measure
- Growth charts for specific age comparisons (see Appendix 5)

Subjective Data: Focus Questions

Inquire about child's development milestones (see Appendix 2).
Inquire about immunizations (see Appendix 3).
Inquire about parent–child relationships (see Appendix 2).

Objective Data: Assessment Techniques

PROCEDURE	NORMAL VARIATIONS
Observe **physical level of development** and compare with chronological age.	See Appendix 2, Developmental Information—Age 1 Month to 18 Years
Monitor **temperature:**	Temperature fluctuates markedly in infants and young children.
Oral. Caution against biting glass thermometer.	*Infants:* 99.4°F (37.2°C; because of excess heat production) *Children and adolescents:* 98.6°F (37°C)

General Physical Survey

Objective Data: Assessment Techniques (continued)

PROCEDURE	NORMAL VARIATIONS
Note: Take tympanic, axillary, or rectal temperature in children younger than 6 years if they are uncooperative or unconscious. *Rectal.* Position child prone, supine, or sidelying (may use parent's lap). Insert lubricated thermometer no more than 1 inch into rectum. *Tympanic.* Pull pinna down and back. Monitor **pulse:** Take apical (not radial) pulse in children younger than 2 years (Fig. 4–3). Count pulse for 1 full minute.	Awake and resting pulse rates vary with the age of the child: 1 wk–3 mo, 100–160; 3 mo–2 y, 80–150; 2–10 y, 70–110; 10 y–adult, 55–90. Athletic adolescents tend to have lower pulse rates.

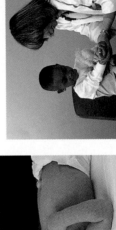 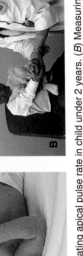

FIGURE 4–3 (*A*) Auscultating apical pulse rate in child under 2 years. (*B*) Measuring radial

General Physical Survey

Objective Data: Assessment Techniques (continued)

PROCEDURE

Monitor **respirations** by observing abdominal movement in infants and young children

Monitor **blood pressure:** Width of cuff should cover two thirds of upper arm or be 20% greater than diameter of the extremity. Length of bladder should encircle without overlapping.

Measure the following and plot on growth chart:

- Height

  Children under 24 months: Measure length from vertex of head to heel in recumbent position

  Children over 24 months: Measure standing height in bare feet.

NORMAL VARIATIONS

Respiratory rates: birth–6 mo, 30–50; 6 mo–2 y, 20–30; 3–10 y, 20–28; 10–18 y, 12–20

Blood pressure rates: *Systolic:* 1–7 years, age in years + 90; 8–18 years, $(2 \times$ age in years$) + 90$; *Diastolic:* 1–5 years, 56; 6–18 years, age in years + 52

- See Appendix 5 for normal height ranges.

Objective Data: Assessment Techniques (continued)

PROCEDURE	NORMAL VARIATIONS
• Weight: For infants and young children, use platform scale.	• See Appendix 5. At 1 year of age, the child's weight is usually three times the birth weight.
• Head circumference (HC) *Children under 24 months:* Measure slightly above eyebrows, pinna of ears over occipital prominence of skull (see Figure 4–4).	• Plot head circumference on standard growth chart (Appendix 5). Head circumference measurement should fall between the 5th and 95th percentiles, and should be comparable with the child's height and weight percentiles. Those greater than 95% may indicate macrocephaly. Those under the 5th percentile may indicate microcephaly. Increased head circumference in children older than 3 years may indicate separation of cranial sutures due to increased intracranial pressure.

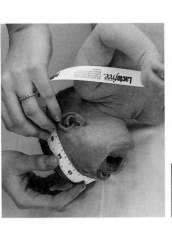

FIGURE 4–4 Measuring the circumference of an infant's head. (© B. Proud.)

GERIATRIC VARIATIONS

- Dress may be heavier because of a decrease in body metabolism and a loss of subcutaneous fat.
- Posture may indicate kyphosis due to osteoporotic thinning and collapse of vertebrae, decreasing height.
- Steps in gait may shorten with decreased speed and arm swing.
- Normal temperature may range from 95.0°F to 97.5°F (35–36.4°C), and thus temperature may not appear to be elevated with an infection.
- Arteries are more rigid, hard, and bent.
- Systolic blood pressure may be increased.
- Systolic murmurs may be present.

CULTURAL VARIATIONS

- Caucasian men tend to be 0.5 inch taller than African American men.
- African American women consistently weigh more than Caucasian women (Overfield, 1995).
- Blood pressure percentiles of prepubertal children in nonindustrialized countries may fall well below Western percentiles.

Possible Collaborative Problems

- Hypertension
- Hypotension
- Infection
- Dysrhythmia

TEACHING TIPS FOR SELECTED NURSING DIAGNOSES AND COLLABORATIVE PROBLEMS

Adult Client

Nursing Diagnosis: Health-Seeking Behaviors (desire to learn more about health promotion)

☐ Teach client self-assessment procedures (eg, breast self-exam, testicular self-exam) and the importance of regular medical checkups. Refer to community wellness resources and support groups as they relate to client.

Collaborative Problem: Potential complication–hypertension

☐ Explain the relationships between body weight, diet, exercise, stress, and blood pressure. Explain the possible effects of a low-fat, low-cholesterol diet along with vigorous exercise in reducing the atherosclerotic process. Explain methods of preparing food low in sodium and fat, and high in potassium. Teach clients who drink alcohol to limit their intake

[See Tables 4–2 and 4–3 for follow-up and referral.]

Pediatric Client

Nursing Diagnosis: Risk for Imbalanced Body Temperature related to febrile illness

☐ Instruct parents on proper method to assess temperature and detect fever. Teach proper method of giving tepid sponge baths and using antipyretics to reduce fever. Explain the use of quiet play and increasing fluids during this time.

Instruct parent to notify physician in case of high fever.

Nursing Diagnosis: Ineffective Protection related to loss of passive immunity of placenta (age 6–12 months)

☐ Instruct parents to clothe infant well to decrease exposure to others with illnesses. Encourage use of good hand-washing techniques and complete immunizations throughout childhood.

Geriatric Client

Collaborative Problem: Potential complication—postural hypotension

⬛ Identify postural hypotension in elderly (difference of 20 mm Hg systolic BP and 10 mm Hg diastolic BP from a lying to a standing position). Instruct client to reduce risk of falls by moving from a lying to a sitting position slowly, then standing for 2–3 minutes before proceeding.

Nursing Diagnosis: Risk for Imbalanced Body Temperature—Hypothermia—related to decreased cardiac output, and decreased subcutaneous tissue secondary to aging processes

⬛ Encourage good heating in homes and added clothing in cold weather. Teach family to observe for signs of hypothermia, including facial edema, pallor, clouding of vision, decreased blood pressure, and decreased heart rate. Refer to community agencies that may provide shelter, clothing, and food when needed.

Skin, Hair, and Nail Assessment

ANATOMY OVERVIEW

The skin is composed of three layers, the epidermis, dermis, and subcutaneous tissue (Fig. 5–1). The skin is a physical barrier that protects the underlying tissues and structures.

Hair consists of layers of keratinized cells found over much of the body except for the lips, nipples, soles of the feet, palms of the hands, labia minora, and penis.

The nails, located on the distal phalanges of fingers and toes, are hard, transparent plates of keratinized epidermal cells that grow from a root underneath the skin fold called the cuticle (Fig. 5–2).

Equipment Needed

- Adequate lighting (natural daylight is best)
- Comfortable room temperature
- Gloves
- Penlight

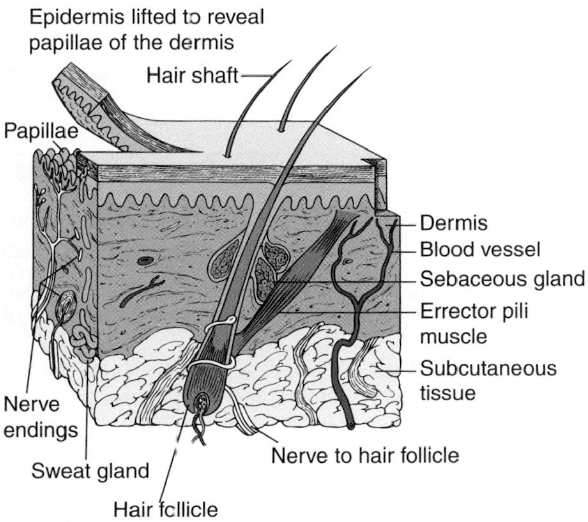

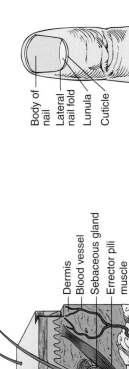

FIGURE 5–2 The nail and related structures.

Body of nail
Lateral nail fold
Lunula
Cuticle

Epidermis lifted to reveal papillae of the dermis
Hair shaft

Dermis
Blood vessel
Sebaceous gland
Errector pili muscle
Subcutaneous tissue

Nerve to hair follicle

Papillae

Nerve endings

Sweat gland

Hair follicle

FIGURE 5–1 The skin and hair follicles and related structures.

- Magnifying glass
- Centimeter rule

Subjective Data: Focus Questions

Skin rashes, lesions, itching, dryness, oiliness, bruising (location; onset; precipitating factors: stress, weather, drugs, exposure to allergens)? Methods of relief (eg, medications, lotions, soaks)? Changes in skin color, lesions, bruising (onset, type of change)? Scalp lesions, itching, infections? History of skin disorders? Surgical excision of skin lesions? Describe. Changes in texture, condition, and amount of hair? Changes in condition of nails and cuticles? Nail breaking, splitting? Cuticle inflammation? Changes in body odor? Skin, hair, and nail care habits; bathing patterns; soaps and lotions used? Shampoo, hair spray, coloring, nail enamels used? Amount of sun/tanning exposure (type of oils and lotions used)? Exposure to chemicals?

RISK FACTORS. Risk for skin cancer related to repeated, intermittent sun exposure with sunburn beginning at early age; use of tanning booths; medical therapies (PUVA and radiation); genetic susceptibility; fair skinned; immunosuppression

Objective Data: Assessment Techniques

Review Figure 5–1 for a diagram of the skin and related structures.

SKIN INSPECTION AND PALPATION

Expose the body part to be inspected (cleanse skin if necessary).

PROCEDURE	NORMAL FINDINGS	DEVIATIONS FROM NORMAL
Inspect skin for the following:		
• Generalized color	• *In white skin:* Light to dark pink	• *In white skin:* Extreme pallor, flushed, bluish (cyanosis).

SKIN INSPECTION AND PALPATION (continued)

PROCEDURE	NORMAL FINDINGS	DEVIATIONS FROM NORMAL
	• *In dark skin*: Light to dark brown, olive	• *In dark skin*: Loss of red tones in pallor; ashen gray in cyanosis. Bluish colored palms, soles, lips, nails, earlobes are seen with cyanosis. Cyanosis is seen in vasoconstriction, myocardial infarction, or pulmonary insufficiency. Pallor is seen in arterial insufficiency and anemia.
• Color variations in patches on body	• *In white skin*: Sun-tanned areas, white patches (vitiligo) • *In dark skin*: Lighter colored palms, soles, nail beds, and lips; black/blue area over lower lumbar area (mongolian spot); frecklelike pigmentation of nail beds and sclerae	• *In white skin*: Generalized pale yellow to pumpkin color (jaundice). • *In dark skin*: Yellow color may appear in sclerae, oral mucous membranes, hard and soft palates, palms, and soles. Increased pigmented areas; decreased pigmented areas; reddened, warm areas (erythema); black and blue marks (ecchymosis); tiny red spots (petechiae). Jaundice is often seen in liver or gallbladder disease, hemolysis, or anemia.
Palpate skin for the following: • Texture	• Smooth, soft	• Rough, thick. Dry skin is seen in hypothyroidism.

SKIN INSPECTION AND PALPATION (continued)

PROCEDURE	NORMAL FINDINGS	DEVIATIONS FROM NORMAL
• Temperature and moisture: feel with back of hand.	• Warm, dry	• Extremely cool or warm, wet, oily. Cold skin is seen in shock, hypotension, arterial insufficiency. Very warm skin is seen in fever and hyperthyroidism.
• Turgor: Pinch up skin on sternum or under clavicle.	• Pinched-up skin returns immediately to original position.	• Pinched-up skin takes 30 seconds or longer to return to original position. Turgor is decreased in dehydration.
• Edema: Press firmly for 5–10 seconds over tibia and ankle.	• No swelling, pitting, or edema	• Swollen, shallow to deep pitting, ascites. Generalized edema is seen in congestive heart failure or kidney disease. Unilateral, localized edema is seen in peripheral vascular problems such as venous stasis, obstruction, or lymphedema.
If a skin lesion is detected, inspect and palpate for size, location, mobility, consistency, and pattern (circular, clustered, or straight-lined).	Silver-pink stretch marks (striae), moles (nevi), freckles, birthmarks	Primary lesions (Fig. 5–3) arise from normal skin owing to disease or irritation. Secondary lesions (Fig. 5–4) arise from changes in primary lesions. Vascular lesions (Fig. 5–5) may be seen with increased venous pressure, aging, liver disease, or pregnancy. Skin cancer can manifest as either primary or secondary lesions.

Nonpalpable Lesion

Macule: Flat and colored
(Example: Freckle, petechia)

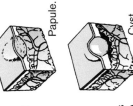

Macule.

Palpable Lesions With Fluid

Vesicle: Elevated and filled with fluid
(Example: Blister)

Nodule, tumor: Elevated and firm, has dimension of depth
(Example: Lipoma)

Pustule: Elevated and filled with pus
(Example: Acne)

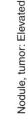

Vesicle.

Bulla.

Tumor.

Pustule.

Palpable Lesions

Papule: Elevated and superficial (Example: Mole)

Cyst: Encapsulated, filled with fluid or semisolid mass
(Example: Epidermoid cyst)

Wheal: Localized edema
(Example: Insect bite)

Papule.

Cyst.

Wheal.

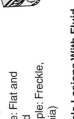
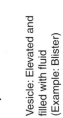
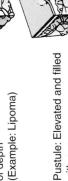

FIGURE 5–3 Primary skin lesions.

Ulcer: Skin surface loss, often bleeds

Atrophy: Thin, shiny taut skin

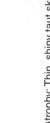

Crust: Dried pus or blood

Lichenification: Thickened, roughened skin

Scale: Thin, flaky skin

Keloid: Hypertrophied scar

FIGURE 5-4 Secondary skin lesions (changes in primary lesions).

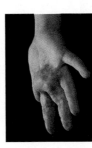

Spider vein: Bluish; may have radiating legs; seen mostly on legs

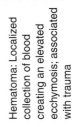

Ecchymosis: Round or irregular macular lesion; larger than petechia; color varies and changes black, yellow, and green

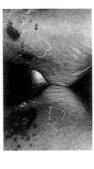

Hematoma: Localized collection of blood creating an elevated ecchymosis; associated with trauma

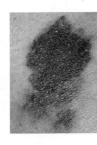

Cherry angioma: Ruby red; flat or raised

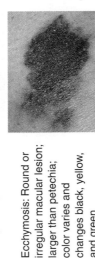

Spider angioma: Bright red with radiating legs; pulsating seen on center of lesion, or legs, or arms, and upper trunk; blanches when pressure is applied to center

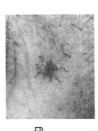
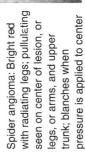
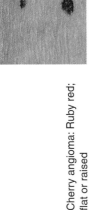

Petechia: Round red or purple macule

FIGURE 5–5 Vascular lesions.

HAIR INSPECTION AND PALPATION

PROCEDURE	NORMAL FINDINGS	DEVIATIONS FROM NORMAL
Inspect and palpate hair for the following:		
• Color	• Varies	• Patchy gray areas are seen in nutritional deficiencies. Copper-red hair in an African American child may indicate severe malnutrition.
• Amount and distribution	• Vary	• Sudden loss of hair (alopecia) or increase in facial hair in females (hirsutism). Hirsutism is seen in Cushing syndrome; general hair loss seen in infections, nutritional deficiencies, hormonal disorders, some types of chemotherapy, or radiation therapy; patchy loss seen with scale infection, and lupus erythematosus.
• Texture	• Fine to coarse, pliant	• Change in texture, brittle. Dull, dry hair is seen in hypothyroidism and malnutrition.
• Presence of parasites	• None	• Lice (body or head), eggs attached to hair shaft, usually accompanied by severe itching.

SCALP INSPECTION AND PALPATION

PROCEDURE	NORMAL FINDINGS	DEVIATIONS FROM NORMAL
Inspect and palpate scalp for the following:		
• Symmetry	• Symmetrical	• Asymmetrical
• Texture	• Smooth, firm	• Bumpy, scaly, excoriated. Scaly, dry flakes are seen in dermatitis; gray scaly patches are seen in fungal infections; dandruff seen with psoriasis.
• Lesions	• None	• Open or closed lesions

NAIL INSPECTION AND PALPATION

PROCEDURE	NORMAL FINDINGS	DEVIATIONS FROM NORMAL
Inspect and palpate nails for the following:		
• Color	• Pink nail bed *In dark skin:* may have small or large pigmented deposits, streaks, freckles	• Pale or cyanotic nails are seen in hypoxia or anemia; yellow discoloration seen in fungal infections or psoriasis; splinter hemorrhages (vertical lines) seen in trauma;

NAIL INSPECTION AND PALPATION (continued)

PROCEDURE	NORMAL FINDINGS	DEVIATIONS FROM NORMAL
		Beau's lines (horizontal) seen in acute trauma; nail pitting seen in psoriasis. 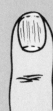 Splinter hemorrhages 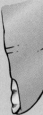 Beau's lines (acute illness)

NAIL INSPECTION AND PALPATION (continued)

PROCEDURE	NORMAL FINDINGS	DEVIATIONS FROM NORMAL
• Shape	• Round nail with 160° nail base	• Clubbing: 180° or more nail base is seen with hypoxia. Spoon nails occur with iron deficiency anemia.

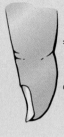

160°

Normal angle

Spoon nails
(iron deficiency anemia)

180°

Early clubbing
(oxygen deficiency)

>180°

Late clubbing
(oxygen deficiency)

Skin, Hair, and Nail Assessment

NAIL INSPECTION AND PALPATION (continued)

PROCEDURE	NORMAL FINDINGS	DEVIATIONS FROM NORMAL
• Texture	• Nail is round, hard, immobile *In dark skin:* may be thick	• Thickened nails are seen with decreased circulation.
• Condition of nail bed	• Smooth, firm, and pink	• Paronychia (inflamed nail head) indicates infection. Onycholysis (detached nail plate from nail bed) indicates infection or trauma.

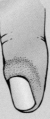

Paronychia (local infection)

PEDIATRIC VARIATIONS

Subjective Data: Focus Questions

Skin eruptions or rashes and relationship to any allergies (eg, food, formula, type of diapers used, diaper creams, soaps, dust)? Bathing routines and soap used? Play injuries (cuts, abrasions, bruises)? Indicators of physical abuse (bruises)? Exposure to communicable diseases? Exposure to pets, stuffed animals? Eczema (onset; precipitating factors; treatment)? Acne (during adolescence; location: face, back, chest; onset; precipitating factors; treatment)? Excessive nail biting? Twirling of hair? History of communicable diseases? Immunization history (see Appendix 3)?

Objective Data: Assessment Techniques

PROCEDURE	NORMAL FINDINGS	DEVIATIONS FROM NORMAL
Inspect the following:		
• Skin color	• Infant's skin is lighter shade than parents'; Mongolian spot is common hyperpigmentation variation in blacks, Native Americans, Latin Americans, and Asians. Body piercing may be cultural or a fad. Excessive piercing or tattooing that is "homemade" may increase risk for hepatitis B or HIV from infected needles.	• Yellow skin is seen in jaundice or with ingestion of too many yellow/orange vegetables.

Objective Data: Assessment Techniques (continued)

PROCEDURE	NORMAL FINDINGS	DEVIATIONS FROM NORMAL
• Oiliness and acne	• Adolescents have increased sebaceous gland activity.	• Cystic acne
• Skin lesions	• None	• Crusted or ruptured vesicles are seen in impetigo. Pruritic macular–papular skin eruptions that become vesicular are seen in chicken pox. Pink to red macular–papular rash is seen in measles.
• Hand creases: Assess dermatoglyphics by inspecting flexion creases in palm.	• Three flexion creases present in palm	• More or fewer than three flexion creases with varied pattern in palm; eg, one horizontal crease in palm (Simian crease)

Skin, Hair, and Nail Assessment

Objective Data: Assessment Techniques (continued)

PROCEDURE	NORMAL FINDINGS	DEVIATIONS FROM NORMAL

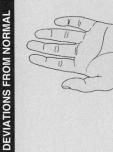

Normal creases
• Lustrous, strong, elastic

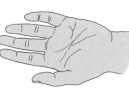

Simian creases

• Hair

GERIATRIC VARIATIONS

Skin
- Thinning epithelium
- Wrinkles, decreased turgor and elasticity
- Dry, itchy skin due to decrease in activity of eccrine and sebaceous glands
- Seborrheic or senile keratosis (tan to black macular–papular lesions on neck, chest, or back)
- Senile lentigines ("liver spots" or "age spots"—flat brown maculae on hands, arms, neck, face)
- Cherry angiomas (small, round, red elevated spots)
- Senile purpura (vivid purple patches)
- Acrochordons (soft, light-pink to brown skin tags)
- Prominent veins due to thinning epithelium

Hair
- Loss of pigment; fine, brittle texture
- Alopecia, especially in men; sparse body hair
- Coarse facial hair, especially in women
- Decreased axillary, pubic, and extremity hair

Nails
- Thickened, yellow, brittle nails
- Ingrown toenails

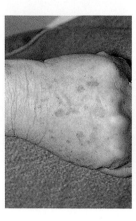

Solar lentigines are common on aging skin.

CULTURAL VARIATIONS

- Infants and newborns of African American, Native American, or Asian descent often have mongolian spots, a blue-black or purple macular area on buttocks and sacrum; sometimes this pattern appears on the abdomen, thighs, or upper extremities.

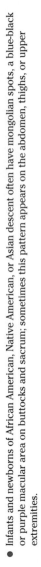
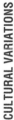

- Dark-skinned clients tend to have lighter colored palms, soles, nail beds, and lips. They may also have frecklelike pigmentation of nail beds and sclera. Nails may also be thick.
- Females of certain cultural groups shave or pluck pubic hair.
- Pallor is assessed in the dark-skinned client by observing the absence of underlying red tones. (Brown skin appears yellow-brown; black skin appears ashen-gray.)
- Erythema is detected by palpation of increased warmth of skin in dark-skinned clients.
- Cyanosis is detected in dark-skinned clients by observing the lips and tongue, which become ashen-gray.
- Inspect for petechiae in the oral mucosa or conjunctiva of the dark-skinned client, because they are difficult to see in dark-pigmented areas; also observe the sclerae, hard palate, palms, and soles for jaundice.
- Presence of body piercing may be a fad or a cultural norm.

Possible Collaborative Problems

Skin infections	Burns	Allergic reactions (skin)
Skin rashes	Graft rejection	Insect/animal bite
Skin lesions	Hemorrhage	

TEACHING TIPS FOR SELECTED NURSING DIAGNOSES

Adult Client

Nursing Diagnosis: Readiness for Enhanced Skin Integrity
- Teach client that regular exercise improves circulation and oxygenation of skin.
- Encourage protective clothing and boots when walking in wooded areas.

- Reduce sun exposure.
- Always use sunscreen (SPF 15 or higher) when sun exposure is anticipated.

- Wear long-sleeved shirts and wide-brimmed hats.
- Avoid sunburns.
- Avoid intermittent tanning.
- Understand the link between sun exposure and skin cancer and the accumulating effects of sun exposure on developing cancers.
- Teach self skin assessment (Appendix 6). If there is anything unusual, seek professional advice as soon as possible.

Nursing Diagnosis: Ineffective Health Maintenance related to lack of hygienic care of skin, hair, and nails, and/or excessive piercing/tattooing performed with "homemade" materials

☐ Assess hair, nail, and skin care, and instruct client on appropriate hygiene measures as necessary (eg, use mild soap, lotion for dry skin; wash oily areas with warm soap and water three times a day.)

Teach dangers of hepatitis B and HIV when using contaminated needles.

Nursing Diagnosis: Risk for Impaired Skin Integrity related to prolonged sun exposure

☐ Caution client against prolonged sun exposure or tanning lamp, and instruct that proper use of sunscreen agents can decrease the risk of skin pathologies. Teach client to report a change in the size or appearance of a mole, nodule, pigmented area, new growth on the skin; to limit or avoid sun exposure between 10 AM and 4 PM, when the sun's ultraviolet rays are strongest; to use a sunscreen with a solar protection factor (SPF) of at least 15; to wear protective clothing and hats (American Cancer Society, 2003).

Nursing Diagnosis: Risk for Impaired Nail Integrity related to prolonged use of nail polish

☐ Caution client of potential nail damage caused by prolonged use of nail polish.

Pediatric Client

Nursing Diagnosis: Risk for Impaired Skin Integrity: "diaper rash" related to parental knowledge deficit of skin care for diapered infant or child

☐ Inform parents of products available for treatment of rash and importance of frequent diaper changes and cleansing of skin with mild soap (eg, Ivory or Dove).

Nursing Diagnosis: Impaired Skin Integrity: acne related to developmental changes

☐ Teach adolescents proper skin cleansing and the significance of adequate rest, moderate exercise, and balanced diet.

Geriatric Client

Nursing Diagnosis: Risk for Impaired Skin Integrity related to immobility, decreased production of natural oils, and to thinning skin

☐ Teach client and family the benefits of turning of client, range-of-motion (ROM) exercises, massage, and cleaning of skin for reducing risk of skin breakdown. Teach family and client how to observe for reddened pressure areas. Encourage the use of lotions to replace skin oils. Massage skin with lotions. Instruct client to decrease the frequency of baths and use a humidifier during the cold seasons. Explain the effects of proper nutrition and adequate fluids on skin integrity.

Nursing Diagnosis: Risk for Impaired Tissue Integrity related to thickened, dried toenails

☐ Instruct client to soak nails 15 minutes in warm water prior to cutting. Use good scissors and lighting. Refer to podiatrist as necessary. Ascertain whether shoes fit correctly.

Head, Neck, and Cervical Lymph Node Assessment

ANATOMY OVERVIEW

The framework of the head is the skull, which can be divided into two subsections, the cranium and the face (Fig. 6–1).

The structure of the neck is composed of muscles, ligaments, and the cervical vertebrae. Contained within the neck are the hyoid bone, several major blood vessels, the larynx, trachea, and the thyroid gland (Fig. 6–2).

The sternomastoid (sternocleidomastoid) and trapezius muscles are two of the paired muscles that allow movement and provide support to the head and neck (Fig. 6–3).

The thyroid gland is the largest endocrine gland in the body. The first upper tracheal ring, called the cricoid cartilage has a small notch in it. The thyroid cartilage (Adam's apple) is larger and located just above the cricoid cartilage. The hyoid bone, which is attached to the tongue, lies above the thyroid cartilage and under the mandible (see Fig. 6–2).

Several lymph nodes are located in the head and neck (Fig. 6–4).

Equipment Needed

- Clean gloves
- Small cup of water for client during thyroid exam

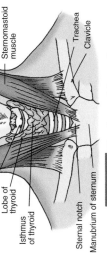

FIGURE 6-2 Structures of the neck.

Hyoid bone

Sternomastoid muscle

Trachea

Clavicle

Thyroid cartilage

Cricoid cartilage

Lobe of thyroid

Isthmus of thyroid

Sternal notch

Manubrium of sternum

Head, Neck, and Cervical Lymph Node Assessment

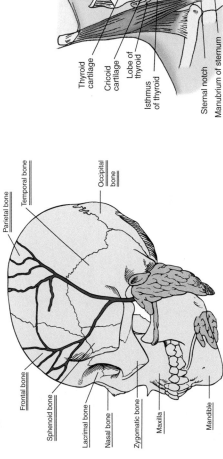

FIGURE 6-1 Bones and sutures of the skull (face and cranium).

Parietal bone

Temporal bone

Occipital bone

Frontal bone

Sphenoid bone

Lacrimal bone

Nasal bone

Zygomatic bone

Maxilla

Mandible

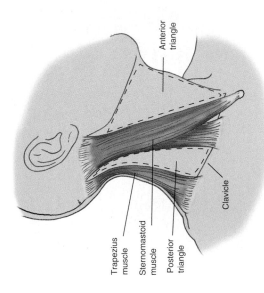

Trapezius
muscle

Sternomastoid
muscle

Posterior
triangle

Clavicle

Anterior
triangle

FIGURE 6-3 Neck muscles and landmarks.

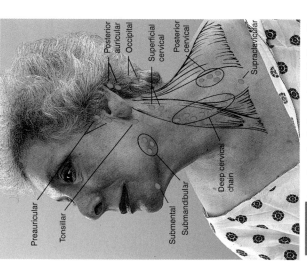

FIGURE 6–4 Lymph nodes in the neck. (© B. Proud.)

Subjective Data: Focus Questions

Lumps (onset, location, size, texture)? Limited movement of neck? Describe. Facial pain/neck pain/headaches (location, onset, duration, precipitating factors, relief)? Prior neck injuries (date, related to work, recreation, treatment)? Prior radiation therapy to head or neck? Prior thyroid surgery? Family history of head/neck cancer, migraines? Head and neck self-care: posture; use of helmet, seat belts, tobacco products?

RISK FACTORS. For head injury: high-risk sports, lack of protective devices (eg, seatbelts, helmet). For thyroid disease: radiation to upper body, family history. For lymphatic enlargement: immunosuppression, chronic disease, malnutrition.

Objective Data: Assessment Techniques

See Figures 6–1 to 6–4 for diagrams of the anatomy of the head, neck, and lymph nodes.

SCALP, FACE, AND NECK INSPECTION AND PALPATION

PROCEDURE	NORMAL FINDINGS	DEVIATIONS FROM NORMAL
*Inspect and palpate **scalp** for the following:*		
• Size	• Varies somewhat	• Extremely large or small. Scalp is thick in acromegaly (increase in growth hormones); large, acorn-shaped in Paget disease.
• Shape	• Symmetrical and round	• Asymmetrical

SCALP, FACE, AND NECK INSPECTION AND PALPATION (continued)

PROCEDURE	NORMAL FINDINGS	DEVIATIONS FROM NORMAL
• Consistency	• Hard and smooth	• Bumpy or soft. Lumps or lesions are seen in cancer and trauma.
Observe **face** *for the following:*		
• Symmetry	• Symmetrical	• Asymmetrical. Face is asymmetrical with parotid gland enlargement or Bell palsy, mask face in Parkinson disease.

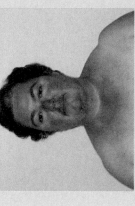

A moon-shaped face with reddened cheeks and increased facial hair may indicate Cushing's syndrome.

Head, Neck, and Cervical Lymph Node Assessment

SCALP, FACE, AND NECK INSPECTION AND PALPATION (continued)

PROCEDURE	NORMAL FINDINGS	DEVIATIONS FROM NORMAL
• Facial features	• Features vary • Symmetrical, centered head position	• Distorted features: mask face in Parkinson disease; tightened, hard face in scleroderma; sunken, hollow face in cachexia; swollen face in nephrotic syndrome; moon shape with red cheeks, facial hair in Cushing's syndrome (see Fig. 6-1).
*Observe **neck** for the following:* • Appearance	• Smooth, controlled movements; range of motion (ROM) from upright position:	• Asymmetrical head position, masses or scars present. Swelling is seen in cancer, enlarged thyroid, or inflamed lymph nodes.
• Movement	Flexion = 45° Extension = 55° Lateral abduction = 40° Rotation = 70°	• Rigid, jerky movements; ROM less than normal values; pain on movement. Limited ROM, stiffness, and rigidity are seen with muscle spasms, inflammation, meningitis, cervical arthritis.

TRACHEA, THYROID, AND LYMPH NODE PALPATION

Palpate first the trachea, then the thyroid using the guidelines described in Figure 6-5. After the thyroid, palpate the cervical lymph nodes.

1. Stand behind client and position your hands with thumbs on nape of client's neck.
2. Ask client to flex neck forward and to the right, and use fingers of your left hand to displace thyroid to the right.
3. Palpate the right lobe using your right fingers while client swallows—offer small sips of water.
4. Repeat procedure to examine the left lobe.
(Note: Ability to see or palpate the thyroid varies considerably with client thyroid size and body fluid.)

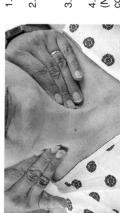

FIGURE 6-5 Palpating the thyroid. (© B. Proud.)

TRACHEA, THYROID, AND LYMPH NODE PALPATION (continued)

PROCEDURE	NORMAL FINDINGS	DEVIATIONS FROM NORMAL
Palpate **trachea** for position and landmarks (tracheal rings, cricoid and thyroid cartilage) (see Fig. 6–2 for location).	Midline position; symmetrical; landmarks identifiable	Asymmetrical. Position deviates from the midline with tumor, enlarged thyroid, aortic aneurysm, pneumothorax, atelectasis, or fibrosis.
Palpate **thyroid** *(see Fig. 6–5) for the following:*		
• Position	• Midline	• Deviates from the midline if obscured by masses or growths
• Characteristics, landmarks	• Smooth, firm, nontender	• Enlarged lobes, irregular consistency, tender or irregular consistency, tender on palpation. Diffuse enlargement is seen in hyperthyroidism, Graves disease, or endemic goiter; rapid enlargement of a single nodule suggests malignancy.
Note: *Ability to see or palpate the thyroid varies considerably with client's thyroid size and body build.*		
Palpate **cervical lymph nodes** *(see Figure 6–4 for location) for the following:*		
• Size and shape	• Cervical lymph nodes are usually not palpable. If palpable, they should be 1 cm or less and round.	• Enlarged nodes with irregular borders. Enlarged nodes greater than 1 cm are seen in acute or chronic infection, autoimmune disorders, or metastatic disease; hard, fixed, enlarged, unilateral nodes seen in

TRACHEA, THYROID, AND LYMPH NODE PALPATION (continued)

PROCEDURE	NORMAL FINDINGS	DEVIATIONS FROM NORMAL
• Delineation • Mobility • Consistency • Tenderness	• Discrete • Mobile • Soft • Nontender	metastasis; tender, enlarged nodes seen in acute infections; enlarged occipital nodes seen in HIV infection. • Confluent • Fixed to tissue • Hard, firm • Client verbalizes pain on palpation. 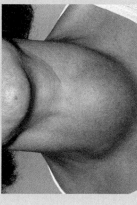 Diffuse enlargement of the thyroid gland.

PEDIATRIC VARIATIONS

PROCEDURE	NORMAL FINDINGS	DEVIATIONS FROM NORMAL
Observe **head shape, size** (see Appendix 5 for head circumference norms), **and symmetry.**	Normocephalic and symmetrical, features appropriate for size. Head may have odd shape due to molding during birth.	Uneven molding, asymmetrical masses, enlarged head. Hydrocephalus is seen with increased cerebrospinal fluid. Microcephaly is a head circumference less than norms.
Observe **head control.**	Holds head erect in midline by 4 months; moves head up and down, side to side	Resistance to movement (head lag after 6 months seen with cerebral injury)
Palpate **skull and fontanelles** (Fig. 6–6) very gently when infant is quiet in sitting position.	Smooth, fused except for fontanelles	Ecchymotic areas on scalp; loss of hair in spots; posterior fontanelle (triangular) open after 2 months of age, anterior fontanelle open after 12–18 months of age. Bulging fontanelle is seen in increased intracranial pressure; depressed fontanelles seen in dehydration or malnutrition; delayed fusion of fontanelles seen with hydrocephalus, Down syndrome, hypothyroidism, or rickets; third fontanel seen in Down syndrome; limited ROM seen in torticollis (wryneck).

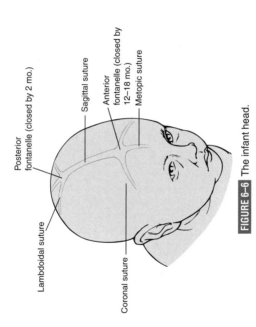

FIGURE 6-6 The infant head.

Posterior fontanelle (closed by 2 mo.)

Sagittal suture

Anterior fontanelle (closed by 12–18 mo.)

Metopic suture

Lambdoidal suture

Coronal suture

PEDIATRIC VARIATIONS (continued)

PROCEDURE	NORMAL FINDINGS	DEVIATIONS FROM NORMAL
Palpate **neck** for lymph nodes.	Moderate number of small (> 3 mm), shotty, firm lymph nodes in child (age 3–12 years)	Diffuse large lymph nodes, asymmetrical placement. Enlarging supraclavicular lymph nodes are seen with Hodgkin disease.

GERIATRIC VARIATIONS

- Bones of face and nose are more angular in appearance.
- Muscle atrophy and loss of fat cause shortening of neck.

Possible Collaborative Problems

Lymphedema
Hypercalcemia
Hypocalcemia

TEACHING TIPS FOR SELECTED NURSING DIAGNOSES

Adult Client

Nursing Diagnosis: Risk for Injury to Head and Neck related to poor posture
☑ Teach correct posture and body mechanics for lifting and pushing.

Nursing Diagnosis: Risk for Injury to Head and Neck related to not wearing protective devices (eg, head gear during contact sports, seatbelts, eye goggles).
☑ Teach risk reduction tips:
- Use safe driving techniques.
- Wear protective gear such as helmets and seatbelts, especially when riding a bicycle or motorcycle.
- Avoid violent or potentially violent environments when possible.
  - Modify one's residence to prevent falls.
  - Avoid dangerous contact sports likely to cause brain injury; wear protective equipment when engaging in such activity.

Pediatric and Adolescent Clients

Nursing Diagnosis: Risk for Injury related to open fontanelles
☑ Teach parents normal development of fontanelles and how to protect infants from pressure and injury.

Nursing Diagnosis: Ineffective Health Maintenance related to a knowledge deficit on the effects of smokeless tobacco
☑ Teach that "dipping snuff" is highly addictive and increases the risk of cheek and gum cancer nearly 50-fold among long-term snuff users. Explain that this is *not* a healthy substitute for smoking cigarettes (*American Cancer Society,* 2000).

Nursing Diagnosis: Risk for Injury to Teeth and Oral Mucous Membrane related to tongue piercing and wearing metal balls
☑ Teach risks of teeth chipping, and hepatitis B and HIV virus when done with contaminated needles.

Head, Neck, and Cervical Lymph Node Assessment

CHAPTER 7

Mouth, Oropharynx, Nose, and Sinus Assessment

ANATOMY OVERVIEW

The mouth or oral cavity is formed by the lips, cheeks, hard and soft palates, uvula, and the tongue and its muscles (Fig. 7–1).

Contained within the mouth are the tongue, teeth, gums, and the openings of the salivary glands (parotid, submandibular, and sublingual). The gums (gingiva) are covered by mucous membrane and normally hold 32 permanent teeth in the adult (Fig. 7–2).

Three pairs of salivary glands secrete saliva (watery, serous fluid containing salts, mucus, and salivary amylase) into the mouth (Fig. 7–3): submandibular glands, and the sublingual glands.

The throat (pharynx), located behind the mouth and nose, serves as a muscular passage for food and air. The upper part of the throat is the nasopharynx. Below the nasopharynx lies the oropharynx, and below the oropharynx lies the laryngopharynx. (Fig. 7–4).

The superior, middle, and inferior turbinates are bony lobes, sometimes called conchae, that project from the lateral walls of the nasal cavity. These three turbinates serve to increase the surface area that is exposed to incoming air (see Fig. 7–4).

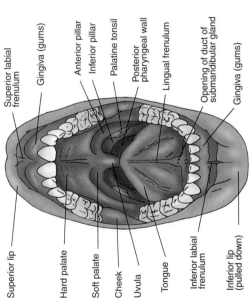

FIGURE 7–1 Structures of the mouth.

Superior labial frenulum

Gingiva (gums)

Anterior pillar

Inferior pillar

Palatine tonsil

Posterior pharyngeal wall

Lingual frenulum

Opening of duct of submandibular gland

Gingiva (gums)

Superior lip

Hard palate

Soft palate

Cheek

Uvula

Tongue

Inferior labial frenulum

Inferior lip (pulled down)

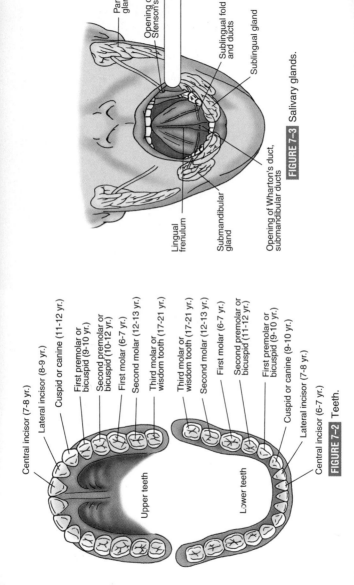

Central incisor (7-8 yr.)
Lateral incisor (8-9 yr.)
Cuspid or canine (11-12 yr.)
First premolar or bicuspid (9-10 yr.)
Second premolar or bicuspid (10-12 yr.)
First molar (6-7 yr.)
Second molar (12-13 yr.)
Third molar or wisdom tooth (17-21 yr.)

Upper teeth

Lower teeth

Third molar or wisdom tooth (17-21 yr.)
Second molar (12-13 yr.)
First molar (6-7 yr.)
Second premolar or bicuspid (11-12 yr.)
First premolar or bicuspid (9-10 yr.)
Cuspid or canine (9-10 yr.)
Lateral incisor (7-8 yr.)
Central incisor (6-7 yr.)

FIGURE 7-2 Teeth.

Parotid gland
Opening of Stenson's duct
Sublingual fold and ducts
Sublingual gland
Submandibular gland
Opening of Wharton's duct, submandibular ducts
Lingual frenulum

FIGURE 7-3 Salivary glands.

Mouth, Oropharynx, Nose, and Sinus Assessment

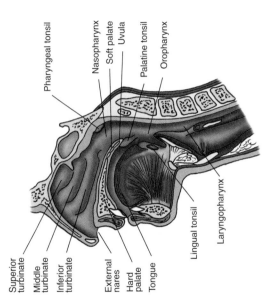

Pharyngeal tonsil

Nasopharynx
Soft palate
Uvula

Palatine tonsil

Oropharynx

Superior
turbinate

Middle
turbinate

Inferior
turbinate

External
nares

Hard
palate

Tongue

Lingual tonsil

Laryngopharynx

FIGURE 7–4 Nasal cavity and throat structures.

MOUTH AND OROPHARYNX ASSESSMENT

Equipment Needed

- Penlight
- Tongue blade
- Small gauze (2 × 2-inch)
- Clean gloves

Subjective Data: Focus Questions

Prior dental problems? Dentures? Lip or oral lesions? Redness or swelling (location, occurrence, relief)? Sore throat? Dysphagia? Hoarseness? History of mouth, nose, or throat cancer in family? Smoking or use of smokeless tobacco? Dental care practices? Brushing, flossing, dental checkups?

RISK FACTORS. Risk for oral cancer related to smoking or use of smokeless tobacco; family history; alcoholism; working with wood, nickel refining, or textile fibers.

Objective Data: Assessment Techniques

Review Figures 7–1 through 7–4 for diagrams of the mouth, oropharynx, and nose.

INSPECTION AND PALPATION

PROCEDURE	NORMAL FINDINGS	DEVIATIONS FROM NORMAL
Inspect **open and closed mouth** *for symmetry and alignment*	Lips and surrounding tissue relatively symmetrical in net position and with smiling, drooping. No lesions, swelling, drooping. Upper teeth resting on top of lower teeth with upper incisors slightly overriding lower ones	Asymmetrical mouth may indicate neurological condition (eg, Bell palsy, stroke), tumors, infections, or dental abnormalities or poorly fitting dentures. Malocclusion of teeth, separation of individual teeth, or protrusion of upper or lower incisors
Wearing gloves, inspect and palpate **lips** *for the following:* • Color	• *In white skin:* Pink *In dark skin:* May have bluish hue or frecklelike pigmentation	• Cyanotic, pale lips in shock or anemia; reddish in ketoacidosis or carbon monoxide poisoning
• Consistency	• Moist, smooth with no lesions	• Dry, cracked; nodules, fissures, or lesions present; cheilosis (cracking in the corners) seen in riboflavin deficiencies; broken vesicles with crusting in herpes simplex type 1; scaly nodular lesions or ulcers occur with lip carcinoma
Note: Ask client to remove any dentures or dental appliances prior to continuing examination.		

INSPECTION AND PALPATION (continued)

PROCEDURE	NORMAL FINDINGS	DEVIATIONS FROM NORMAL
Wearing gloves, inspect and palpate **buccal mucosa** *for the following:* • Color • Consistency	• Pink (increased pigmentation often noted in dark-skinned clients) • Smooth, moist, without lesions	• Pale, cyanotic, or reddened mucosa • Ulcers, dry mucosa, bleeding, or white patches (leukoplakia) that do not scrape off are precancerous; white, curdy patches that scrape off and bleed indicate thrush; red spots over red mucosa (Koplik spots) indicate measles. Canker sores (painful vesicles that erupt) are seen with allergies and stress.

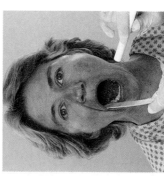

Inspecting the buccal mucosa.
(© B. Proud.)

INSPECTION AND PALPATION (continued)

PROCEDURE	NORMAL FINDINGS	DEVIATIONS FROM NORMAL
• Landmarks	• Parotid duct (Stensen duct) openings are seen as small papillae located near upper second molar	• Elevated, markedly reddened area near upper second molar
Wearing gloves, retract client's lips to inspect and palpate **gums** *for the following:*		
• Color	• Pink	• Pale, markedly reddened. Swollen gums that bleed are seen with gingivitis; recessed red gums with tooth loss seen with periodontitis, bluish black gum line present in lead poisoning. 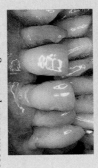 Receding gums (periodontitis). (Courtesy of Dr. Michael Bennett.)

Mouth, Oropharynx, Nose, and Sinus Assessment

INSPECTION AND PALPATION (continued)

PROCEDURE	NORMAL FINDINGS	DEVIATIONS FROM NORMAL
• Consistency	• Moist, clearly defined margins	• Dry, edema, ulcers, bleeding, white patches, tenderness
*Wearing gloves, inspect and palpate **teeth** for the following:*		
• Number (see Fig. 7–2)	• 32 teeth	• Missing teeth
• Position and condition	• Stable fixation, smooth surfaces and edges	• Loose or broken teeth, jagged edges, dental caries
• Color	• Pearly white and shiny	• Darkened, brown, or chalky white discoloration. Teeth may be yellow-brown in clients who use excessive coffee, tea, tobacco, or fluoride. Chalky white area is seen with beginning cavity.

INSPECTION AND PALPATION (continued)

PROCEDURE	NORMAL FINDINGS	DEVIATIONS FROM NORMAL
*Inspect protruded **tongue** for:* • Symmetry and texture	• Moist; papillae present; symmetrical appearance; midline fissures present. *Common variations:* Fissured, geographic tongue	• Dry; nodules, ulcers present; papillae or fissures absent; asymmetrical. Deep fissures are seen in dehydration; black, hairy tongue with use of some antibiotics; smooth, red, shiny tongue seen in niacin or vitamin B_{12} deficiency.

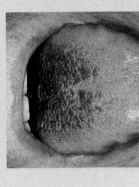

Black hairy tongue. (Courtesy of Dr. Michael Bennett.)

Mouth, Oropharynx, Nose, and Sinus Assessment

INSPECTION AND PALPATION (continued)

PROCEDURE	NORMAL FINDINGS	DEVIATIONS FROM NORMAL
• Movement • Color	• Smooth • Pink	• Jerky or unilateral movement • Markedly reddened; white patches; pale
Inspect ventral surface of the tongue and mouth floor for the following: • Color	• Pink, slightly pale	• Markedly reddened, cyanotic, or extreme pallor
• Landmarks	• Submandibular duct openings (Wharton ducts) are located on both sides of the frenulum. Tongue is free of lesions or increased redness; frenulum is centered (see Fig. 7–3).	• Lesions, ulcers, nodules, or hypertrophied duct openings are present on either side of the frenulum.

INSPECTION AND PALPATION (continued)

PROCEDURE	NORMAL FINDINGS	DEVIATIONS FROM NORMAL
*Inspect and palpate **sides of tongue** for color and lesions*	Pink, smooth, moist; no lesions	White or reddened areas, ulcerations, or indurations present. Leukoplakia indicates precancerous lesions; may see canker sores. 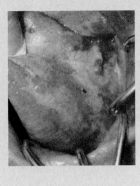 Leukoplakia (ventral surface).
*Inspect **hard and soft palate** (see Fig. 7–3) for the following:* • Color	• *Hard palate:* Pale *Soft palate:* Pink	• Extreme pallor, white patches, or markedly reddened areas

INSPECTION AND PALPATION (continued)

PROCEDURE	NORMAL FINDINGS	DEVIATIONS FROM NORMAL
• Consistency		• *Hard palate:* Firm with irregular transverse rugae; *common variation:* palatine torus (bony protuberance) on hard palate *Soft palate:* Spongy texture with symmetrical elevation or phonation • Softened tissue over hard palate; lesions present; absence of elevation; soft palate asymmetrical elevation with phonation. Thick, white plaques are seen in *Candida* infection; deep, purple lesions may indicate Kaposi sarcoma. 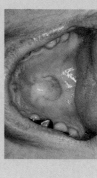 Torus palatinus. (Courtesy of Dr. Michael Bennett.)

INSPECTION AND PALPATION (continued)

PROCEDURE	NORMAL FINDINGS	DEVIATIONS FROM NORMAL
*Inspect **oropharynx** (see Fig. 7–1) for the following:*		
• Color	• Pink	• Markedly reddened with exudate seen in pharyngitis; yellow mucus seen with postnasal sinus drainage
• Landmarks	• Tonsillar pillars symmetrical; tonsils present (unless surgically removed) and without exudate; uvula at midline and rises on phonation	• Enlarged tonsils (tonsils are red, enlarged, and covered with exudate in tonsillitis); see tonsillitis grading scale (Fig. 7–5); asymmetrical; uvula deviates from midline; edema, ulcers, lesions.

In a client who has both tonsils and a sore throat, tonsilitis can be identified and ranked with a grading scale from 1 to 4 as follows:

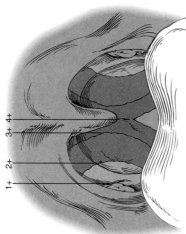

1+   Tonsils are visible.

2+   Tonsils are midway between tonsillar pillars and uvula.

3+   Tonsils touch the uvula.

4+   Tonsils touch each other.

FIGURE 7–5   Detecting and grading tonsilitis.

PEDIATRIC VARIATIONS

Subjective Data: Focus Questions

Number of teeth, time of eruptions? Thumb sucking, use of pacifier (type)? Sore throats? Use of bottle? Fluoridated water?

Objective Data: Assessment Techniques

Observe for eruption of deciduous teeth (Fig. 7–6).
Observe for eruption of permanent teeth (see Fig. 7–2).
Inspect dental caries; may be due to bottle caries syndrome.
Note: A sucking pad inside upper lip of infant may be apparent due to sucking friction.
Tonsils reach adult size by age 6 years and continue to grow. By age 10 to 12 years, they are twice the adult size. By the end of adolescence they begin to atrophy back to normal adult size.

GERIATRIC VARIATIONS

- Worn teeth, abraded enamel, and yellowing teeth
- Gums recede and undergo fibrotic changes.
- Poor-fitting dentures may cause facial asymmetry and poor eating habits.
- Oral mucosa is drier owing to decreased production of saliva.
- Tongue may be fissured and have varicose veins on ventral surface.
- Decreased taste sensations due to a decrease in number of taste buds

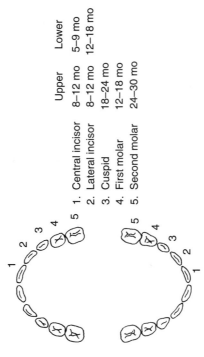

	Upper	Lower
1. Central incisor	8–12 mo	5–9 mo
2. Lateral incisor	8–12 mo	12–18 mo
3. Cuspid	18–24 mo	
4. First molar	12–18 mo	
5. Second molar	24–30 mo	

FIGURE 7–6 Timetable for eruption of deciduous teeth.

CULTURAL VARIATIONS

- Dark-skinned clients may have lips with bluish hue or frecklelike pigmentation.
- Some groups have reduced teeth number; Australian aborigines have four extra molars.
- Dark-skinned clients may have dark pigment or freckling on side or ventral surface of tongue and floor of mouth; hard and soft palate may also be darkly pigmented.
- Some groups (especially Asians) may have mandibular torus (lump) on inner mandible near second premolar.
- Native Americans and Asians may have a split uvula.

Possible Collaborative Problems

Stomatitis
Gingivitis
Oral lesions
Periodontal (gum) disease (periodontitis)

TEACHING TIPS FOR SELECTED NURSING DIAGNOSES AND COLLABORATIVE PROBLEMS

Adult Client

Nursing Diagnosis: Impaired Oral Mucous Membrane related to inadequate mouth care

Instruct client on proper brushing and flossing. (Client should brush teeth at least twice a day, and floss once a day to remove plaque from under gum line and sides of teeth.)

Recommend a toothbrush with soft rounded end or polished bristles, to be replaced every 2–3 months when frayed, in addition to an "American Dental Association–accepted" fluoride toothpaste and mouth rinse. Explain the role of fluoride in decreasing tooth decay. Refer to dentist for fluoride protection advice if client's water supply is not fluoridated. Explain the significance of a well-balanced diet in decreasing tooth decay and periodontal (gum) disease. Dry mouth can cause problems with oral health. Refer to dentist or physician for possible recommendation of artificial saliva or fluoride mouth rinse.

Collaborative Problem: Potential complication: Periodontal (gum) disease

Teach client warning signs:

- Gums that bleed with brushing
- Red, swollen, tender gums or gums that pull away from teeth
- Pus between teeth and gums
- Loose or separating teeth
- Change in position of teeth or denture fit.
- Persistent bad breath

Teach prevention:

- Brush and floss every day
- Schedule regular dental visits (American Dental Association, 1999).

Collaborative Problem: Potential complication: Oral cancer

Teach client warning signs:

- Sore in mouth that does not heal
- White scaly patches in mouth
- Swelling or lumps in mouth/throat/on lips
- Numbness or pain in mouth/throat/on lips
- Repeated bleeding in mouth
- Difficulty chewing, swallowing, speaking, or moving tongue or jaw
- Change in bite

Teach client to

- Stop smoking
- Limit alcohol consumption
- Eat a healthy, balanced diet

Pediatric Client

Nursing Diagnosis. Impaired Dentition related to lack of proper mouth care

◻ Instruct parents not to put child to bed with a bottle filled with formula, milk, juices, or sugar water, because these liquids pool around teeth and promote decay. Use only water in bottles when putting child to bed, to prevent so-called baby bottle tooth decay. Teach the importance of fluoride in drinking water and proper nutrition to prevent decay. Fluoride drops are recommended for infants and fluoride tablets for children up through age 14 years if adequate fluoride is not in water. Refer child who sucks thumb past age 4 years. Explain the benefits of using a small, cool spoon rubbed over gums or using teething rings during teething period. Instruct parents to start brushing child's teeth with eruption of first tooth. Begin flossing when primary teeth have erupted (2–2½ years.) Parents should be taught to brush and floss child's teeth until child can be taught to do this alone (approximately age 5 years for brushing and age 8 years for flossing). Encourage a dental exam by a dentist when child is between 6 and 12 months of age.

Nursing Diagnosis: Risk for Injury to teeth related to developmental age and play activities

◻ In case of broken or knocked-out tooth, instruct parent to rinse the tooth in cool water (do not scrub it); when possible, insert back in socket and hold in place. If this cannot be done, put tooth in cup of milk or water, or wrap it in wet cloth and take child to dentist at once for possible replacement. Recommend use of mouth guards to prevent injuries in contact sports.

Geriatric Client

Nursing Diagnosis: Imbalanced Nutrition: Less Than Body Requirements related to decreased appetite secondary to decreased senses of taste and smell

◻ Explore food preferences with client and use visual appeal of food to enhance appetite.

NOSE AND SINUS ASSESSMENT

Equipment Needed

- Penlight
- Nasal speculum or otoscope with short, broad-tipped speculum

Subjective Data: Focus Questions

Change in ability to smell? Nosebleeds? Difficulty breathing through nostrils? Past sinus infections? Past oral, nasal, or sinus surgery? Trauma? Obstructed nares? Use of nasal sprays? Frequent infections? Allergies? Headaches located in sinus areas? Postnasal drip?

Objective Data: Assessment Techniques

See Figure 7–1 for a diagram of the nasal cavity.

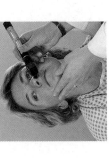

INSPECTION

The external nose is inspected; then the internal nose is inspected, using the following guidelines.

Guidelines for Using Nasal Speculum

- Tilt client's head back to facilitate speculum insertion and visualization.
- Hold speculum in hand and brace your index finger against the client's nose.
- Insert the speculum tip approximately 1 cm and dilate the naris as much as possible.
- Use the other hand to position client's head and hold penlight.

INSPECTION

PROCEDURE	NORMAL FINDINGS	DEVIATIONS FROM NORMAL
Observe **external nose** for the following:		
• Skin appearance	• *Color:* Same as face *Consistency:* Smooth	• Nodules, lesions, erythema, visible vasculature
• Shape	• Symmetrical appearance	• Asymmetry
• Nares	• Symmetrical appearance; no changes in nares with respiration; dry with no crusting; septum midline	• Asymmetry; flaring nares; discharge, crusting; displaced septum
Inspect **internal nose** for the following:		
• Appearance	• Mucosa pink and moist with uniform color and no lesions	• Mucosa markedly red, dry, or cracked; areas of discoloration; polyps; masses. Mucosa is swollen, pale pink or bluish gray with allergies; nasal mucosa red and swollen with upper respiratory infection; ulcers seen with trauma, infection, nose-picking, or cocaine use; polyps seen with chronic allergies.

INSPECTION (continued)

PROCEDURE	NORMAL FINDINGS	DEVIATIONS FROM NORMAL
• Landmarks: Turbinates, septum (Fig. 7–7)	• Turbinates and middle meatus visible and same color as mucosa, moist and free of lesions; septum symmetrical and uniform without lesion	• Turbinates are not visible owing to edema or occlusion; turbinates pale or markedly reddened; polyps, lesions, copious discharge, bleeding, perforation, deviation present.
Assess function of nose for patency (with client's mouth closed and one naris occluded, feel for air).	Air is felt being exhaled through opposite naris; noiseless	Noisy or obstructed exhalation when mouth is closed and one naris is occluded

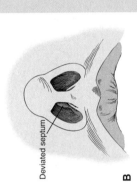

Middle turbinate
Inferior turbinate

Deviated septum

A　　　　　**B**

FIGURE 7–7 Structures of the internal nose. (*A*) Normal internal nose. (*B*) Deviated septum.

PALPATION

PROCEDURE	NORMAL FINDINGS	DEVIATIONS FROM NORMAL
Palpate **external nose** for firmness.	Solid placement; no nodules, masses, or pain reported on palpation	Unstable placement; nodules or masses present; client verbalizes pain on palpation. Nasal tenderness is seen with local infection.
Palpate **sinuses**, both frontal and maxillary (Fig. 7–8), for tenderness.	Nontender on palpation	Client verbalizes pain or discomfort on palpation with allergies or sinus infection.

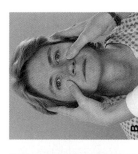

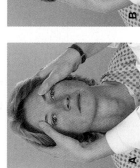

FIGURE 7-8 Palpation of frontal and maxillary sinuses. (*A*) The frontal sinuses. (*B*) The maxillary sinuses. (© B. Proud.)

PERCUSSION

PROCEDURE	NORMAL FINDINGS	DEVIATIONS FROM NORMAL
Percuss sinuses for resonance.	Hollow tone elicited	Flat, dull tone elicited; client expresses pain on percussion.

GERIATRIC VARIATIONS

- Decreased senses of taste and smell due to progressive atrophy of olfactory bulbs

Possible Collaborative Problem

Nosebleed

TEACHING TIPS FOR SELECTED NURSING DIAGNOSES AND COLLABORATIVE PROBLEMS

Adult Client

Nursing Diagnosis: Ineffective Health Maintenance related to a lack of information regarding over-the-counter nasal medications

☒ Instruct client on use, proper dosage, and effects of overuse of nasal sprays.

Collaborative Problem: Potential complication: Nosebleed

☒ Instruct client to apply pressure for 5 minutes while breathing through mouth and leaning forward. Caution against blowing nose for several hours afterward. Refer as necessary.

Pediatric Client

Nursing Diagnosis: Risk for Injury related to insertion of foreign bodies into nasal cavity

☒ Caution and give instructions to parents about child's interest in inserting objects into body openings such as the nose. Instruct on common objects to remove from child's reach.

8

Eye Assessment

ANATOMY OVERVIEW

External Structures of the Eye

The *eyelids* (upper and lower) are two movable structures composed of skin and two types of muscle—striated and smooth (Fig. 8–1). The palpebral conjunctiva lines the inside of the eyelids, and the bulbar conjunctiva covers most of the anterior eye, merging with the cornea at the limbus.

The *lacrimal apparatus* consists of glands and ducts that serve to lubricate the eye (Fig. 8–2). The *lacrimal gland*, located in the upper outer corner of the orbital cavity just above the eye, is responsible for tear production. Tears are channeled into the *nasolacrimal sac*, through the *nasolacrimal duct*. They drain into the nasal meatus.

The *extraocular muscles* are the six muscles attached to the outer surface of each eyeball (Fig. 8–3).

Internal Structures of the Eye

The eyeball is composed of three separate coats or layers (Fig. 8–4). The outermost layer consists of the *sclera* and *cornea*.

The *iris* is a circular disc of muscle that contains pigments that determine eye color. The central aperture of the iris is called the pupil.

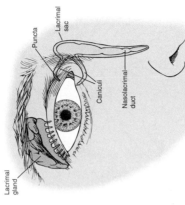

FIGURE 8-2 The lacrimal apparatus consists of tear (lacrimal) glands and ducts.

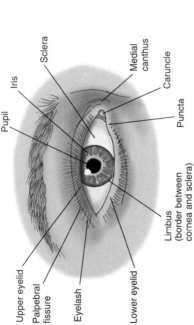

FIGURE 8-1 Eyelids are structured to protect the eyes from foreign matter, distribute tears, and shield the eye from excessive light.

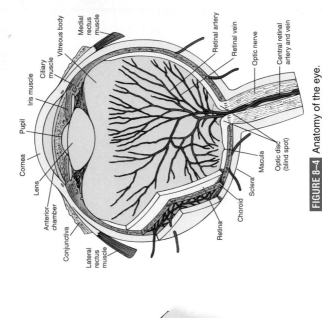

FIGURE 8-3 Extraocular muscles control the direction of eye movement.

Superior oblique

Superior rectus

Medial rectus

Lateral rectus

Inferior rectus

Inferior oblique

FIGURE 8-4 Anatomy of the eye.

Medial rectus muscle

Vitreous body

Ciliary muscle

Iris muscle

Pupil

Cornea

Lens

Anterior chamber

Conjunctiva

Lateral rectus muscle

Retinal artery

Retinal vein

Optic nerve

Central retinal artery and vein

Optic disc (blind spot)

Macula

Sclera

Choroid

Retina

The *lens* is a biconvex, transparent, avascular, encapsulated structure located immediately posterior to the iris.

The innermost layer, the *retina*, extends only to the ciliary body anteriorly and consists of numerous layers of nerve cells, including the cells commonly called rods and cones.

The *optic disc* is a cream-colored, circular area located on the retina toward the medial or nasal side of the eye (Fig. 8–5). A small circular area that appears slightly depressed is referred to as the *physiological cup*.

The *retinal vessels* can be readily viewed with the aid of an ophthalmoscope. Four sets of *arterioles* and *venules* travel through the optic disc, bifurcate, and extend to the periphery of the fundus. Vessels are dark red and grow progressively narrower as they extend out to the peripheral areas. A retinal depression known as the fovea centralis is located adjacent to the optic disc in the temporal section of the fundus (see Fig. 8–5). This area is surrounded by the macula, which appears darker than the rest of the fundus.

Equipment Needed

- Eye chart (Snellen or handheld Rosenbaum)
- Near-vision chart or newsprint
- Cover card or occluder
- Penlight
- Ophthalmoscope
- Ruler

Subjective Data: Focus Questions

Recent changes in vision? (Spots? Floaters? Blind spots? Halos? Rings? Difficulty with night vision? Double vision? Blurred vision? Strabismus?) Eye pain? Redness or swelling? Eye discharge? Excessive watering or tearing? History of prior eye surgery? Trauma? Use of corrective glasses or contact lenses? Date of last eye exam? Eye care habits? (Use of sunglasses? Safety glasses? Work around chemicals, sparks, smokes, fumes, or dust?) Have visual changes affected work or ability to care for self?

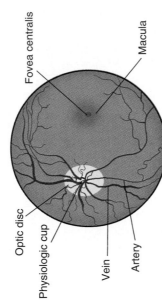

Fovea centralis

Macula

Optic disc

Physiologic cup

Vein

Artery

FIGURE 8–5 Normal ocular fundus. (© 1994, CMSP.)

RISK FACTORS. Risk for glaucoma related to diabetes mellitus, myopia, older than 75 years, or family history of glaucoma. Risk for cataracts related to increasing age, ultraviolet light exposure, diabetes mellitus, smoking, alcohol use, diet low in antioxidant vitamins.

Objective Data: Assessment Techniques

Review Figure 8–1 through 8–5 for diagrams of the anatomy of the internal and external eye structures.

Client should be seated comfortably in a well-lighted room that can be darkened for ophthalmic examination. First, the external eye structures are examined. Then eye function is tested, followed by the ophthalmic examination, using the following guidelines:

EXTERNAL EYE EXAMINATION

PROCEDURE	NORMAL FINDINGS	DEVIATIONS FROM NORMAL
Inspect eyelids and lashes (see *Figure 8–1*) for the following: • Position and appearance	• Lid margins moist and pink; lashes short, evenly spaced and curled outward; lower margins at bottom edge of iris; upper margins of lid cover approximately 2 mm of iris	• Crusting; scales; lashes absent or curled inward; edema or xanthelasma present; itching; ulcerative lesions; asymmetry of lids; weak muscles See Box 8-1 for illustrations of the following: *Ectropion:* Lower lids turn outward. *Entropion:* Lower lids turn inward. *Chalazion:* Inflammation of meibomian glands

BOX 8-1. External Eye Examination: Deviations from Normal

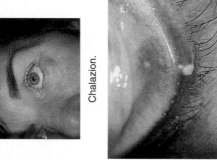

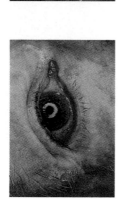

Ectropion.

Chalazion.

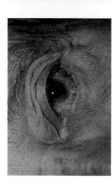

Entropion.

Hordeolum [stye].

BOX 8-1. (*continued*)

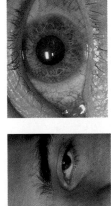

Conjunctivitis. (© 1995 Dr. P. Marazzi/Science Photo Library/CMSP.)

Ptosis.

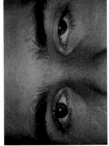

Blepharitis.

BOX 8–1. (*continued*)

Mydriasis.

Miosis.

Anisocoria.

EXTERNAL EYE EXAMINATION (continued)

PROCEDURE	NORMAL FINDINGS	DEVIATIONS FROM NORMAL
		Hordeolum: Stye or inflammation of glands in lid
		Blepharitis: Waxy white scales (seborrheic) or inflammation of hair follicles (*Staphylococcus*)
		Prosis: Drooping of lids; seen with oculomotor nerve damage, myasthenia gravis. Protrusion of eyeballs with retracted lids seen with hyperthyroidism
• Blinking	• Blinking symmetrical, involuntary, at approximately 15 blinks/min	• Asymmetrical blink, incomplete closure, rapid blinking
Inspect **conjunctiva** (bulbar and palpebral) **and sclera** for clarity and appearance by separating lids with thumb and index finger and asking the client to look up, down, and to either side.	Bulbar conjunctiva is clear with tiny vessels visible; palpebral conjunctiva is pink with no discharge; sclera is blue-white	Lesions, nodules, discharge, crusting, foreign body present. Marked redness of the conjunctiva is seen with conjunctivitis (see Box 8-1). Sclera with petechiae; marked jaundice
Inspect **cornea** (using oblique lighting) for appearance.	Transparent, smooth, moist	Lesions, opacities, irregular light reflections, or foreign body present. Rough or dry cornea is seen with trauma or allergic responses.

Eye Assessment

EXTERNAL EYE EXAMINATION (continued)

PROCEDURE	NORMAL FINDINGS	DEVIATIONS FROM NORMAL
*Inspect **iris and pupil** for the following:*		
• Shape	• Round	• Irregular. Miosis is constricted, fixed pupils; mydriasis (see Box 8-1).
• Equality	• Equal	• Unequal; anisocoria is abnormal when difference in pupil size becomes greater during pupillary reaction tests (see Box 8-1).
• Color (iris)	• Uniform color	• Inconsistent color
Inspect **lens** for clarity.	• Clear	Cloudy; opacities are seen with cataracts (see page 139).
*Inspect and palpate **lacrimal apparatus** (see Figure 8–2) for the following:*		
• Appearance	• Puncta (small elevations on the nasal side of the upper and lower lids), mucosa pink	• Puncta markedly reddened and edematous with infection, blockage, or inflammation
• Response to pressure applied at nasal side of lower orbital rim	• No tenderness or discharge noted when pressure is applied	• Fluid or purulent discharge expressed with pain on palpation with duct blockage

EYE FUNCTION TESTING

PROCEDURE	NORMAL FINDINGS	DEVIATIONS FROM NORMAL
Check **visual acuity:** • Check distance vision with Snellen chart 20 feet from client. 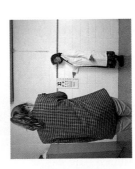	• 20/20 OD and OS with no hesitation, frowning, or squinting	• Any letters missed on 20/20 line or above; client reads chart by leaning forward, with head tilted, or squinting. *Myopia*, impaired far vision, occurs when second number is larger than first number (eg, 20/40).
• Check near vision with newspaper approximately 14 inches from client's head	• Client reads print at 14 inches without difficulty.	• Client reads print by holding it closer or farther away than 14 inches. *Presbyopia*, impaired near vision, is seen when client moves reading material farther away to read owing to decreased accommodation of lenses.

EYE FUNCTION TESTING (continued)

PROCEDURE	NORMAL FINDINGS	DEVIATIONS FROM NORMAL
Check **peripheral vision:** Face client at a distance of 2–3 feet; client and examiner look directly ahead and cover eye directly opposite each other.	Client and examiner report seeing object at the same time as it approaches from the periphery.	With reduced peripheral vision, client does not report seeing object at the same time as the examiner.
Check **accommodation** (Fig. 8–6): Ask client to stare at an object 3–4 feet away, and move object in toward client's nose.	Pupils converge and constrict as object moves in toward the nose; pupil responses are uniform.	Pupils do not converge or constrict. Pupil responses are unequal.

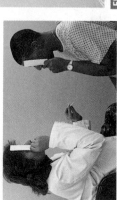

FIGURE 8–6 Testing accommodation of pupils. (© B. Proud.)

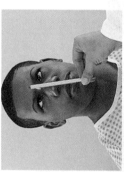

Checking peripheral vision. (© B. Proud.)

EYE FUNCTION TESTING (continued)

PROCEDURE	NORMAL FINDINGS	DEVIATIONS FROM NORMAL
Check extraocular movements (Fig. 8–7): Ask client to follow object as it is moved in six cardinal fields.	Both eyes move in a smooth, coordinated manner in all directions	Jerky eye movements (nystagmus) are seen with inner ear disorders, multiple sclerosis, brain lesions, or narcotics use; failure to follow object with one or both eyes indicates muscle weakness or cranial nerve dysfunction.

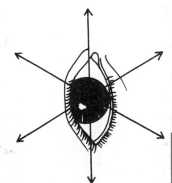

FIGURE 8–7 Six cardinal fields for checking extraocular movements.

EYE FUNCTION TESTING (continued)

PROCEDURE	NORMAL FINDINGS	DEVIATIONS FROM NORMAL
Check response to light: • Check corneal light reflex by asking client to look straight ahead and then shining light toward facial midline.	• Reflections of light noted at same location on both eyes	• Light reflections noted at different areas on both eyes occur with deviation in alignment of eyes due to muscle weakness or paralysis.
• Check direct pupil response by asking client to look straight ahead and approaching each eye from the client's side with a penlight.	• Illuminated pupils constrict.	• Illuminated pupils fail to constrict.
• Check consensual pupil response by asking client to look straight ahead and approaching each eye from the client's side with a penlight.	• Pupil opposite the one illuminated constricts simultaneously.	• Pupil opposite the one illuminated fails to constrict; monocular blindness is seen when light directed to blind eye results in no response in either pupil.
Check for **abnormal eye movement** using cover-uncover test (Fig. 8–8): 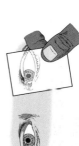	Uncovered eye does not move as opposite eye is covered. 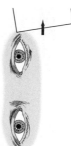	Uncovered eye moves to focus when opposite eye is covered. Covered eye moves to 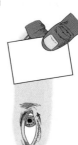

FIGURE 8–8 Cover test abnormalities.

EYE FUNCTION TESTING (continued)

PROCEDURE	NORMAL FINDINGS	DEVIATIONS FROM NORMAL
Ask client to look straight ahead, covering one eye with a cover card, and observe uncovered eye for movement.	Covered eye does not move as cover is removed.	focus when cover is removed. These findings are seen with eye muscle weakness and deviation in alignment of eyes. *Esotropia* is turning in of eyes, *exotropia* is turning outward of eyes, and *strabismus* is constant malalignment of eyes.

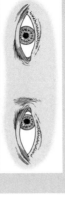
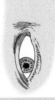

Strabismus (or tropia).

Ophthalmic Examination

Use ophthalmoscope according to the following guidelines:

Guidelines for Using the Ophthalmoscope

The examiner can rotate the lenses that are labeled with a negative or positive number. Red numbers indicate a negative diopter and are used for myopic (nearsighted) clients. Black numbers indicate a positive diopter and are used for hyperopic (farsighted) clients. The zero lens is used if neither the examiner nor the client has a refractive error.

1. Turn ophthalmoscope on and select the aperture with the large, round beam of white light.

2. Ask the client to remove glasses. Remove your glasses. Contact lenses can be left in the eyes of the client or examiner.

3. Ask the client to fix gaze on an object that is straight ahead and slightly upward.

4. Darken the room to allow pupils to dilate.

5. Hold the ophthalmoscope in your right hand with your index finger on the lens wheel and place the instrument to your right eye (braced between the eyebrow and nose). Examine the client's right eye. Use your left hand and left eye to examine the client's left eye.

6. Begin about 10–15 inches from the client at a 15° angle to the client's side.

7. Keep focused on the red reflex as you move in closer, then rotate the diopter setting to see the optic disc.

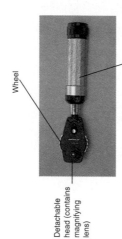

Ophthalmoscope.

Wheel

Body (contains light source)

Detachable head (contains magnifying lens)

Eye Assessment

Ophthalmic Examination (continued)

PROCEDURE	NORMAL FINDINGS	DEVIATIONS FROM NORMAL
Inspect **red reflex** for shape and color.	Red reflex is round, bright, with red-orange glow	Red reflex has decreased color or abnormal shape; dark spots are seen with cataracts. 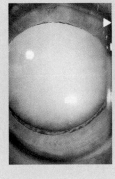 Nuclear cataracts appear gray when seen with a flashlight; they appear as a black spot against the red reflex when seen through an ophthalmoscope.

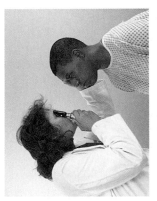

Inspecting the red reflex. (© B. Proud.)

Ophthalmic Examination (continued)

PROCEDURE	NORMAL FINDINGS	DEVIATIONS FROM NORMAL
*Inspect **optic disc** (see Fig. 8–5) for the following:*		
• Shape	• Round or slightly oval disc with sharply defined margins	• Irregularly shaped disc, blurred margins. A swollen disc with blurred margins is papilledema and is seen with hypertension or increased intracranial pressure. Optic atrophy is a white-colored disc without vessels and is seen with the death of optic nerves. 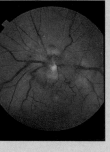 Papilledema.
• Color	• Creamy pink (lighter than retina)	• Pallor of entire disc or one section

Ophthalmic Examination (continued)

PROCEDURE	NORMAL FINDINGS	DEVIATIONS FROM NORMAL
• Size	• Approximately 1.5 mm size, symmetrical in both eyes	• Size of disc not equal in both eyes
• Physiological cup	• Small area is noted as paler than disc located just temporal of center of disc; occupies $\frac{4}{10}$ to $\frac{5}{10}$ of the diameter of the disc.	• Cup location and size are not symmetrical in both eyes; cup occupies more than $\frac{5}{10}$ diameter of the disc.
Inspect **retinal vessels** *for the following:*		
• Appearance	• *Arteries:* Light red and smaller than veins *Veins:* Darker in color and larger than arteries	• Arteries less than $\frac{2}{3}$ size of veins; arteries pale • Arterioles widen and have copper color in hypertension; with long-standing hypertension arterioles have silver color.
• Distribution	• Vessels regular in shape and decreasing in size as they branch and move toward the periphery; crossing of arteries and veins show no changes in the diameter of the underlying vessel.	• Vessels irregular in shape and uneven in distribution; narrowing of underlying vessels at crossings of arteries and veins; abnormal arteriole venous crossings are seen with hypertension and arteriosclerosis.
Inspect **retinal background** for appearance	Fine texture with pink, uniform color	Pallor of the fundus; soft or hard exudates (cotton-wool patches) seen in hyperten-

Ophthalmic Examination (continued)

PROCEDURE	NORMAL FINDINGS	DEVIATIONS FROM NORMAL
Inspect **macula** for appearance	Darker than remainder of retina; fovea seen as a tiny bright light in the center of macula	sion and diabetes; red spots or streaks may be microaneurysms or hemorrhages. Abnormalities in color or vessels; lesions present. Clumped pigment is seen with detached retinas or injuries.

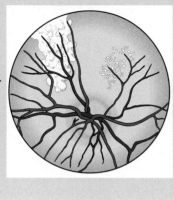

Exudates.

Ophthalmic Examination (continued)

DEVIATIONS FROM NORMAL

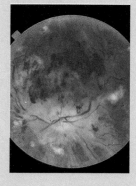

Retinal hemorrhages.

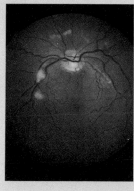

Cotton wool patches.

Objective Data: Assessment Techniques

Explain procedure to decrease child's fear when room is darkened.

PROCEDURE	NORMAL FINDINGS	DEVIATIONS FROM NORMAL
Inspect **placement of light** on cornea	Light falls symmetrically within each pupil.	Asymmetrical location of light reflection on pupil signals strabismus.
Observe **placement and alignment of eyes** *by doing the following:* • Measure inner canthal distance.	• Average distance 3 cm (1.2 in)	• Wide-set eyes, upward slant, and thick epicanthal folds may suggest Down syndrome. • Presence of upward slant in non-Asians
• Assess palpebral slant.	• Outer canthus aligns with tips of pinna (except in Asian children). 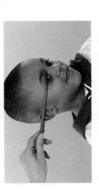 Outer canthus is in alignment with the tip of the pinna. (© B. Proud.)	• Upper lid lies above iris ("setting-sun" sign) suggests hydrocephalus. Black and white speckling of iris (Brushfield spots) seen in Down syndrome

PEDIATRIC VARIATIONS (continued)

PROCEDURE	NORMAL FINDINGS	DEVIATIONS FROM NORMAL
• Observe placement of lids.	• With eye open, lids lie between upper iris and pupil.	
Inspect **iris.**	Color varies from brown to green to blue.	
Inspect **lacrimal apparatus.**	Lacrimal meatus not present until 3 months of age	
Perform **visual acuity tests.** Use E chart for preschoolers.	Children can differentiate colors by age 5 years	A 1-line difference indicates visual impairment and should be referred; may be due to congenital defects, chronic disease, or refractive errors.

GERIATRIC VARIATIONS

External eye examination reveals the following:

- Conjunctiva thins and becomes yellowish.
- White ring around iris (arcus senilis)—does not affect vision
- Dry eyes due to decreased tear production
- Drooping eyelids (senile ptosis)
- Entropion and ectropion common in the older adult
- Clouding of lens (cataracts)
- Yellowish nodules on bulbar conjunctiva (pinguecula) common

Visual examination reveals the following:

- Presbyopia (decreased near vision due to decreased elasticity of lens) common in clients older than 45 years
- Slowed pupillary response and slowed accommodation
- Poorer night vision and decreased tolerance to glare

Visual field examination reveals the following:

- Decreased peripheral vision
- Difficulty differentiating blues from greens

Funduscopic examination reveals the following:

- Pale, narrowed arterioles

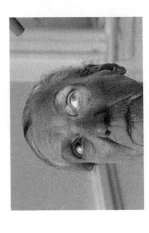

Observe the pupils. With a penlight or similar device, test pupillary reaction to light. (© B. Proud.)

CULTURAL VARIATIONS

- Asians and members of some other groups may have common variation of epicanthal folds or narrowed palpebral fissures.
- Dark-skinned clients may have sclera with yellow or pigmented freckles.

Possible Collaborative Problems

Visual changes	Glaucoma
Eye infections	Impaired functioning of lacrimal apparatus
Cataracts	Corneal abrasions

TEACHING TIPS FOR SELECTED NURSING DIAGNOSES

Adult Client

Nursing Diagnosis: Ineffective Health Maintenance related to lack of knowledge of necessity for eye examinations

Recommend the following guidelines for frequency of eye exams for individuals without risk factors:

Age	Frequency
≥ 65	Every 1–2 years
40–64	Every 2–4 years
20–39	At least once during period

(Reprinted with permission from the American Academy of Ophthalmology [1996]. *Comprehensive adult eye evaluation, preferred practice patterns.* San Francisco.)

See Table 8–1 for guidelines for patients with risk factors.

TABLE 8–1 FREQUENCY OF COMPREHENSIVE EYE EVALUATION FOR PATIENTS WITH RISK FACTORS

Condition/Risk Factor	Frequency of Evaluation
Diabetes without retinopathy	
Onset after age 30	Once a year
Onset before age 30	5 years after onset and yearly thereafter
Pregnancy	Prior to conception or early in the first trimester; every 3 months thereafter
Risk factors for glaucoma (individuals of African descent, family history of glaucoma)	
Age 65 or older	Every 1–2 years
Age 40–64	Every 2–4 years
Age 20–39	Every 3–5 years

(Reprinted with permission from the American Academy of Ophthalmology (1996). *Comprehensive adult eye evaluation, preferred practice patterns*. San Francisco.)

Nursing Diagnosis: Ineffective Health Maintenance related to inadequate knowledge of eye infection care

☐ Instruct client on proper administration of eye drops and ointments. Discuss proper cleansing from inner to outer canthus and changing of cleansing cloth to prevent cross-contamination (from eye to eye).

Pediatric Client

Nursing Diagnosis: Readiness for Enhanced Knowledge of Eye Care During the Growing Years

☐ *In the newborn nursery.* Pediatricians or family physicians should examine all infants; ophthalmologists should examine all high-risk infants.

By age 6 months. Pediatricians, family physicians, or ophthalmologists should screen all infants.

At age 3½ years. Pediatricians, family physicians, or ophthalmologists should examine all children. Focus should be on visual acuity.

At age 5 years. Pediatricians, family physicians, or ophthalmologists should evaluate vision and alignment. Further screening should be done at routine school checks or after the appearance of symptoms.

(Reprinted from American Academy of Ophthalmology [1996]. *Policy statement: Vision screening for infants and children.* San Francisco.)

Geriatric Client

Nursing Diagnosis: Ineffective Protection related to decreased tear production secondary to the aging process

☐ Instruct client on the use of artificial tears as necessary.

Nursing Diagnosis: Ineffective Protection related to impaired vision secondary to the aging process

☐ Explore with client aids for independent living (eg, magnifying glasses, cane). Encourage further evaluation if necessary. Instruct family to keep furniture in same place and to provide better lighting. Provide community resources (eg, "talking" books and magazines available in libraries).

Adults age 65 years or older should have an ophthalmological eye examination at least every 2 years. To promote this goal, the National Eye Care Project is a nationwide outreach program sponsored by the American Academy of Ophthalmology as a public service. It is designed to help the disadvantaged elderly obtain medical eye care. The toll-free phone number is 1-800-222-EYES. To be eligible, a person must be a US citizen or legal resident, age 65 years or older, who does not have access to an ophthalmologist he or she may have seen in the past.

Clients should wear sunglasses and hats in the sun. This is important because even on bright cloudy days, ultraviolet light can penetrate clouds. Squinting does not eliminate ultraviolet light entering the eye.

Adults with diabetes mellitus should have an ophthalmologic eye examination at the time of diagnosis and at medically appropriate intervals thereafter.

Adults with risk factors such as family history of glaucoma, cataract, retinal detachment, or degenerative eye disease should seek more frequent care, especially if they experience any of the following problems:

- Blurry vision uncorrectable by lenses
- Distorted or double vision
- Dimming of vision that comes and goes, or sudden loss of vision
- Red eye
- Pain in or around the eye
- Excessive tearing or discharge from the eye
- Swelling of the eyelids or protrusion of the eye
- New floaters or flashes of light
- Loss of side vision
- Crossed, turned, or wandering eye
- Halos (colored rays or circles around lights)

(Reprinted with permission from the American Academy of Ophthalmology [1991]. *Eye care for the elderly*. San Francisco.)

9 Ear Assessment

ANATOMY OVERVIEW

The external ear is composed of the auricle or pinna and the external auditory canal (Fig. 9–1). A translucent, pearly gray, concave membrane, the tympanic membrane, or eardrum, serves as a partition stretched across the inner end of the auditory canal, separating it from the middle ear. The distinct landmarks (Fig. 9–2) of the tympanic membrane include:

- Handle and short process of the malleus
- Umbo
- Cone of light
- Pars flaccida
- Pars tensa

The middle ear, or tympanic cavity, is a small, air-filled chamber in the temporal bone. It is separated from the external ear by the eardrum and from the inner ear by a bony partition containing two openings, the round and oval windows. The middle ear cavity contains three auditory ossicles: The malleus, the incus, and the stapes (see Fig. 9–1).

The inner ear, or labyrinth, is fluid filled and is made up of the bony labyrinth and an inner membranous labyrinth. The bony labyrinth has three parts: the cochlea, the vestibule, and the semicircular canals.

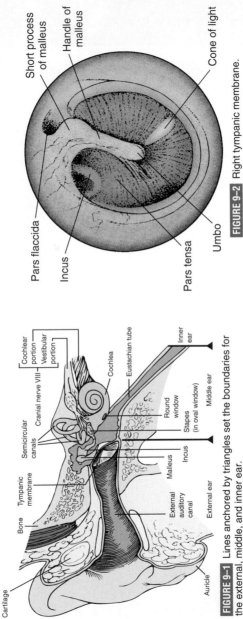

FIGURE 9-2 Right tympanic membrane.

Short process of malleus

Handle of malleus

Cone of light

Pars flaccida

Incus

Pars tensa

Umbo

Cochlear portion
Vestibular portion
Cranial nerve VIII

Cochlea

Eustachian tube

Inner ear

Semicircular canals

Round window

Stapes (in oval window)

Middle ear

Malleus

Incus

Tympanic membrane

Bone

External auditory canal

External ear

Cartilage

Auricle

FIGURE 9-1 Lines anchored by triangles set the boundaries for the external, middle, and inner ear.

Equipment Needed

- Otoscope with good batteries (pneumatic bulb device for young children)
- Tuning fork (512 and 1024 Hz)

Subjective Data: Focus Questions

Recent changes in hearing? All or some sounds affected? Ear drainage? Type? Ear pain? Occurrence? Relief? Associated factors such as sore throat, sinus infection, or gum/teeth problems? Ringing or cracking in ears (tinnitus)? Dizziness, unbalanced or spinning (vertigo)? History of prior ear surgery? Trauma? Use of ototoxic medications? Last hearing examination?

RISK FACTORS. Risk for hearing loss related to genetic predisposition, congenital anomalies, loud noises, ototoxic medications, aging (presbycusis).

Objective Data: Assessment Techniques

Review Figures 9–1 to 9–2 for the anatomy of the external, middle, and inner ear.

Client should be comfortably seated in such a way that you can easily visualize both ears. First examine the external ear, then examine the ear canal and tympanic membrane with the otoscope, and finally assess hearing function.

PROCEDURE	NORMAL FINDINGS	DEVIATIONS FROM NORMAL
Inspect **external ear** *(Fig. 9–3) for the following:*		
• Size and shape	• Ears of equal size and similar appearance	• Ears of unequal size or configuration (smaller than 4 cm or larger than 10 cm)

Ear Assessment

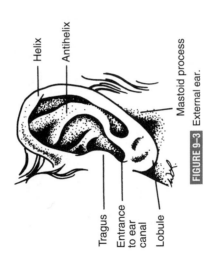

Helix

Antihelix

Mastoid process

Tragus

Entrance
to ear
canal

Lobule

FIGURE 9–3 External ear.

Objective Data: Assessment Techniques (continued)

PROCEDURE	NORMAL FINDINGS	DEVIATIONS FROM NORMAL
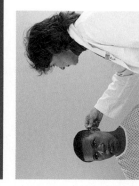 Inspecting the external ear. (© B. Proud.)		
• Position	• Alignment of pinna with corner of eye and within 10° angle of vertical position	• Pinna positioned below a line from corner of eye, or unequal alignment. Malaligned or low-set ears are seen with chromosomal defects or genitourinary disorders.
• Lesions and discolorations	• Skin smooth and without nodules; color pink	• Erythema, edema, nodules, or areas of discoloration. Postauricular cysts are seen with blocked sebaceous glands;

Ear Assessment

Objective Data: Assessment Techniques (continued)

PROCEDURE	NORMAL FINDINGS	DEVIATIONS FROM NORMAL
Palpate **external ear.** (See Fig. 9–3)	Nontender auricle, tragus	ulcerated crusted nodules may be malignant; pale-blue color seen in frostbite. Painful auricle or tragus associated with otitis externa or postauricular cyst. Tenderness behind ear is associated with otitis media.
Palpate **mastoid process** for the following: • Tenderness • Temperature • Edema	• No tenderness or pain when palpated • Warm • Mastoid process easily palpated	• Pain on palpation of mastoid process with mastoiditis • Erythema • Actual process difficult to palpate; ear displaced outward owing to edema
Inspect **auditory canal** using otoscope (Fig. 9–4) for the following: • Cerumen	• *Color:* Black, dark red, gray or brown *Consistency:* Waxy, flaky, soft or hard *Odor:* None	• Impacted cerumen (obstructs visualization of membrane); bloody purulent discharge is seen in otitis media with perforated eardrum; foul-smelling discharge associated with otitis externa or impacted foreign body.

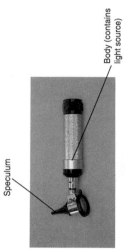

Body (contains light source)

Speculum

FIGURE 9-4 Otoscope.

Objective Data: Assessment Techniques (continued)

PROCEDURE	NORMAL FINDINGS	DEVIATIONS FROM NORMAL
• Appearance	• Canal walls pink and uniform with tympanic membrane (TM) visible	Build-up of cerumen in ear canal. • Lesions, foreign body, erythema, or edema present in canal. Red, swollen canals are seen with otitis media; polyps (Box 9-2) or nonmalignant nodular swellings can block the view of the eardrum.

Objective Data: Assessment Techniques (continued)

PROCEDURE	NORMAL FINDINGS	DEVIATIONS FROM NORMAL
• Tenderness	• Little or no discomfort on manipulation of pinna; inner two thirds of canal very tender if touched with speculum	• Moderate to severe pain when pinna is moved or otoscope speculum is inserted
*Inspect **tympanic membrane** (TM), using otoscope (Box 9–1), for the following:* • Color	• Pearly gray, shiny, and translucent	• Dull appearance: blue (blood) or pink/red (inflammation). Red, bulging TM is seen with acute otitis media (see Box 9-2); yellow bulging TM seen with serous otitis media; blue or dark color seen in trauma when there is blood behind the TM.

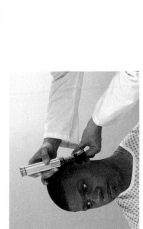

Inspecting the external canal and tympanic membrane. (© B. Prouc.)

BOX 9-1. Using Otoscope to Inspect Tympanic Membrane

1. Ask clients to sit comfortably with the back straight and the head tilted slightly away from you toward their opposite shoulder.

2. Choose the largest speculum that fits comfortably into the ear canal (usually 5 mm in the adult) and attach it to the otoscope. Hold otoscope in your dominant hand and turn the otoscope light to "on."

3. Use thumb and fingers of your opposite hand to grasp client's auricle firmly but gently. Pull out, up, and back to straighten the external auditory canal. Do not alter this position during the exam.

4. Grasp the otoscope handle between your thumb and fingers. Hold otoscope up or down, whichever is comfortable for you.

5. Steady your hand holding the otoscope against the client's head or face.

6. Insert the speculum gently down and forward into the ear canal (approximately 0.5 inch). Be careful not to touch the inner portion of the sensitive canal wall.

7. Position your eye against the lens.

BOX 9–2. Ear Assessment: Deviations from Normal

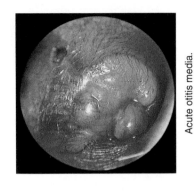

Acute otitis media.

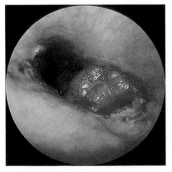

Polyp.

BOX 9–2. (*continued*)

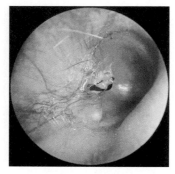

Scarred tympanic membrane.

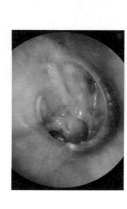

Perforated tympanic membrane.
(© 1992 Science Photo
Library/CMSP.)

Objective Data: Assessment Techniques (continued)

PROCEDURE	NORMAL FINDINGS	DEVIATIONS FROM NORMAL
• Consistency	• Intact; may show movement when swallowing	• *Perforations, scarring* (see Box 9-2), or immobility. White spots are seen with scarring of the TM.
• Landmarks (see Figure 9–2)	• Cone of light, umbo, handle of malleus and short process of malleus easily visualized	• Retracted TM accentuates landmarks; bulging TM partially occludes landmarks. Prominent landmarks indicate TM retraction due to negative pressure from obstructed eustachian tube, whereas obscured landmarks indicate thickened TM due to chronic otitis media.
Assess **auditory function** *for the following:*		
• Gross hearing ability: Whisper words 1–2 feet behind client; hold watch 1–2 inches from client's ear.	• Client is able to hear whispered words from 1–2 feet; able to hear watch tick from 1–2 inches.	• Client is unable to hear whispered words or watch tick; unequal response.
• Lateralization of sound—Weber test: Place activated tuning fork on center top of client's head (Fig. 9–5A).	• Vibration heard equally in both ears	• Vibratory sound lateralized to poor ear in conductive loss and to good ear in sensorineural loss.

Ear Assessment

Objective Data: Assessment Techniques (continued)

PROCEDURE	NORMAL FINDINGS	DEVIATIONS FROM NORMAL
• Comparison of air conduction (AC) to bone conduction (BC)—Rinne test: Place tuning fork on mastoid process until no longer heard, then move it to front of ear (Fig. 9–5B, C).	• AC > BC (AC is twice as long as BC)	• BC ≥ AC Bone conduction heard longer than or equal to air conduction in conductive loss; AC longer than, but not twice as long as, BC in sensorineural loss.

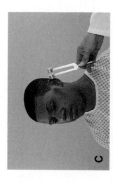

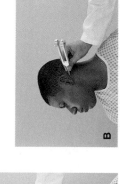

FIGURE 9–5 Using a tuning fork to assess auditory function. (A) Weber test. (B) Rinne test: bone conduction. (C) Rinne test: air conduction. (© B. Proud.)

Objective Data: Assessment Techniques (continued)

PROCEDURE	NORMAL FINDINGS	DEVIATIONS FROM NORMAL
Perform **Romberg test for equilibrium** by having client stand with feet together first with eyes open, then with eyes closed (put your arms around client to prevent fall).	Client stands straight with minimal swaying.	Client sways and moves feet apart to prevent fall—may indicate vestibular disorder.

PEDIATRIC VARIATIONS

Objective Data: Assessment Techniques

PROCEDURE	NORMAL FINDINGS	DEVIATIONS FROM NORMAL
Observe for **placement and alignment of pinna.**	Pinna slightly crosses the horizontal line (Fig. 9–6A), extends slightly forward from skull symmetrically.	Pinna falls below horizontal line (Fig. 9–6B); low ears with vertical alignment greater than 10° angle suggest mental retardation or congenital syndrome; abnormal shape indicates renal pathology.

Ear Assessment

PEDIATRIC VARIATIONS (continued)

PROCEDURE	NORMAL FINDINGS	DEVIATIONS FROM NORMAL
Note on otoscopic exam: For examination of infants and young children, restraint may be necessary to accomplish a safe, effective assessment (Fig. 9–7). In infants and young children, examination with the otoscope should be last in the assessment because this part of the examination is often distressing to clients of this age group.		
Observe **inner canal.**		
Child younger than 3 years. Restrain; pull pinna downward and backward.		
Child older than 3 years. Pull pinna upward and backward.		
Inspect **TM** using otoscope with pneumatic device.	TM moves with introduction of air	TM does not move with introduction of air.

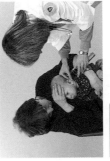

FIGURE 9–7 Child being restrained in the upright position. (© B. Proud.)

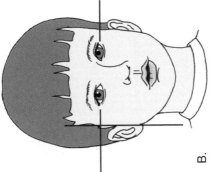

A.   B.

FIGURE 9-6 Placement and alignment of pinna in children. (*A*) Normal. (*B*) Low-set ears with alignment greater than 10° angle.

GERIATRIC VARIATIONS

- Elongated lobule with linear wrinkles
- Tuft of wirelike hair may be present at entrance of ear canal.
- More cerumen buildup; drier; harder cerumen due to rigid cilia in ear canal
- Perception of consonants (Z, T, F, G) and high-frequency sounds (S, Sh, Ph, K) decreases.
- Dull, retracted TM—may be cloudy with more prominent landmarks owing to normal aging process
- Diminished hearing acuity (presbycusis)

CULTURAL VARIATIONS

- Ear wax varies. Dry, gray, flaky wax is usual in Asians and Native Americans. Light-honey to orange to dark-brown wax is most common in African Americans and Caucasians.

Possible Collaborative Problems

Otitis media: acute, chronic, serous otitis externa
Perforated tympanic membrane
Hearing impairment

TEACHING TIPS FOR SELECTED NURSING DIAGNOSES

Adult Client

Nursing Diagnosis: Risk for Disturbed Sensory Perception (hearing) related to working in loud, noisy environment

Teach client to wear protective hearing device when in environment with loud noises such as music, loud engines, aircraft, explosives, or firearms.

Nursing Diagnosis: **Risk for Injury** related to decreased auditory perception

☐ Teach safety measures (eg, burglar alarms, lights on telephone and alarms, phone designed for hearing impaired). Explore availability of resources for hearing aids, and refer client to reading materials or sign language learning if appropriate. Encourage client to ask others to repeat what is not heard.

Nursing Diagnosis: **Readiness for Enhanced Auditory Perception**

☐ Teach client to cleanse ears with damp cloth and to avoid use of cotton-tipped applicators for cleaning internal auditory canal. Encourage use of sunscreen on external ear. Teach client to shake head to remove water in ear and to dry ear after swimming to prevent swimmer's ear.

Pediatric Client

Nursing Diagnosis: **Risk for Injury** related to attempts to insert foreign objects in ear

☐ Teach parents and child (as appropriate for age) dangers of insertion of foreign objects in ear. Teach parents to avoid toys with small, removable parts. Also, teach parents to avoid putting infant to bed with bottle filled with formula, juices, or sugar water, because this can settle in the oral pharynx and provide medium for bacterial growth and cause middle ear infections. Encourage yearly ear screening with physical examination during growing years.

Geriatric Client

Nursing Diagnosis: **Disturbed Sensory Perception (auditory)** related to aging process

☐ Speak clearly, and allow client to see your lips. Speak within distance of 3–6 feet.

Thoracic and Lung Assessment

ANATOMY OVERVIEW

Thorax

The term *thorax* identifies the portion of the body extending from the base of the neck superiorly to the level of the diaphragm inferiorly. This thoracic cage is constructed of the sternum, 12 pairs of ribs, 12 thoracic vertebrae, muscles, and cartilage. The thorax consists of the anterior thoracic cage (Fig. 10–1) and the posterior thoracic cage (Fig. 10–2).

The sternum, or breastbone, lies in the center of the chest anteriorly and is divided into three parts: The manubrium, the body, and the xiphoid process. The clavicles (collar bones) extend from the manubrium to the acromion of the scapula. The manubrium connects laterally with the clavicles and the first two pairs of ribs. A U-shaped indentation located on the superior border of the manubrium is an important landmark known as the *suprasternal notch*. A few centimeters below the suprasternal notch, a bony ridge can be palpated at the point where the manubrium articulates with the body of the sternum. This landmark, is referred to as the *sternal angle* (or angle of Louis).

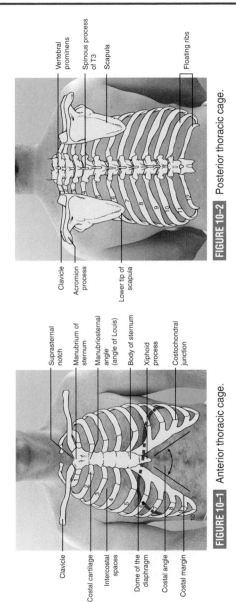

Vertebral prominens

Spinous process of T3

Scapula

Floating ribs

Clavicle

Acromion process

Lower tip of scapula

FIGURE 10–2 Posterior thoracic cage.

Suprasternal notch

Manubrium of sternum

Manubriosternal angle (angle of Louis)

Body of sternum

Xiphoid process

Costochondral junction

Clavicle

Costal cartilage

Intercostal spaces

Dome of the diaphragm

Costal angle

Costal margin

FIGURE 10–1 Anterior thoracic cage.

Ribs (seven through ten) connect to the cartilages of the pair lying superior to them rather than to the sternum (see Fig. 10–1). This configuration forms an angle between the right and left costal margins meeting at the level of the xiphoid process, referred to as the *costal angle*.

Each pair of ribs articulates with its respective thoracic vertebra. The spinous process of the seventh cervical vertebra (C7), also called the *vertebra prominens*, can be easily felt with the client's neck flexed. The lower tip of each scapula is at the level of the seventh or eighth rib when the client's arms are at his or her side (see Fig. 10–2).

To describe a location around the circumference of the chest wall, imaginary lines running vertically on the chest wall are used. On the anterior chest, these lines are known as the *midsternal line* and the *right and left midclavicular lines* (Fig. 10–3A).

The posterior thorax includes the vertebral (or spinal) line and the right and left scapular lines, which extend through the inferior angle of the scapulae when the arms are at the client's side (Fig. 10–3B).

The lateral aspect of the thorax is divided into three parallel lines. The *midaxillary line* runs from the apex of the axillae to the level of the 12th rib. The *anterior axillary line* extends from the anterior axillary fold along the anterolateral aspect of the thorax, whereas the *posterior axillary line* runs from the posterior axillary fold down the posterolateral aspect of the chest wall (Fig. 10–3C).

Thoracic Cavity

The thoracic cavity consists of the mediastinum and the lungs.

The lungs are two cone-shaped, elastic structures suspended within the thoracic cavity. The *apex* of each lung extends slightly above the clavicle, whereas the *base* is at the level of the diaphragm. At the point of the midclavicular line on the anterior surface of the thorax, the lung extends to approximately the sixth rib. Laterally, lung tissue reaches the level of the eighth rib, and, posteriorly, the lung base is at about the tenth rib (Fig. 10–4).

The thoracic cavity is lined by a thin, double-layered serous membrane collectively referred to as the pleura (Fig. 10–5). The *parietal pleura* lines the chest cavity, whereas the *visceral pleura* covers the external surfaces of the lungs. The *pleural space* lies between the two pleural layers.

The trachea lies anterior to the esophagus and is approximately 10 to 12 cm long in an adult (see Fig. 10–5). At the level of the sternal angle, the trachea bifurcates into the right and left main bronchi.

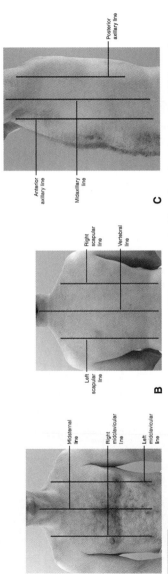

FIGURE 10-3 (*A*) Anterior vertical lines, imaginary landmarks. (*B*) Posterior vertical lines, imaginary landmarks. (*C*) Lateral vertical lines, imaginary landmarks.

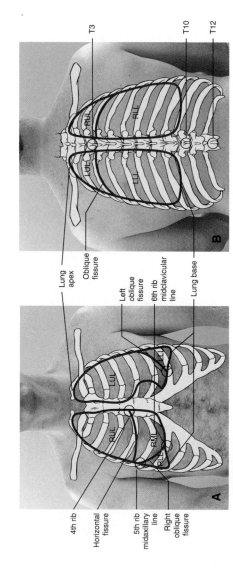

FIGURE 10–4 (*A*) Anterior view of lung position. (*B*) Posterior view of lung position. *(continued)*

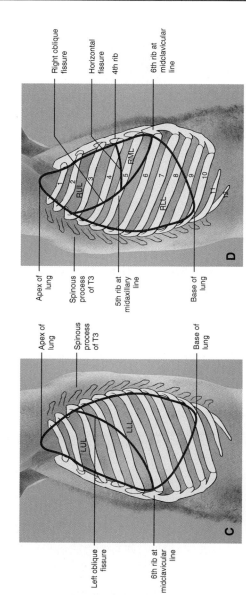

FIGURE 10–4 *(continued)* (*C*) Lateral view of left lung position. (*D*) Lateral view of right lung position.

Labels for (*D*) Lateral view of right lung position:
- Right oblique fissure
- Horizontal fissure
- 4th rib
- 6th rib at midclavicular line
- Apex of lung
- Spinous process of T3
- 5th rib at midaxillary line
- Base of lung
- RUL
- RML
- RLL

Labels for (*C*) Lateral view of left lung position:
- Apex of lung
- Spinous process of T3
- Base of lung
- Left oblique fissure
- 6th rib at midclavicular line
- LUL
- LLL

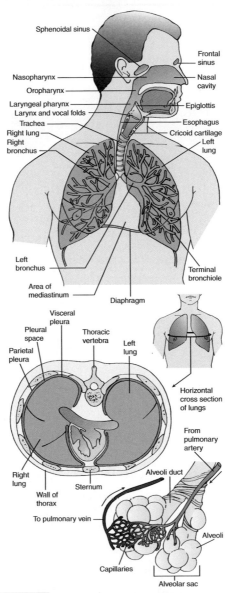

FIGURE 10–5 Major structures of the respiratory system.

Inspired air travels through the trachea into the main bronchi and continues through the system as the bronchi repeatedly bifurcate into smaller passageways known as *bronchioles*. Eventually, the bronchioles terminate at the alveolar ducts, and air is channeled into the alveolar sacs, which contain the alveoli (see Fig. 10–5).

Equipment Needed

● Stethoscope
● Tape measure with centimeters
● Marking pen

Subjective Data: Focus Questions

Difficulty breathing? Timing? Associated factors? Precipitating factors? Relieving factors? Difficulty breathing when sleeping? Use of more than one pillow to sleep? Coughing (productive, nonproductive)? Sputum (type and amount)? Allergies? Dyspnea or shortness of breath (at rest or on exertion)? Chest pain? Location, timing? Associated factors? Precipitating factors? Relieving factors? History of asthma, bronchitis, emphysema, tuberculosis? Exposure to environmental inhalants (chemicals, fumes)? History of smoking (amount and length of time)? Efforts to quit?

RISK FACTORS. Risk for respiratory disease related to smoking, immobilization or sedentary lifestyle, aging, environmental exposures, and morbid obesity; risk for lung cancer related to cigarette smoking and genetic predisposition.

Objective Data: Assessment Techniques

Review Figures 10–1 through 10–5 for anatomy of the thorax and lungs. Expose anterior, posterior, and lateral chest with patient in sitting position. Locate landmarks (see Fig. 10–3).

INSPECTION

Inspect anterior, posterior, and lateral thorax for the following:

PROCEDURE	NORMAL FINDINGS	DEVIATIONS FROM NORMAL
• Color	• Pink	• Pallor, cyanosis
• Intercostal spaces	• Even and relaxed	• Bulging, retracting
• Chest symmetry	• Equal	• Unequal
• Rib slope	• Less than 90° downward	• Horizontal or ≥ 90°
• Respiration patterns (rate, rhythm, depth) (Table 10–1)	• Even, 12–20/min, unlabored	• Uneven, labored, <12/min or >20/min, shallow, deep
• Anterior-posterior to lateral diameter	• 1:2 ratio	• >1:2 ratio (barrel chest seen in emphysema) or <1:2 ratio
• Shape and position of sternum	• Level with ribs	• Depressed or projecting
• Position of trachea	• Midline	• Deviated to one side
• Chest expansion	• 3 inches with deep inspiration	• Less than 3 inches with deep inspiration. Decreased chest excursion is seen with chronic obstructive pulmonary disease.

PALPATION

Drape anterior chest and use finger pads or palms to palpate posterior chest. Have client fold arms across anterior chest and lean forward to increase area of lungs. First palpate, percuss, and auscultate the posterior lungs and thorax while the client is sitting. Then palpate, percuss, and auscultate lateral lungs and thorax while the client is in the supine position.

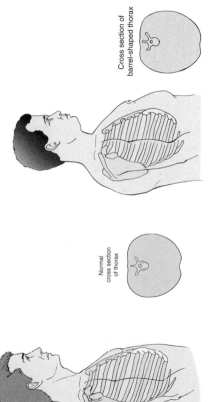

Cross section of thorax.

Cross section of barrel-shaped thorax.

TABLE 10-1 RESPIRATION PATTERNS

Type	Description	Pattern	Clinical Indication
Normal	12 to 20/min and regular	◇◇◇◇◇	Normal breathing pattern
Tachypnea	>24/min and shallow	∿∿∿∿∿∿∿	May be a normal response to fever, anxiety, or exercise. Can occur with respiratory insufficiency, alkalosis, pneumonia, or pleurisy
Bradypnea	<10/min and regular	◇◇◇	May be normal in well-conditioned athletes. Can occur with medication-induced depression of the respiratory center, diabetic coma, neurological damage
Hyperventilation	Increased rate and increased depth	∿∿∿∿∿∿∿∿	Usually occurs with extreme exercise, fear, or anxiety. Kussmaul's respirations are a type of hyperventilation associated with diabetic keto-acidosis. Other causes of hyperventilation include disorders of the central nervous system, an overdose of the drug salicylate, or severe anxiety.

Hypoventilation	Decreased rate, decreased depth, irregular pattern	Usually associated with overdose of narcotics or anesthetics
Cheyne–Stokes respiration	Regular pattern characterized by alternating periods of deep, rapid breathing followed by periods of apnea	May result from severe congestive heart failure, drug overdose, increased intracranial pressure, or renal failure May be noted in elderly persons during sleep, not related to any disease process
Biot's respiration	Irregular pattern characterized by varying depth and rate of respirations followed by periods of apnea	May be seen with meningitis or severe brain damage

PALPATION (continued)

PROCEDURE	NORMAL FINDINGS	DEVIATIONS FROM NORMAL
Palpate thorax at three levels for the following:		
• Sensation	• No pain or tenderness	• Pain, tenderness. Pain over thorax is seen with inflamed fibrous connective tissue; pain over intercostal area seen with inflamed pleura.
• Vocal fremitus as client says "99"	• Vibration decreased over periphery of lungs and increased over major airways	• Vibration increased over lung with consolidation; vibration decreased over airway with obstruction, pleural effusion, or pneumothorax
Palpate thorax for thoracic expansion by the following methods:	2- to 3-inch symmetrical thoracic expansion	Less than 2- to 3-inch thoracic expansion; asymmetrical expansion seen with atelectasis or pneumonia
• Place hands on posterior thorax at level of 10th vertebra. Gently press skin between thumbs and have client take deep breath. Observe thumb movement (Fig. 10–6A).	• Symmetrical expansion (thumbs move apart equal distance in both directions).	• Asymmetrical expansion (thumb movement apart is unequal).
• Anteriorly, press skin together at lower sternum and have patient take deep breath. Observe thumb movement (Fig. 10–6B).	• Symmetrical expansion (thumbs move apart equal distance in both directions).	• Asymmetrical expansion (thumb movement apart is unequal).

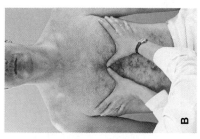

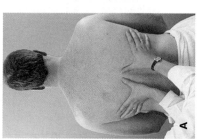

FIGURE 10-6 Palpation of thoracic expansion. (*A*) Posterior. (*B*) Anterior. (© B. Proud.)

PERCUSSION

Use mediate percussion over shoulder apices and intercostal spaces. Compare both for symmetry of percussion notes, while moving from apex to base of lungs as illustrated (see Fig. 10–7).

PROCEDURE	NORMAL FINDINGS	DEVIATIONS FROM NORMAL
Percuss over shoulder apices and at posterior, anterior, and lateral intercostal spaces as illustrated (see Fig. 10–4 to determine which lung areas are being percussed.	Resonance	Hyperresonance is heard over emphysematous lungs; dullness heard over solid masses or fluid, eg, in lobar pneumonia, pleural effusion, or tumor.
Percuss for posterior, diaphragmatic excursions bilaterally, as illustrated (Fig. 10–8).	Diaphragm descends 3–6 cm from T10 (with full expiration held) to T12 (with full inspiration held).	Diaphragm descends less than 3 cm owing to atelectasis of lower lobes, emphysema, ascites, or tumors.

AUSCULTATION

Using diaphragm of stethoscope, exert firm pressure over intercostal space. Instruct client to take slow, deep breaths through the mouth. Listen for two full breaths and compare symmetrical sides of thorax while moving stethoscope from apex to base of lungs.

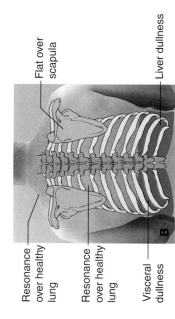

Flat over scapula

Resonance over healthy lung

Resonance over healthy lung

Liver dullness

Visceral dullness

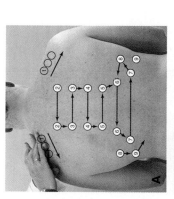

FIGURE 10–7 Intercostal landmarks for percussion and auscultation of thorax. (*A*) Posterior. (*B*) Normal percussive notes (posterior). (*continued*)

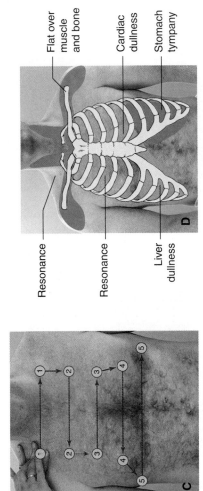

Resonance

Flat over muscle and bone

Resonance

Cardiac dullness

Liver dullness

Stomach tympany

FIGURE 10-7 *(continued)* (*C*) Anterior. (*D*) Normal percussive notes (anterior).

Thoracic and Lung Assessment

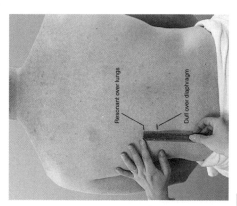

Resonant over lungs

Dull over diaphragm

FIGURE 10-8 Percussing bilaterally for diaphragmatic excursions.

AUSCULTATION (continued)

PROCEDURE	NORMAL FINDINGS	DEVIATIONS FROM NORMAL
*Auscultate **breath sounds** over the following:* • Trachea 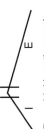	• Bronchial (loud, tubular) breath sounds heard over trachea; expiration longer than inspiration; short silence between inspiration and expiration 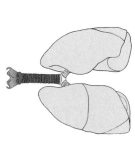 Bronchial breath sounds	• Bronchial sounds heard over lung periphery
• Large-stem bronchi	• Bronchovesicular breath sounds heard over mainstem bronchi: below clavicles and between scapulae (inspiratory phase equal to expiratory phase)	• Bronchovesicular breath sounds heard over lung periphery

AUSCULTATION (continued)

PROCEDURE	NORMAL FINDINGS	DEVIATIONS FROM NORMAL
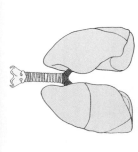	Bronchovesicular breath sounds	Decreased breath sounds with obstruction, pleural thickening, pleural effusion, or pneumothorax
• Lung periphery	• Vesicular (low, soft, breezy) breath sounds heard over lung periphery (inspiration longer than expiration)	
Auscultate breath sounds for **adventitious sounds** (crackles, wheezes). If an abnormal sound is heard, ask client to cough. Note if adventitious sound is still present or if it cleared with cough.	Lungs clear to auscultation on inspiration and expiration	Crackles usually are auscultated during inspiration. They occur late in inspiration with pneumonia and congestive heart failure; occur early in inspiration with bronchitis, asthma, and emphysema. Fine crackles are popping, high-pitched, and

Thoracic and Lung Assessment

AUSCULTATION (continued)

PROCEDURE	NORMAL FINDINGS	DEVIATIONS FROM NORMAL

Vesicular breath sounds

I   E

Crackles (fine)

Crackles (coarse)

AUSCULTATION (continued)

DEVIATIONS FROM NORMAL

very brief (5–10 msec). Coarse crackles are bubbling sounds, lower in pitch, and not quite so brief (20–30 msec). Heard with pneumonia, pulmonary and edema, and fibrosis. Sibilant wheezes (high-pitched musical sounds) are heard on inspiration or expiration in acute asthma and chronic emphysema. Sonorous wheezes are low-pitched moaning sounds heard mostly on expiration in bronchitis, single obstruction and snoring before sleep apnea.

Wheeze (sibilant)

Wheeze (sonorous)

AUSCULTATION (continued)

PROCEDURE	NORMAL FINDINGS	DEVIATIONS FROM NORMAL
*Auscultate for **altered voice sounds** over lung periphery where any previous lung abnormality is noted.*		
• Bronchophony (client says "99" while examiner auscultates).	• Sounds muffled	• Sounds loud and clear over consolidation from pneumonia, atelectasis, or tumor
• Whispered pectoriloquy (client whispers "one, two, three" while examiner auscultates).	• Sounds muffled	• Sounds loud and clear over areas of consolidation
• Egophony (client says "ee" while examiner auscultates).	• Sounds like muffled "ee"	• Sounds like "ay" over areas of consolidation or compression

Adapted from Bickley, L. S. (1999). *Bates' guide to physical examination and history taking*. 7th ed. Philadelphia: Lippincott Williams & Wilkins.

PEDIATRIC VARIATIONS

Subjective Data: Focus Questions

History of wheezing, asthma, or other breathing problems? Exposure to passive smoke? Occurrence of sudden infant death syndrome (SIDS) in family? Frequent colds or congestion?

Objective Data: Assessment Techniques

Inspection

In infants, anteroposterior (AP) diameter is equal to transverse diameter (1:1)—shape is nearly circular. By age 5 to 6 years, the AP diameter reaches that of the adult 1:2 or 5:7 ratio. Chest wall is thin with bony and cartilaginous rib cage soft and pliant.

Respirations should be unlabored and quiet; rate varies according to age (Table 10–2).

TABLE 10-2 RESPIRATORY RATES IN CHILDREN	
Age	**Respiratory Rate (breaths/min)**
Newborn	30–60
Early childhood	20–40
Late childhood	15–25
Age 14 years	14–20

Adapted from Bickley, L. S. (1999). *Bates' guide to physical examination and history taking,* 7th ed. Philadelphia: Lippincott Williams & Wilkins.

Percussion

In infants and young children, normally hyperresonant throughout because of thinness of chest wall. Any decrease in resonance is equal to dullness in the adult.

Auscultation

Bell or small diaphragm should be used to localize findings, especially in infants and young children. Breath sounds will be louder and harsher owing to close proximity to origin of sounds from thin chest wall. Wheezes and rhonchi occur more frequently in infants and young children.

GERIATRIC VARIATIONS

- Increase in normal respiratory rate (16–25)
- Loss of elasticity, fewer functional capillaries, and loss of lung resiliency
- Decreased ability to cough effectively due to weaker muscles and rigid thoracic wall
- Accentuated dorsal curve (kyphosis) of thoracic spine
- Sternum and ribs may be more prominent owing to loss of subcutaneous fat
- Decreased thoracic expansion due to calcification of costal cartilages and loss of the accessory musculature
- Increased diaphragmatic breathing due to anatomic changes
- Hyperresonance of thorax due to age-related emphysemic changes
- Decreased breath sounds and increased retention of mucus due to decreased pulmonary function
- Increased AP diameter (up to 5:7 AP-to-transverse diameter ratio) due to loss of resiliency and loss of skeletal muscle strength
- Resonance of percussive may increase

CULTURAL VARIATIONS

- Thoracic cavity size varies among cultural groups. The tendency is for Caucasians to have larger thoraxes than blacks, Asians, and Native Americans.

Possible Collaborative Problems

Respiratory insufficiency/failure
Pneumonia
Pulmonary edema
Airway obstruction/atelectasis
Laryngeal edema
Pleural effusion
Atelectasis
Asthma
Chronic obstructive pulmonary disease

Oxygen toxicity
Carbon dioxide toxicity
Pneumothorax
Respiratory acidosis
Respiratory alkalosis
Tracheal necrosis
Tracheobronchial constriction

TEACHING TIPS FOR SELECTED NURSING DIAGNOSES

Adult Client

Nursing Diagnosis: Readiness for Enhanced Respiratory Function

Encourage client to participate in a daily exercise program and to eat a healthy low-cholesterol diet with adequate vitamin E and lutein. Provide client with information on the risks of secondhand smoke and how to decrease one's exposure. The Indoor Air Quality Information Hotline provides free information (phone 1-800-438-4318). Encourage client not to start smoking and to limit exposure to air pollution and dangerous substances.

Nursing Diagnosis: Ineffective Airway Clearance related to shallow coughing and thickened mucus

☐ Instruct client on effective deep breathing and coughing. Encourage liquid intake of 2–3 quarts/day. Caution client to use protective measures to prevent spread of infections.

Nursing Diagnosis: Impaired Gas Exchange related to chronic lung tissue damage

☐ Teach client diaphragmatic and pursed-lip breathing.

Nursing Diagnosis: Ineffective Airway Clearance related to chronic allergy

☐ Provide literature on environmental control. Assess whether client has kit to deal with emergencies (eg, bee stings). If allergy is produced by unknown food, assist client with keeping a diary of allergy attacks to determine cause.

Nursing Diagnosis: Ineffective Breathing Pattern: hyperventilation related to hypoxia and lack of knowledge of controlled breathing techniques

☐ Teach client how to become aware of breathing patterns and how to assess what aggravates hyperventilation (eg, fatigue, stress). Teach controlled breathing techniques.

Nursing Diagnosis: Impaired Gas Exchange related to smoking and/or frequent exposure to air pollution or dangerous substances

☐ Explain effects of smoking and how it is a primary risk factor for lung cancer. Assess client's desire to quit and refer to community agencies for self help on smoking cessation programs. Discuss alternate methods of coping. Wear mask if job requires exposure to dangerous inhalants

Pediatric Client

Nursing Diagnosis: Ineffective Airway Clearance related to bronchospasm and increased pulmonary secretions

☐ Postural drainage and percussion may be used with children of various ages. Teach parents safety measures when using vaporizers. Teach alternate ways of humidifying air. For example, have parent run hot water in shower and close bathroom door. Sit with child in this room for approximately 10 minutes to liquefy secretions by steam (child must not be left alone in room). Teach parents the importance of throat cultures for upper respiratory infections to identify streptococcal infections. *If child has asthma:* Asthma attacks decrease with increasing age of child. Assist parents with letting child have more independence and avoiding overprotection. Teach family how to decrease allergens (eg, dust) in home by using smooth surfaces that are easy to clean.

Geriatric Client

Nursing Diagnosis: Impaired Gas Exchange related to poor muscle tone and decreased ability to remove secretions

Teach client the importance of mobility and exercise to maintain adequate respiratory hygiene. Encourage client to discuss consideration of the flu shot with the physician.

11

Cardiac Assessment

ANATOMY OVERVIEW

Heart and Great Vessels

The heart is a hollow, muscular, four-chambered organ located in the middle of the thoracic cavity between the lungs in the space called the *mediastinum*. It is about the size of a clenched fist and weighs approximately 255 g (9 oz) in women and 310 g (10.9 oz) in men. The heart extends vertically from the second to the fifth intercostal space (ICS) and horizontally from the right edge of the sternum to the left midclavicular line (MCL). The heart can be described as an inverted cone. The upper portion, near the second ICS, is the base, and the lower portion, near the fifth ICS and the left MCL, is the apex. The anterior chest area that overlies the heart and great vessels is called the *precordium* (Fig. 11–1).

The large veins and arteries leading directly to and away from the heart are referred to as the *great vessels*. The *superior and inferior vena cava* return blood to the right atrium from the upper and lower torso, respectively. The *pulmonary artery* exits the right ventricle, bifurcates, and carries blood to the lungs. The *pulmonary veins* (two from each lung) return oxygenated blood to the left atrium. The *aorta* transports oxygenated blood from the ventricle to the body (Fig. 11–2).

The heart consists of four chambers or cavities: two upper chambers, the *right and left atria*, and two lower chambers, the *right and left ventricles*. The entrance and exit of each ventricle are protected by one-way valves that direct the flow of blood through the heart. The *atrioventricular* (AV) valves are located at the entrance into the ventricles. There are two AV

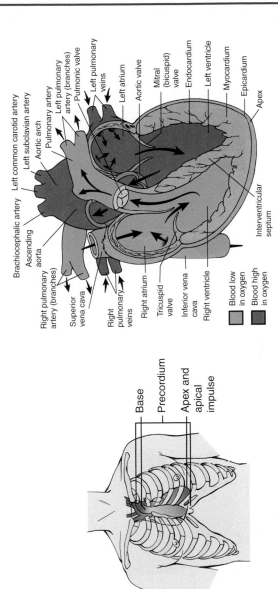

FIGURE 11–2 Heart chambers, valves, and direction of circulatory flow.

Left common carotid artery
Left subclavian artery
Aortic arch
Pulmonary artery
Left pulmonary artery (branches)
Pulmonic valve
Left pulmonary veins
Left atrium
Aortic valve
Mitral (bicuspid) valve
Endocardium
Left ventricle
Myocardium
Epicardium
Apex
Interventricular septum
Right ventricle
Tricuspid valve
Inferior vena cava
Right atrium
Right pulmonary veins
Superior vena cava
Right pulmonary artery (branches)
Ascending aorta
Brachiocephalic artery

Blood low in oxygen
Blood high in oxygen

Base
Precordium
Apex and apical impulse

FIGURE 11–1 The heart and major blood vessels lie centrally in the chest behind the protective sternum.

valves: the tricuspid valve and the bicuspid, which is also called the *mitral valve*. The tricuspid valve is composed of three cusps or flaps and is located between the right atrium and the right ventricle; the bicuspid (mitral) valve is composed of two cusps or flaps and is located between the left atrium and the left ventricle.

Open AV valves allow blood to flow from the atria into the ventricles. However, as the ventricles begin to contract, the AV valves snap shut, preventing the regurgitation of blood into the atria.

The *semilunar valves* are located at the exit of each ventricle at the beginning of the great vessels. Each valve has three cusps or flaps that look like half-moons; hence the name "semilunar." There are two semilunar valves: the pulmonic valve is located at the entrance of the pulmonary artery as it exits the right ventricle, and the aortic valve is located at the beginning of the ascending aorta (see Fig. 11–2).

Production of Heart Sounds

Heart sounds are produced by valve closure. The opening of valves is silent. Normal heart sounds, characterized as "lub dubb" (S_1 and S_2), and, occasionally, extra heart sounds and murmurs can be auscultated with a stethoscope over the precordium, the area of the anterior chest overlying the heart and great vessels.

The first heart sound (S_1) is the result of closure of the AV valves—the mitral and tricuspid valves. S_1 correlates with the beginning of systole (Fig. 11–3). If heard as two sounds, the first component represents mitral valve closure (M_1), and the second component represents tricuspid closure (T_1).

The second heart sound (S_2) results from closure of the semilunar valves (aortic and pulmonic) and correlates with the beginning of diastole. S_2 ("dubb") is also usually heard as one sound but may be heard as two sounds. If S_2 is heard as two sounds, the first component represents aortic valve closure (A_2) and the second component represents pulmonic valve closure (P_2).

Equipment Needed

- Ruler with centimeters
- Marking pen
- Stethoscope with bell and diaphragm
- Alcohol swab to clean ear and end pieces

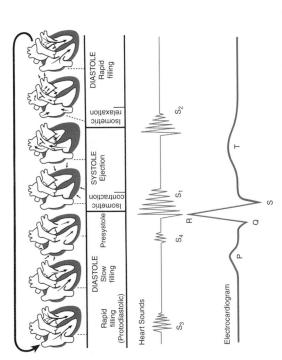

FIGURE 11–3 The cardiac cycle consists of filling and ejection. Heart sounds S_2, S_3, and S_4 are associated with diastole, whereas S_1 is associated with systole. The electrical activity of the heart is measured throughout diastole and systole by electrocardiography.

Subjective Data: Focus Questions

Chest pain—Location? Radiation? Quality? Rating on scale of 1 to 10 (10 being the worst)? Duration? What brings it on? What relieves it? Are there any other associated symptoms, such as nausea, vomiting, sweating? Irregular heartbeat, palpitations? Does your heart pound or beat too fast? Does your heart skip or jump? Dizziness? Swollen ankles? History of heart defect? Murmur? Heart surgery? Smoking? Packs per day? Over how many years? Family history of heart disease? Activities of daily living—Diet? Alcohol consumption? Usual exercise? Daily stressors? Forms of relaxation?

RISK FACTORS. Risk for coronary heart disease related to hypertension, increased low-density lipoprotein cholesterol and decreased high-density lipoprotein cholesterol, diabetes mellitus, minimal exercise, cigarette smoking, diet high in fat, postmenopausal without estrogen replacement (in females), family history, and upper body obesity.

Objective Data: Assessment Techniques

See Figure 11–2 for a diagram of the heart chambers, valves, and circulation.

INSPECTION

Inspect chest to identify landmarks that aid in assessment of the heart. Check for visibility of point of maximum impulse (PMI) and any abnormal pulsations.

PROCEDURE	NORMAL FINDINGS	DEVIATIONS FROM NORMAL
Inspect the following: • Intercostal space (ICS): Locate by finding the sternal angle, which is felt as a ridge in the sternum approximately 2 inches below the	• Small apical impulse (≤2.5 cm) at or medial to left midclavicular line at fourth or fifth ICS. May not be visible in client with large chest.	• Impulses lateral to midclavicular line; pulsations (heaves or lifts) other than the apical pulsation are considered abnormal, and may be seen with an enlarged

INSPECTION (continued)

PROCEDURE	NORMAL FINDINGS	DEVIATIONS FROM NORMAL
sternal notch (Fig. 11–4). The adjacent rib is the second rib with the second ICS directly below it. Other ICSs can be identified by counting from the second ICS. The fifth ICS is at the junction of the sternum and the xiphoid process. • Midsternal line (MSL): Imaginary line extending down the chest through the middle of the sternum. It divides the anterior chest in half (see Fig. 11–4). • Midclavicular line (MCL): Imaginary line extending from the middle of the clavicle down the chest, dividing the left or right anterior chest into two parts (see Fig. 11–4). • Anterior axillary line (AAL): Imaginary line extending along the lateral wall of the anterior chest and even with the anterior axillary fold (see Fig. 11–4).		left ventricle due to work overload; apical impulse on right side of chest. Bulging and/or prominent pulsations (>3 cm) at the PMI. • Prominent impulse at right sternal border in pulmonic or aortic area.

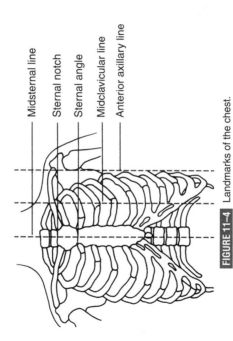

Midsternal line
Sternal notch
Sternal angle
Midclavicular line
Anterior axillary line

FIGURE 11–4 Landmarks of the chest.

PALPATION

The client should be lying down. Palpate using the fingertips and palmar surfaces of fingers in an organized fashion, beginning in the aortic area and moving down the chest toward the tricuspid area (Fig. 11–5).

PROCEDURE	NORMAL FINDINGS	DEVIATIONS FROM NORMAL
Palpate the following: • Aortic area: Palpate second ICS at right sternal border (see Fig. 11–5). • Pulmonic area: Palpate second ICS at left sternal border (see Fig. 11–5). • Erb's point: Palpate third ICS at left sternal border (see Fig. 11–5). • Tricuspid area: Palpate fifth ICS at lower left sternal border (see Fig. 11–5).	• No vibrations or pulsations are palpated in aortic, pulmonic, or tricuspid area.	• Thrill, which feels similar to a purring cat, or pulsation in any of these areas except the mitral area is usually associated with a grade 4 or higher murmur.
• Mitral area: Palpate fifth ICS at the left MCL. This is also called the PMI (see Fig. 11–5). If this pulsation cannot be palpated, have the client assume a left lateral position. This displaces the heart toward the left chest wall and relocates the apical impulse farther to the left.	• PMI is felt as a pulsation and is approximately the size of a nickel. May not palpate in large chest.	• No pulsation. If area of pulsation is the size of a quarter or larger, displaced, more forceful, or of longer duration, cardiac enlargement should be suspected.

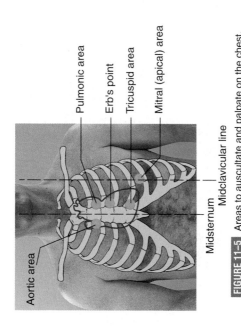

Aortic area

Pulmonic area

Erb's point

Tricuspid area

Mitral (apical) area

Midsternum

Midclavicular line

FIGURE 11-5 Areas to auscultate and palpate on the chest.

Cardiac Assessment

PALPATION (continued)

PROCEDURE

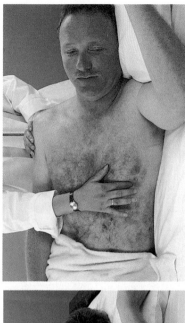

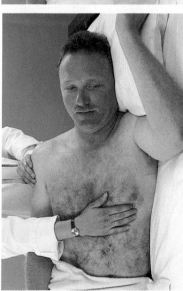

Locate the apical impulse with the palmar surface (*left*), then palpate the apical pulse with the fingerpad (*right*). (© B. Proud.)

PERCUSSION

Percussion may be done to define cardiac borders by identifying areas of dullness, but it is generally unreliable. Size of heart can be more accurately determined by chest x-ray.

AUSCULTATION

Auscultate in an orderly, systematic fashion beginning with the aortic area. Move across and then down the chest. Focus on one sound at a time. Auscultate each area with the stethoscope diaphragm applied firmly to the chest. Repeat the sequence using the stethoscope bell applied lightly to the chest. Auscultate with the client in the supine position. Then listen specifically over the apex with the bell while client is in the left lateral position. Assist client to a sitting position, and auscultate the pericardium with the diaphragm. Then have client lean forward and exhale while you listen over the aortic area with the diaphragm.

PROCEDURE	NORMAL FINDINGS	DEVIATIONS FROM NORMAL
Auscultate to identify the **first heart sound** (S_1), or "lub," and the **second heart sound** (S_2), or "dubb" (Fig. 11–6).	S_1 follows the long diastolic pause and precedes the short systolic pause and corresponds to each carotid pulsation. S_2 follows the short systolic phase and precedes the long diastolic phase.	
Auscultate for **rate and rhythm.**	*Rate:* 60–100 bpm *Rhythm:* regular	Bradycardia (heart rate <60); tachycardia (heart rate >100) may result in decreased cardiac output; irregular rhythms

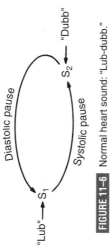

FIGURE 11–6 Normal heart sound: "Lub-dubb."

AUSCULTATION (continued)

PROCEDURE	NORMAL FINDINGS	DEVIATIONS FROM NORMAL
		(eg, premature beats of atrial or ventricular premature contractions, atrial flutter and atrial fibrillation with varying block) need to be referred.
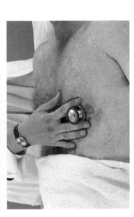 Auscultating S₁. (© B. Proud.) If irregular rhythm is detected, auscultate for **pulse rate deficit** by comparing the radial pulse with the apical pulse for a full minute.	Radial and apical pulse should be identical.	A pulse deficit (difference between radial and apical pulses) may indicate atrial fibrillation, atrial flutter, premature ventricular contractions, and varying degrees of heart block.

AUSCULTATION (continued)

PROCEDURE	NORMAL FINDINGS	DEVIATIONS FROM NORMAL
Auscultate and focus on each sound and pause individually:	Crisp, distinct sound heard in each area but loudest at mitral and tricuspid areas	Split sound in middle-aged and older adults
• Auscultate S₁; Heard best with diaphragm.	• May become softer with inspiration. Split S₁ is normal in children, young adults, and pregnant women.	
• Auscultate S₂; Heard best with diaphragm	• Crisp, distinct sound heard loudest at the aortic and pulmonic areas. Split S₂ may be normal in adults if heard only during inspiration.	• Split sound heard equally during inspiration and expiration
• Auscultate systolic pause space: Heard between S₁ and S₂ (see Fig. 11–6).	• Silent pause—should hear distinct end of S₁ and beginning of S₂ with nothing in between	• *Murmur:* Swishing sound heard at beginning, middle, or end of systolic pause (note intensity, pitch, and quality—Table 11–1). *Click:* Sharp, high-pitched snapping sound heard immediately after S₁ or in the middle of the systolic pause
• Auscultate diastolic pause space: Heard between S₂ and the next S₁ (see Fig. 11–6).	• Silent pause—should hear distinct end of S₂ and distinct beginning of next S₁	• *Murmur:* Swishing sound heard at beginning, middle, or end of diastolic pause (note intensity, pitch, and quality—Table 11–1).

Cardiac Assessment

TABLE 11-1 CLASSIFICATION FOR INTENSITY, PITCH, AND QUALITY OF MURMURS

Intensity
Grade 1—Very faint, heard only after the listener has "tuned in;" may not be heard in all positions
Grade 2—Quiet, but heard immediately upon placing stethoscope on the chest
Grade 3—Moderately loud
Grade 4—Loud with palpable thrill
Grade 5—Very loud, may be heard with stethoscope partly off the chest ⎫ Associated with thrills
Grade 6—May be heard with stethoscope entirely off the chest ⎭

Pitch
High, medium, or low

Quality
Blowing, rumbling, harsh, or musical

Adapted from Bickley, L. S. (2003). *Bates' guide to physical examination and history taking* (8th ed). Philadelphia: Lippincott Williams & Wilkins.

AUSCULTATION (continued)

PROCEDURE	NORMAL FINDINGS	DEVIATIONS FROM NORMAL
		Snap: High-pitched snapping sound heard after S_2 during the diastolic pause in the mitral or tricuspid area
• Auscultate S_3 with bell of stethoscope: Low, faint sound occurring at the beginning of the diastolic pause (Fig. 11–7).	• S_3 auscultated in children and young adults but disappears upon standing or sitting up; heard in people with a high cardiac output, and in women in the third trimester of pregnancy	• S_3 auscultated in adults or that continues with standing or sitting in children and young adults; also called ventricular gallop (has rhythm of the word "Kentucky"); may be heard with ischemic heart disease, myocardial failure, volume overload of the ventricle from valvular disease; may be earliest sign of heart failure.
• Auscultate S_4: Soft, low-pitched sound heard best with client in supine or left lateral position with stethoscope bell (Fig. 11–8).	• Auscultated in trained athletes and some older clients, especially after exercise	• Auscultated in adults; also called atrial gallop (has rhythm of the word "Tennessee") and is associated with coronary artery disease, hypertension, aortic and pulmonic stenosis, and acute myocardial infarction.

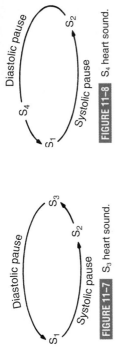

Diastolic pause

S₃

S₂

Systolic pause

S₁

FIGURE 11–7 S₃ heart sound.

Diastolic pause

S₄

S₂

Systolic pause

S₁

FIGURE 11–8 S₄ heart sound.

Subjective Data: Focus Questions

In addition to the focus questions for adults, inquire about the following: Mother's use of therapeutic drugs or drug abuse during pregnancy? Poor weight gain? Signs of delayed development (eg, slowed social development, language development, or motor skills)? Difficulty in feeding (breast, bottle, acceptance of new foods)? Inability to tolerate physical activity or play with peers? Excessive irritability or crying? Squatting behavior? Circumoral cyanosis or central cyanosis?

Objective Data: Assessment Techniques

PROCEDURE	NORMAL FINDINGS AND VARIATIONS
Inspect **chest wall** in semi-Fowler position from an angle for PMI.	PMI easily visible because heart is larger in proportion to chest size (Fig. 11–9). Heart lies more horizontally up to age 5 to 6 years. Thus, the PMI may be lateral to the MCL.
Palpate **peripheral pulse points** in relation to apical pulse and to each other: Femoral, radial, brachial, and carotid.	Symmetrical and equal rate, strength, and rhythm.
Percuss **heart size.** (*Note:* This is rarely done owing to inaccuracy of the method.)	Percussion area is slightly larger because of horizontal position and overlying thymus gland.
Auscultate **S₁** and **S₂** at pulmonic area (Erb's point).	S_1 is louder than S_2, or S_2 is louder than S_1. Splitting of S_2 is heard best at Erb's point (25–33% of all children). This is a frequent site of innocent murmurs (grade 3 or lower), which are common throughout childhood. They are of short duration with no transmission to other areas, are low pitched, musical, or of groaning quality that is variable in intensity in relation to position, respiration, activity, fever, and anemia with no other associated signs of heart disease. Other murmurs may indicate pathology.

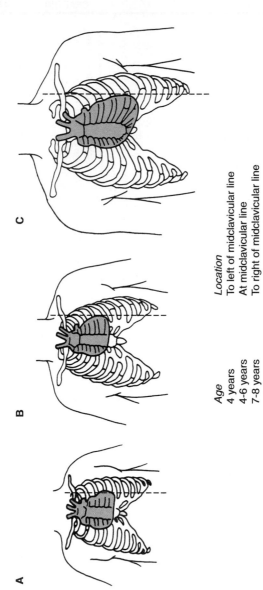

Age	Location
4 years	To left of midclavicular line
4-6 years	At midclavicular line
7-8 years	To right of midclavicular line

FIGURE 11–9 Location of apex of heart in (*A*) infant, (*B*) child, and (*C*) adult.

Objective Data: Assessment Techniques (continued)

PROCEDURE	NORMAL FINDINGS AND VARIATIONS
• Tricuspid area • Mitral area • Sinus arrhythmia	• S_1 louder, preceding S_2. • S_1 loudest. • Varies with respiration; very common and disappears with age.
• Rate	• See Table 11–2 for normal pediatric pulse rates.

TABLE 11–2   AVERAGE HEART RATE OF INFANTS AND CHILDREN AT REST

Age	Average Rate (beats per minute)	±2 Standard Deviations
Birth	140	90–190
First 6 months	130	80–180
6–12 months	115	75–155
1–2 years	110	70–150
2–6 years	103	68–138
6–10 years	95	65–125
10–14 years	85	55–115

From Bickley, L. S. (2003). *Bates' guide to physical examination and history taking* (8th ed.). Philadelphia: Lippincott Williams & Wilkins.

Cardiac Assessment

GERIATRIC VARIATIONS

- Thickening of heart walls.
- Decreased elasticity of heart and arteries; reduced pumping ability of heart.
- Decreased cardiac output and cardiac reserve.
- Apical impulse may be difficult to palpate owing to increase in anteroposterior diameter of chest.
- Location of heart sounds and PMI may be varied owing to kyphosis or scoliosis.
- Early and soft systolic murmurs are common.
- Atrial fibrillations often occur.
- Reduced maximum heart rate.

CULTURAL VARIATIONS

- African Americans have higher HDL levels, but higher lifestyle risk factors for CHD than white Americans.
- African Americans have higher rates of hypertension, stroke, and CHD than white Americans. Hypertension in U.S. black women has a higher incidence, earlier onset, and higher mortality than in white women [Overfield, 1995; Gillum, 1996].

Possible Collaborative Problems

Decreased cardiac output   Congenital heart disease
Congestive heart failure   Endocarditis
Myocardial ischemia   Angina
Cardiogenic shock   Dysrhythmia

TEACHING TIPS FOR SELECTED NURSING DIAGNOSES

Adult Client

Nursing Diagnosis: Fear related to perceived increased risk of heart disease and family history of heart disease

Explain what you are doing when auscultating so client won't become alarmed by the amount of time you are taking. Explain that vigorous exercise (20–30 minutes three times a week) may decrease serum triglycerides and cholesterol, and therefore may prevent heart disease by increasing the working capabilities of the body and heart capillaries. Advise client to have a complete physical examination prior to starting a new fitness program.

Nursing Diagnosis: Ineffective Therapeutic Regimen Management related to knowledge deficit: Taking pulse in order to assess heart rate prior to taking cardiac medications

☐ Teach client correct method for taking pulse. Instruct on heart rate necessary for taking prescribed medication.

Nursing Diagnosis: Ineffective Sexuality Patterns related to fear of injury post myocardial infarction

☐ Instruct client to discuss limitations on sexual activities as recommended by physician. (Usually, a client can safely engage in sexual intercourse by the time he or she is permitted to walk up a flight of stairs.)

Nursing Diagnosis: Ineffective Therapeutic Regimen Management related to knowledge deficit: Optimal diet for preventing coronary heart disease

☐ Teach client the following dietary and lifestyle guidelines (American Heart Association, 2000):

- Elimination of cigarette smoking.
- Appropriate levels of caloric intake and physical activity to prevent obesity and reduce weight if already overweight.
- Consumption of 30% or less of the day's total calories from fat.
- Limit saturated fats, trans fatty foods, and cholesterol (full-fat dairy products, fatty meat, tropical oils, partially hydrogenated vegetable oils, and egg yolks).
- Sodium intake should not exceed 6 g/day.
- Consumption of 55 to 60% of calories as complex carbohydrates.
- For those who drink and for whom alcohol (ethanol) is not contraindicated, consumption should not exceed two drinks for a man and one drink for a woman per day. "One drink" means no more than 1/2 oz of pure alcohol. (1 oz of 100-proof whisky, 4 oz of wine, or 12 oz of beer contains 1/2 oz of ethanol).

Nursing Diagnosis: Ineffective Cardiopulmonary Tissue Perfusion related to excessive activity and congestive heart failure

☐ Teach client to follow physician's activity recommendations. Teach client to cluster low-energy tasks (walk to bathroom, brush teeth, gather clothes, return to chair before putting on clothes). Teach client to space higher energy tasks with adequate rest periods. Teach client to take radial pulse and follow physician's recommendations for maximum pulse rate with activity.

Nursing Diagnosis: Readiness for Enhanced activity–exercise pattern

☐ Teach client to seek physician's recommendation regarding an exercise plan and describe the following guidelines for healthy individuals (American Heart Association, 2004):

● Walk or do other physical activity for at least 30 minutes on most days. To lose weight, do enough activity to use more calories than you eat every day. May need to increase physical activity to 60 minutes most days of the week.
● Exercise only when feeling well. Wait until symptoms and signs of a cold or the flu (including fever) have been absent 2 days or more before resuming activity.
● Do not exercise vigorously soon after eating. Wait at least 2 hours.
● Adjust exercise to the weather. Exercise should be adjusted to environmental conditions. Special precautions are necessary when exercising in hot weather. If air temperature is >70°F (21.1°C), slow pace, be alert for signs of heat injury, and drink adequate fluids to maintain hydration. If air temperature is >80°F (26.6°C), exercise in early morning or late afternoon to avoid the heat. Air-conditioned shopping malls are popular for walking.
● Slow down for hills. When ascending hills, decrease speed to avoid overexertion.
● Wear proper clothing and shoes. Dress in loose-fitting, comfortable clothes made of porous material appropriate for the weather. Use sweat suits only for warmth.
● Understand personal limitations. Everyone should have periodic medical examinations. When under a physician's care, ask if there are activity limitations.

- Select appropriate exercises. Cardiovascular (aerobic) exercises should be a major component of activities. Flexibility and strengthening exercises, however, should also be considered for a well-rounded program.
- Be alert for symptoms. If the following symptoms occur, contact a physician before continuing exercise. Although any symptom should be clarified, these are particularly important: discomfort in upper body, including the chest, arm, neck, or jaw, during exercise; faintness accompanying exercise; shortness of breath during exercise; discomfort in bones and joints either during or after exercise. There may be slight muscle soreness when beginning exercise, but if back or joint pain develops discontinue exercise until after evaluation by physician.
- Watch for the following signs of overexercising: inability to finish; inability to converse during the activity; faintness or nausea after exercise; chronic fatigue; sleeplessness; aches and pains in joints. Although there may be some muscle discomfort, joints should not hurt or feel stiff.
- Start slowly and progress gradually. Allow time to adapt.

Peripheral Vascular Assessment

ANATOMY OVERVIEW

Arteries

Arteries are the blood vessels that carry oxygenated, nutrient-rich blood from the heart to the capillaries. The brachial artery is the major artery that supplies the arm. The brachial artery divides near the elbow to become the radial artery (extending down the thumb side of the arm) and the ulnar artery (extending down the little finger side of the arm). Both of these arteries provide blood to the hand (Fig. 12–1).

The femoral artery is the major supplier of blood to the legs. This artery travels down the front of the thigh and then crosses to the back of the thigh, where it is termed the popliteal artery. The popliteal artery divides below the knee into anterior and posterior branches. The anterior branch descends down the top of the foot, where it becomes the dorsalis pedis artery (see Fig. 12–1).

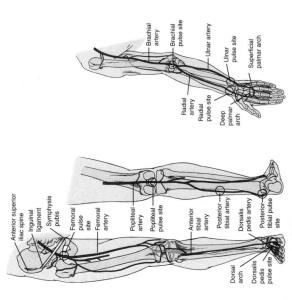

FIGURE 12–1 Major arteries of the arms and legs.

Brachial artery
Brachial pulse site
Ulnar artery
Radial artery
Radial pulse site
Ulnar pulse site
Deep palmar arch
Superficial palmar arch

Anterior superior iliac spine
Inguinal ligament
Symphysis pubis
Femoral pulse site
Femoral artery
Popliteal artery
Popliteal pulse site
Anterior tibial artery
Posterior tibial artery
Dorsalis pedis artery
Posterior tibial pulse site
Dorsal arch
Dorsalis pedis pulse site

Veins

Veins are the blood vessels that carry deoxygenated, nutrient-depleted, waste-laden blood from the tissues back to the heart. The veins of the arms, upper trunk, head, and neck carry blood to the superior vena cava, where it passes into the right atrium. Blood from the lower trunk and legs drains upward into the inferior vena cava.

There are three types of veins: deep veins, superficial veins, and perforator (or communicator) veins. The two deep veins in the leg are the femoral vein in the upper thigh and the popliteal vein located behind the knee.

The superficial veins are the great and small saphenous veins. The great saphenous vein is the longest of all veins and it extends from the medial dorsal aspect of the foot, crosses over the medial malleolus, and continues across the thigh to the medial aspect of the groin, where it joins the femoral vein. The small saphenous vein begins at the lateral dorsal aspect of the foot, travels up behind the lateral malleolus on the back of the leg, and joins the popliteal vein. The perforator veins connect the superficial veins with the deep veins (Fig. 12–2).

Equipment Needed

- Stethoscope
- Sphygmomanometer
- Doppler
- Tape measure (paper)
- Cotton (to detect light touch)
- Paper clip (tip used to detect sharp sensation—safer than pin tip)
- Tuning fork (to detect vibratory sensation)

Subjective Data: Focus Questions

Any changes in skin color, texture, or temperature? Pain in calves, feet, buttocks, or legs? What aggravates the pain? Walking? Sitting for long periods? Standing for long periods? Does it awaken you? What relieves the pain? Elevating legs?

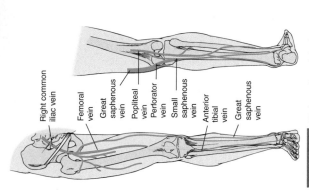

Right common
iliac vein

Femoral
vein

Great
saphenous
vein

Popliteal
vein

Perforator
vein

Small
saphenous
vein

Anterior
tibial
vein

Great
saphenous
vein

FIGURE 12-2 Major veins of the legs.

Rest? Lying down? Is there associated coldness, cyanosis, edema, varicosities, paresthesia, or tingling in legs or feet? Any leg veins that are ropelike, bulging, or contorted? Any sores on legs? Location? Size? Appearance? Length of time? If client is male: Any changes in sexual activity? History of heart or blood vessel surgery? Family history of diabetes, hypertension, coronary artery disease, or elevated cholesterol or triglyceride levels? Is client taking any drugs that may mimic arterial insufficiency? Self-care activities: Does client have well-fitting shoes? Does client wear constricting garments or hosiery? In what type of chair does client usually sit? Does client cross legs frequently? What amount and type of exercise does the client do? Does client smoke? Amount and for how long?

RISK FACTORS. Risk for arterial peripheral vascular disease related to tobacco smoking, age over 50 years, family history of peripheral vascular disease, hypertension, coronary or peripheral vascular disease, or male sex.

Risk for venous peripheral vascular disease related to pregnancy, job with prolonged standing, limited physical activity/poor physical fitness, congenital or acquired vein wall weakness, female sex, increasing age, genetics (eg, non–African American), obesity, lack of dietary fiber, use of constricting corsets/clothes.

Objective Data: Assessment Techniques

See Figures 12–1 and 12–2 for diagrams of major arteries and veins.

INSPECTION, PALPATION, AND AUSCULTATION OF CIRCULATION TO ARMS AND NECK

Inspection, palpation, and auscultation are performed together to assess blood pressure and circulation to the upper extremities and neck while the client is in a sitting, then standing, position. A special maneuver (Allen test) is used to detect arterial insufficiency of the hand.

INSPECTION, PALPATION, AND AUSCULTATION OF CIRCULATION TO ARMS AND NECK (continued)

PROCEDURE	NORMAL FINDINGS	DEVIATIONS FROM NORMAL
Palpate brachial artery, then auscultate arterial blood pressure alternately in both arms with client sitting.	May be difference of 5–10 mm Hg between both arms. *Systolic pressure:* <120 mm Hg. *Diastolic pressure:* <80 mm Hg.* (See Table 4–2).	More than 10 mm Hg difference between both arms. *Systolic pressure:* ≥120 mm Hg.* *Diastolic pressure:* ≥80 mm Hg.* (See Table 4–2).
Palpate brachial artery, then auscultate arterial blood pressure alternately in both arms with client standing.	*Systolic pressure:* Difference between arms of 15 mm Hg or less. *Diastolic pressure:* Difference between arms of 5 mm Hg or less.	*Systolic pressure:* Difference between arms of more than 15 mm Hg. *Diastolic pressure:* Difference between arms of more than 5 mm Hg.
Palpate each carotid artery alternately for rate, rhythm, symmetry, strength, and elasticity.	60 to 90 beats per minute; regular, equal, strong, and elastic.	<60 or >90 bpm; irregular, unequal, weak and thready, bounding and firm, inelastic. Pulse inequality may indicate arterial constriction or occlusion in one carotid. Weak pulses occur with hypovolemia, shock, or decreased cardiac output. Loss of elasticity may indicate arteriosclerosis.

*Values may vary with individuals.

INSPECTION, PALPATION, AND AUSCULTATION OF CIRCULATION TO ARMS AND NECK (continued)

PROCEDURE

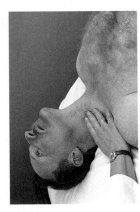

Palpating the carotid artery. (© B. Proud.)

Caution: Use *light* palpation over carotids (one at a time) because increased pressure may stimulate carotid sinus reflex and lower heart rate and blood pressure.

Peripheral Vascular Assessment

INSPECTION, PALPATION, AND AUSCULTATION OF CIRCULATION TO ARMS AND NECK (continued)

PROCEDURE	NORMAL FINDINGS	DEVIATIONS FROM NORMAL
Auscultate carotid arteries with stethoscope bell while patient holds breath.	No sound heard.	Bruit (swishing sound) is caused by turbulent blood flow through a narrowed vessel and is indicative of occlusive arterial disease.

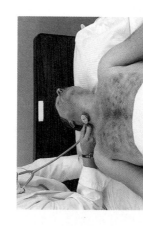

Auscultating the carotid artery. (© B. Proud.)

INSPECTION, PALPATION, AND AUSCULTATION OF CIRCULATION TO ARMS AND NECK (continued)

PROCEDURE	NORMAL FINDINGS	DEVIATIONS FROM NORMAL
Inspect and palpate upper extremities for the following:		
• Color	• Pink; pink or red tones visible under dark pigmentation.	• Pallor, cyanosis, rubor; rapid color changes—pallor, cyanosis, and redness seen with Raynaud disease.
• Temperature	• Warm.	• Cold; cool extremities seen with arterial insufficiency and Raynaud disease.
• Sensation: Scatter stimuli over trunk and upper extremities with client's eyes closed.	• Client can identify light and deep touch; nontender.	• Paresthesia, tenderness, pain; numbness is seen in Raynaud disease.
• Mobility	• Mobile.	• Paralysis.
• Radial pulses (Fig. 12–3)	• Bilateral pulses strong and equal	• Bilateral/unilateral pulses weak, asymmetrical, or absent may indicate partial or complete obstruction; increased radial pulse may indicate hyperkinesis.
• Ulnar pulses (Fig. 12–4)	• Bilateral pulses strong and equal	• Bilateral/unilateral pulses weak, asymmetrical, or absent
If client has weak radial and/or ulnar pulses, perform Allen test, a special maneuver (Fig. 12–5).	Full palm of hand becomes pink with release of ulnar or radial artery	Only half of palm of hand becomes pink with release of ulnar or radial artery; other half of palm remains whitish. Pallor persists with occlusion of ulnar artery.

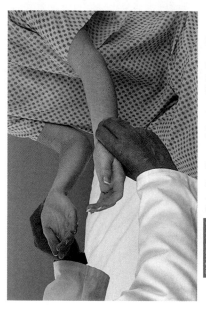

FIGURE 12-3 Palpating the radial pulse. (© B. Proud.)

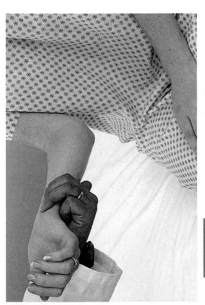

FIGURE 12-4 Palpating the ulnar pulse. (© B. Proud.)

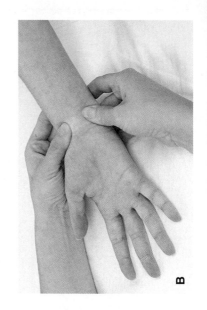

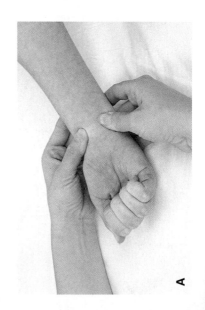

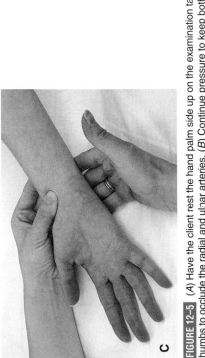

FIGURE 12-5 (A) Have the client rest the hand palm side up on the examination table and then make a fist. Use your thumbs to occlude the radial and ulnar arteries. (B) Continue pressure to keep both arteries occluded, and have the client release the fist. Note that the palm remains pale. (C) Release the pressure on the ulnar artery and watch for color to return to hand. To assess radial patency, repeat the procedure as before, but at the last step, release pressure on the radial artery. (© B. Proud.)

INSPECTION AND PALPATION OF JUGULAR VENOUS PRESSURE AND CIRCULATION OF LOWER EXTREMITIES

Inspection and palpation are performed together to assess the jugular venous pressure and circulation of the lower extremities with the client in a supine position. Finally, special maneuvers are performed to detect venous and arterial insufficiencies of the legs.

PROCEDURE	NORMAL FINDINGS	DEVIATIONS FROM NORMAL
Inspect jugular veins with head elevated 45°. Identify the highest point of venous wave (Fig. 12–6) in relation to the sternal angle. Measure in centimeters or inches.	Pulsation height ≤1 inch (3 cm)	Pulsation height >1 inch (3 cm). Fully distended veins with torso elevated are seen with increased central venous pressure that may be due to right ventricular failure, pulmonary hypertension, pulmonary edema, or cardiac tamponade.
Inspect and palpate legs for the following:		
• Color	• Pink; pink or red tones visible under dark pigmentation	• Pallor, cyanosis, rubor; pallor on elevation and rubor on dependency suggest arterial insufficiency; rusty or brownish pigmentation around ankles indicates venous insufficiency.

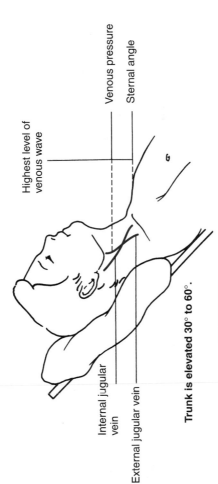

Highest level of venous wave

Venous pressure

Sternal angle

Internal jugular vein

External jugular vein

Trunk is elevated 30° to 60°.

FIGURE 12–6 Inspection of jugular vein.

INSPECTION AND PALPATION OF JUGULAR VENOUS PRESSURE AND CIRCULATION OF LOWER EXTREMITIES (continued)

PROCEDURE	NORMAL FINDINGS	DEVIATIONS FROM NORMAL
• Temperature	• Warm	• Cold; coolness in one leg suggests arterial insufficiency; increased warmth in leg may be due to thrombophlebitis; bilateral coolness in feet and legs suggests cold room, recent cigarette smoking, or anxiety.
• Sensation: Scatter stimuli with client's eyes closed.	• Client can identify light and deep touch; nontender.	• Paresthesia, tenderness, pain.
• Mobility	• Mobile.	• Paralysis.
• Superficial veins	• Slight venous distention with standing that collapses with elevation	• Severe venous distention and bulging are seen with varicose veins due to incompetent valves, vein wall weakness, or venous obstruction; superficial vein thrombophlebitis is characterized by redness, thickening, and tenderness along the vein.
• Condition of skin	• Intact	• Lesions
• Edema	• Not present	• Present
• Femoral pulse (Fig. 12–7)	• Bilateral pulses strong and equal	• Bilateral/unilateral pulses weak, asymmetrical, or absent in arterial occlusion

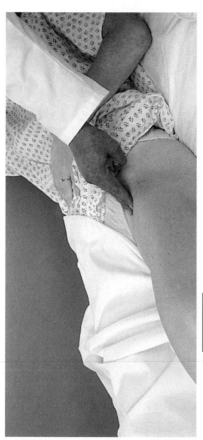

FIGURE 12-7 Palpating the femoral pulses (© B. Proud.)

INSPECTION AND PALPATION OF JUGULAR VENOUS PRESSURE AND CIRCULATION OF LOWER EXTREMITIES (continued)

PROCEDURE	NORMAL FINDINGS	DEVIATIONS FROM NORMAL
• Popliteal pulse: Have client bend knees or, if on table, roll on to stomach and flex leg 90°. Press deeply to feel (Fig. 12–8).	• Bilateral pulses strong and equal, but it is not unusual for popliteal pulse to be difficult or impossible to detect.	• Bilateral/unilateral pulses weak, asymmetrical, or absent may indicate occluded artery.
• Dorsalis pedis pulse: Have client dorsiflex or extend foot (Fig. 12–9).	• Bilateral pulses strong and equal (congenitally absent in 5–10% of population)	• Bilateral/unilateral pulses weak, asymmetrical, or absent may indicate impaired arterial circulation.
• Posterior tibial pulse (located on medial malleolus of ankle; Fig. 12–10).	• Bilateral pulses strong and equal	• Bilateral/unilateral pulses weak or absent may indicate arterial occlusion.

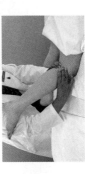
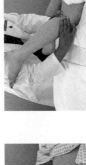

FIGURE 12-8 Palpating the popliteal pulse with the client (*left*) supine and (*right*) prone. If you cannot detect a pulse, try palpating with the client in a prone position. Partially raise the leg and place your fingers deep in the bend of the knee. Repeat palpation in opposite leg and note amplitude bilaterally. (© B. Proud.)

Peripheral Vascular Assessment

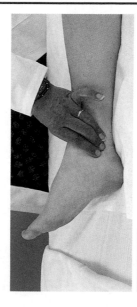

FIGURE 12–10 Palpating the posterior tibial pulse. (© B. Proud.)

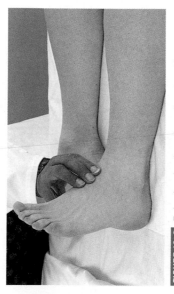

FIGURE 12–9 Palpating the dorsalis pedis pulse. (© B. Proud.)

INSPECTION AND PALPATION OF JUGULAR VENOUS PRESSURE AND CIRCULATION OF LOWER EXTREMITIES (continued)

PROCEDURE	NORMAL FINDINGS	DEVIATIONS FROM NORMAL
Special maneuvers: • Check for deep phlebitis by quickly squeezing calf muscles against tibia.	• Client verbalizes no calf pain.	• Client verbalizes painful calves with deep phlebitis.
• Check Homans sign by extending leg and dorsiflexing foot (Fig. 12–11).	• Client verbalizes no calf soreness or pain.	• Client reports soreness and pain in calf with deep vein thrombosis or superficial thrombophlebitis; further diagnostic testing, however, is needed to confirm diagnosis.

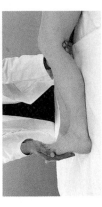
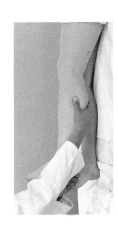

FIGURE 12–11 Elicit Homans sign by (*left*) squeezing the calf muscle and also by (*right*) passive dorsiflexion of the foot. (© B. Proud.)

INSPECTION AND PALPATION OF JUGULAR VENOUS PRESSURE AND CIRCULATION OF LOWER EXTREMITIES (continued)

PROCEDURE	NORMAL FINDINGS	DEVIATIONS FROM NORMAL
• Check for arterial insufficiency (Fig. 12–12) if leg pulses are decreased. Have client lie down on back while you support client's legs 12 inches above heart level. Have client flap feet up and down at ankles for 60 seconds, then sit up and dangle legs.	• Feet pink to slight pale color with this maneuver; pink color returns to tips of toes in 10 seconds; veins on top of feet fill in 15 seconds.	Extensive pallor with this maneuver in arterial insufficiency; toes and feet exhibit rubor (dusky red); venous return to feet is delayed 45 seconds or more in arterial insufficiency.

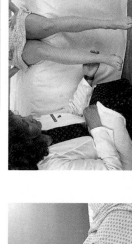

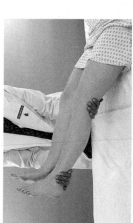

FIGURE 12–12 Testing for arterial insufficiency by (*left*) elevating the legs and then (*right*) having the client dangle the legs. (© B. Proud.)

Peripheral Vascular Assessment

INSPECTION AND PALPATION OF JUGULAR VENOUS PRESSURE AND CIRCULATION OF LOWER EXTREMITIES (continued)

PROCEDURE	NORMAL FINDINGS	DEVIATIONS FROM NORMAL
• Check for competency of valves (Fig. 12–13) (manual compression test) if client has varicose veins—compress dilated veins with one hand while using the other hand to feel pulsations 6–8 inches above the first hand. Repeat in other leg. Compare venous and arterial insufficiency of lower extremities (Table 12–1).	• No pulsation palpated	• Pulsation felt with incompetent valves. **Note:** See Table 12–1 and 12–2 for characteristics of venous and arterial insufficiencies and differentiation of arterial and venous ulcers.

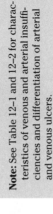

FIGURE 12–13 Performing manual compression to assess competence of venous valves in clients with varicose veins.

TABLE 12-1 COMPARISON OF ARTERIAL AND VENOUS INSUFFICIENCIES

	Arterial Insufficiency	Venous Insufficiency
Pulses	Decreased or absent	Present
Color	Pale on elevation, dusky rubor on dependency	Pink to cyanotic, brown pigment at ankles
Temperature	Cool, cold	Warm
Edema	None	Present
Skin	Shiny skin, thick nails, absence of hair, ulcers on toes, gangrene may develop (Table 12-2)	Ulcers on ankles; discolored, scaly
Sensation	Leg pain aggravated by exercise and relieved with rest; pressure or cramps in buttocks or calves during walking, paresthesias.	Leg pain aggravated by prolonged standing or sitting, relieved by elevation of legs, lying down, or walking; also relieved with use of support hose.

TABLE 12–2 CHARACTERISTICS OF VENOUS AND ARTERIAL LEG ULCERS

Characteristics	Venous Ulcer	Arterial Ulcer
Pulses	Present	Diminished or absent
Capillary refill	<3 seconds	>3 seconds
Skin temperature	Warm/no temperature gradient	Cool/temperature gradient
Ankle–brachial index	0.90–1.0	<0.75
Ulcer location	Typically near medial malleolus	Tips of toes, foot or lateral malleolus
Ulcer margin	Irregular	Rounded and smooth
Ulcer tissue	Dark-red granulation tissue	Black eschar or pale-pink granulation tissue
Ulcer drainage	Moderate to large amount	Minimal
Periulcer skin	Bronze-brown pigmentation, thick, hardened, and indurated	Pale, thin, friable, and shiny; thick toe nails; elevation pallor; dependency rubor
Dermatitis	Frequently occurs	Rarely occurs
Pruritus	Frequently occurs	Rarely occurs
Edema	Moderate to severe	Minimal unless leg constantly in dependent position
Pain	Ulcer often painful, especially if infected	Intermittent claudication or rest pain in foot; ulcer not painful

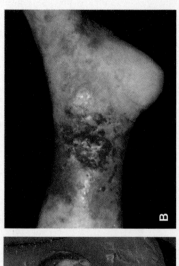

(A) Characteristic ulcer of arterial insufficiency. (© 1994 Michael English, M.D.) (B) Characteristic ulcer of venous insufficiency. (Courtesy of Dermik Laboratories, Inc.)

(Used with permission from Wipke-Tevis, D. D. [1999]. Caring for vascular leg ulcers. *Home Healthcare Nurse 17*[2], 87–95.)

INSPECTION AND PALPATION OF JUGULAR VENOUS PRESSURE AND CIRCULATION OF LOWER EXTREMITIES (continued)

PROCEDURE	NORMAL FINDINGS	DEVIATIONS FROM NORMAL
Auscultation of Arteries		
If arterial insufficiency is found in legs, auscultate over the following areas:		
• Aorta	• No sound	• Bruits
• Renal arteries	• No sound	• Bruits
• Iliac arteries	• No sound	• Bruits
• Femoral arteries (Fig. 12–14)	• No sound	• Bruits

CULTURAL VARIATIONS

Black Africans have fewer valves in the external iliac veins but many more valves lower in the leg than do Caucasians, which may account for a lower prevalence of varicose veins in blacks (1–3%) than in whites (10–18%) [Overfield, 1995].

GERIATRIC VARIATIONS

● Hair loss of lower extremities occurs with aging and may not be an absolute sign of arterial insufficiency.
● Inspect for rigid, tortuous veins and arteries (decreased venous return and competency) because varicosities are common in older adult.

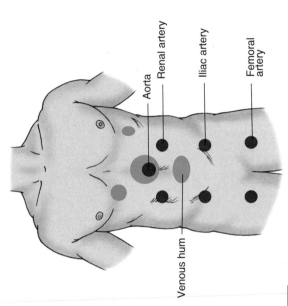

FIGURE 12–14 Vascular sounds and friction rubs can best be heard over these areas.

- Prominent, bulging veins are common. Varicosities are considered a problem only if ulcerations, signs of thrombophlebitis, or cords are present. Cords are nontender, palpable veins having a rubber tubing consistency.
- Blood pressure increases as elasticity decreases in arteries with proportionately greater increase in systolic pressure resulting in a widening of pulse pressure.

Possible Collaborative Problems

Hypertension	Edema
Thrombophlebitis	Gangrene
Arterial insufficiency	Vasospasms
Peripheral neuropathy	Claudication
Thrombosis/emboli	Stasis ulcers
Venous insufficiency	

TEACHING TIPS FOR SELECTED NURSING DIAGNOSES AND COLLABORATIVE PROBLEMS

Adult Client

Nursing Diagnosis: Impaired Skin Integrity related to arterial insufficiency

☐ Instruct client on importance of exercise and diet (eat foods high in protein, vitamins A and C, and zinc to promote healing, unless contraindicated by other therapies) to aid healing of leg ulcers. Explain importance of keeping area clean and dry.

Nursing Diagnosis: Impaired Skin Integrity related to venous insufficiency

☐ Instruct client on importance of rest, avoidance of restrictive clothing, elevation of extremities to reduce edema, and proper diet to aid healing of leg ulcers.

Nursing Diagnosis: Ineffective Peripheral Tissue Perfusion related to venous insufficiency

☐ Teach client how to assess condition of extremities (color, temperature, sensation, movement, swelling). Teach client how to use assessment to determine activity level. Teach methods for accomplishing activities of daily living with restricted activity level.

Nursing Diagnosis: Risk for Peripheral Neurovascular Dysfunction related to increasing peripheral vascular disease

☐ Teach client how to assess condition of extremities (color, temperature, sensation, movement, swelling). Teach client how to modify activities of daily living in order to prevent injury and complications.

Teach client to

- Stop smoking.
- Control hypertension.
- Eat a low-fat diet.
- Increase dietary fiber intake.
- Control high blood sugars of diabetes mellitus.
- Limit alcohol intake.
- Get regular exercise.
- Maintain weight within ideal range for height and body structure.
- Avoid prolonged standing or sitting; modify work and leisure habits to vary position (eg, to reduce risk for hemorrhoids, use squatting position when toileting).
- Avoid constrictive clothing, including girdles, garters for stockings or tightly cuffed knee-high hose, or any items that compress vessels.

Collaborative problem. Potential complication: Hypertension

☐ Explain the effects of diet (low fat and low cholesterol), reduction of stress, vigorous exercise, no smoking, and decreased use of alcohol on promotion of adequate circulation. Blood pressure checks should be done on a regular basis. Refer any client with a reading ≥140/90 mm Hg.

13 Breast Assessment

ANATOMY OVERVIEW

The breasts are paired mammary glands that lie over the muscles of the anterior chest wall, anterior to the pectoralis major and serratus anterior muscles (Fig. 13–1). The male and female breasts are similar until puberty, when female breast tissue enlarges in response to hormones.

For assessment purposes, the breasts are divided into four quadrants by drawing horizontal and vertical imaginary lines that intersect at the nipple (Fig. 13–2).

The skin of the breasts is smooth and varies in color. The nipple contains the tiny openings of the lactiferous ducts. The areola surrounds the nipple and contains elevated sebaceous glands (Montgomery glands).

Female breasts consist of three types of tissue: glandular, fibrous, and fatty (adipose; Fig. 13–3). The amount of glandular, fibrous, and fatty tissue varies according to various factors including the client's age, body build, nutritional status, hormonal cycle, and whether she is pregnant or lactating.

The major axillary lymph nodes consist of the anterior (pectoral), posterior (subscapular), lateral (brachial), and central (midaxillary) nodes, supraclavicular, and infraclavicular (Fig. 13–4).

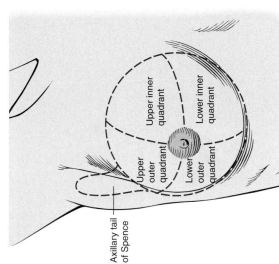

FIGURE 13-2 Breast quadrants. The upper outer quadrant is the area most targeted by breast cancer.

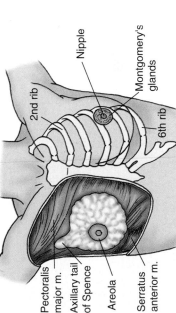

FIGURE 13-1 Anatomic breast landmarks and their position in the thorax.

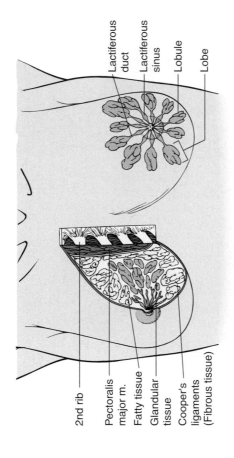

FIGURE 13–3 The internal anatomy of the breast.

Lactiferous duct

Lactiferous sinus

Lobule

Lobe

2nd rib

Pectoralis major m.

Fatty tissue

Glandular tissue

Cooper's ligaments (Fibrous tissue)

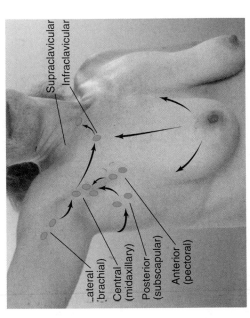

FIGURE 13-4 The lymph nodes drain impurities from the breasts (arrows show direction).

Supraclavicular
Infraclavicular

Lateral
(brachial)
Central
(midaxillary)
Posterior
(subscapular)
Anterior
(pectoral)

Equipment Needed

- Centimeter ruler
- Small pillow
- Breast self-examination brochure
- Gloves and slide for specimen if nipple discharge is present

Subjective Data: Focus Questions

Any lumps or lesions (location, size) or swelling in breasts? Change in size or firmness? Redness, warmth, or dimpling of breasts? Tenderness? Pain? Timing in menstrual cycle? Change in position of nipple or nipple discharge? Age of menstruation? Birth to children and age? Previous breast surgeries? History of breast cancer in family? Self care: Breast self-examination (frequency and time performed)? Use of hormones, birth control, or antidepressants? Exposure to radiation, benzene, or asbestos? Use of alcohol, caffeine? Diet and daily exercise routine? Last breast exam? Last mammogram?

RISK FACTORS. Risk for breast cancer related to increasing age, personal history of breast cancer, family history of breast cancer, early menarche and late menopause, no natural children, first child after age 30 years, and higher education and socioeconomic status.

Objective Data: Assessment Techniques

See Figures 13–1 through 13–8 for illustrations of the breasts and regional lymphatics.

INSPECTION

The breasts should be inspected with client in sitting position with arms at sides, arms overhead, hands pressed on hips, palms pressed together, and arms extended straight ahead as client leans forward (Fig. 13–5). The areolae and nipples should also be inspected.

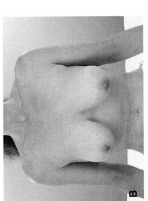

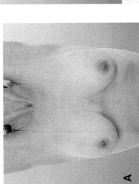

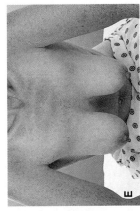

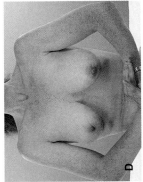

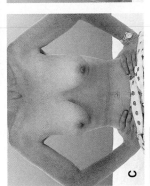

FIGURE 13–5 (*A*) Arms over head. (*B*) Arms at side. (*C*) Arms pressed on hips. (*D*) Hands pressed together. (*E*) Leaning forward, arms extended.

INSPECTION (continued)

PROCEDURE	NORMAL FINDINGS	DEVIATIONS FROM NORMAL
*Observe **breasts** for the following:*		
• Size and symmetry	• Relatively equal with slight variation	• Recent change to unequal size. Recent increase in size of one breast may indicate inflammation or abnormal growth.
• Shape	• Round and pendulous	• Retraction or dimpling may be due to fibrosis and may indicate a malignant tumor.
• Color	• Pink; striae with age and pregnancy	• Redness, inflammation, blue hue, increased venous engorgement
• Skin surface	• Smooth	• Retraction, dimpling, enlarged pores, "peau d'orange" (seen in metastatic breast disease due to edema from blocked lymphatic drainage), edema, lumps, lesions, rashes, ulcers
*Observe **areolae and nipples** for the following:*		
• Size	• Relatively the same, slight variation	• Large variation
• Color	• Pink to dark brown (varies with skin and hair color)	• Inflamed

Breast Assessment

INSPECTION (continued)

DEVIATIONS FROM NORMAL

Retracted breast tissue

Orange peel (peau d'orange) appearance of the breast.

INSPECTION (continued)

PROCEDURE	NORMAL FINDINGS	DEVIATIONS FROM NORMAL
• Shape	• Round, oval, everted	• Inversion, if it occurs after maturation or changes with movement. Recent retraction of previously everted nipple suggests malignancy.
• Discharge	• None; clear yellow 2 days after childbirth	• Foul, purulent, sanguineous drainage. Any spontaneous discharge needs to be referred for further evaluation.
• Texture	• Small Montgomery tubercles present	• Lesions, rashes, ulcers. Peau d'orange skin is seen with carcinoma. Red, scaly, crusty areas are indicative of Paget disease.

PALPATION

Use the flat pads of three fingers to compress tissue against breast wall gently. Palpate with patient sitting. Then have patient lie down and place arm of side being examined over head with small pillow under upper back. Palpate in circular motion starting at the 12-o'clock position and moving in concentric rings inward to areola and nipple (Figure 13–6, *A*). Bimanual palpation may be used in large-breasted clients. A wedge (Figure 13–6, *B*) or vertical (Figure 13–6, *C*) pattern may be used if preferred.

PROCEDURE	NORMAL FINDINGS	DEVIATIONS FROM NORMAL
*Palpate **breasts** for the following:*		
• Temperature	• Warm	• Erythema; heat indicates inflammation if client is not lactating or has not just given birth.
• Elasticity	• Elastic	• Lumpy
• Tenderness	• Nontender; slightly tender (tenderness and fullness may occur before menses).	• Painful
• Masses (note size, shape, mobility, consistency, and location according to quadrant; see Fig. 13–2).	• Bilateral firm inframammary transverse ridge at base of breasts.	• Masses or nodules. Malignant tumors are most often found in upper outer quadrant of breast and are usually unilateral with irregular, poorly delineated borders; hard; nontender; and fixed to underlying tissues. Fibroadenomas (benign) are usually 1–5 cm, round or oval, mobile, firm,

Breast Assessment

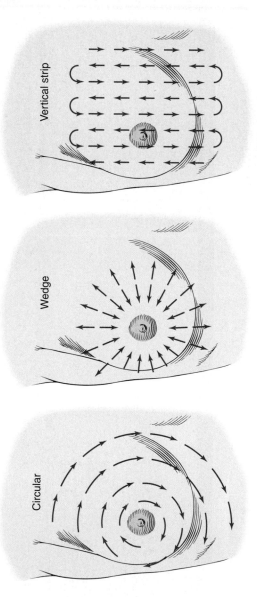

A Circular or clockwise.   B Wedge.   C Vertical strip.

FIGURE 13-6 Patterns for breast palpation. Arrows indicate direction and areas for palpation. (A) Circular or clockwise. (B) Wedge. (C) Vertical strip.

PALPATION (continued)

PROCEDURE	NORMAL FINDINGS	DEVIATIONS FROM NORMAL
Palpate **nipple** gently for discharge.	None: clear yellow 2 days after childbirth.	solid, elastic, nontender, and single or multiple in one or both breasts. Fibrocystic disease (benign) consists of bilateral, multiple, firm, regular, rubbery, mobile nodules with well-demarcated borders (see Fig. 13–7).
		Unilateral serous, serosanguineous, clear, yellow, dark red. Discharge may be seen in endocrine disorders and with some medications, such as antihypertensives, antidepressants, and estrogen. Discharge from one breast may indicate benign intraductal papilloma, fibrocystic disease, or breast cancer.

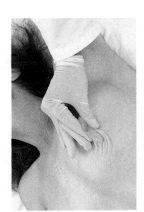

Palpating nipples for masses and discharge.

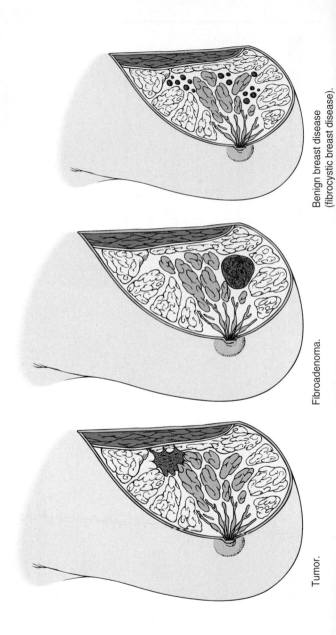

Benign breast disease (fibrocystic breast disease).

Fibroadenoma.

Tumor.

PALPATION (continued)

PROCEDURE	NORMAL FINDINGS	DEVIATIONS FROM NORMAL
Palpate **lymph nodes** in the following areas: supraclavicular, subclavian, intermediate, brachial, scapular, mammary, internal mammary (see Fig. 13–4).	None palpable (<1 cm).	Palpable lymph nodes (>1 cm).

MALE VARIATIONS

Inspect and palpate breast with client seated, arms at sides. Palpate lymph nodes. No swelling, ulcerations, or nodules should be noted. Flat disk of undeveloped breast tissue under nipple is normally palpated. Soft fatty tissue enlargement seen in obesity. Gynecomastia (Fig. 13–8), smooth, firm movable disk of glandular tissue may be seen in one breast during puberty for short time, may be seen in hormonal imbalances (disease or medication induced) and drug abuse. Irregular, hard nodules are seen in malignancy.

PEDIATRIC VARIATIONS

Subjective Data: Focus Questions

Age of menarche? Asymmetrical breast growth? Girls prior to puberty: Pain or discomfort? Boys during adolescence: Abnormal increase in size?

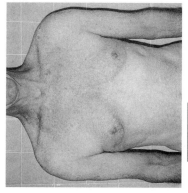

FIGURE 13–8 Gynecomastia.

Objective Data

See normal breast development in Chapter 15, Table 15–1, varies with age. Adolescent breast development is usually seen between age 10 and 13 years and takes about 3 years for full development.

GERIATRIC VARIATIONS

● Breasts pendulous, atrophied, and less firm owing to a decrease in estrogen levels.
● May have smaller, flatter nipples that are less erectile on stimulation. Nipples may retract, but evert with gentle pressure.
● May feel more granular with more fibrotic tissue.

CULTURAL VARIATIONS

Breast cancer rates vary between the U.S. and Europe, with African Americans having the highest age-adjusted death rates. The rates may relate to dry versus wet ear wax also secreted by apocrine glands, active in breast tissue (Overfield, 1995).

Possible Collaborative Problems

Infection (abscess)
Hematoma
Fibrocystic disease
Breast cancer

TEACHING TIPS FOR SELECTED NURSING DIAGNOSES

Adult Client

Nursing Diagnosis: Ineffective Therapeutic Regimen Management related to knowledge deficit of breast self-examination

Assess when and how client examines breasts. Instruct on correct technique and timing. (Breasts should be examined at the same time each month. If client has regular menstrual cycle, she should do examination right after menstruation when breasts are not swollen or tender.)

Reinforce the following American Cancer Society recommendations:

- Monthly breast self-examination for women age 20 years or older
- Breast clinical examination for women age 20 to 39 years every 3 years and every year for women age 40 years and older
- Annual mammography for women age 40 years and older

Advise that cancer of the breast can be treated and often cured if detected early.

Encourage breast-feeding, exercise, and maintaining a healthy body weight.

[American Cancer Society, 2003].

Abdominal Assessment

ANATOMY OVERVIEW

Abdominal Quadrants

The abdomen is divided into four quadrants for purposes of physical examination. These are termed the right upper quadrant (RUQ), right lower quadrant (RLQ), left lower quadrant (LLQ), and left upper quadrant (LUQ) (Fig. 14–1). Note which organs are located within each quadrant (Box 14–1).

Internal Anatomy

Within the abdominal cavity are structures of several different body systems—gastrointestinal, reproductive (female), lymphatic, and urinary. These structures are typically referred to as the abdominal viscera and can be divided into two types—solid viscera and hollow viscera. Solid viscera are those organs that maintain their shape consistently—the liver, pancreas, spleen, ad-renal glands, kidneys, ovaries, and uterus. The hollow viscera consist of structures that change shape depending on their contents. These include the stomach, gallbladder, small intestine, colon, and bladder.

Solid Viscera

The liver is the largest solid organ in the body. It is located below the diaphragm in the RUQ of the abdomen. (Fig. 14–2).
The pancreas, located mostly behind the stomach, deep in the upper abdomen, is normally not palpable (see Fig. 14–2

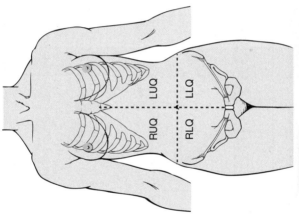

FIGURE 14-1 Abdominal quadrants.

BOX 14–1. Locating Abdominal Structures by Quadrants

RIGHT UPPER
QUADRANT (RUQ)
Ascending and transverse colon
Duodenum
Gallbladder
Hepatic flexure of colon
Liver
Pancreas (head)
Pylorus (the small bowel—or ileum—
traverses all quadrants)
Right adrenal gland
Right kidney (upper pole)
Right ureter

RIGHT LOWER
QUADRANT (RLQ)
Appendix
Ascending colon
Cecum
Right kidney (lower pole)
Right ovary and tube
Right ureter
Right spermatic cord

LEFT UPPER
QUADRANT (LUQ)
Left adrenal gland
Left kidney (upper pole)
Left ureter
Pancreas (body and tail)
Spleen
Splenic flexure of colon
Stomach
Transverse ascending colon

LEFT LOWER
QUADRANT (LLQ)
Left kidney (lower pole)
Left ovary and tube
Left ureter
Left spermatic cord
Sigmoid colon

MIDLINE
Bladder
Uterus
Prostate gland

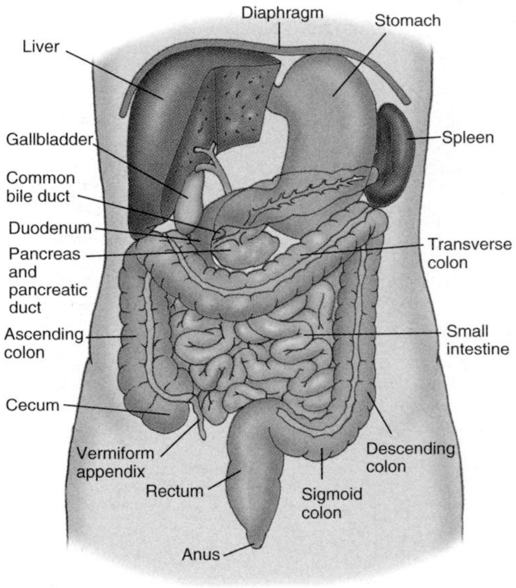

FIGURE 14–2 Abdominal viscera.

and Fig. 14–3). The spleen is approximately 7 cm wide and is located above the left kidney, just below the diaphragm at the level of the ninth, tenth, and eleventh ribs (see Fig. 14–2). This soft, flat structure is normally not palpable. The kidneys are located high and deep under the diaphragm (see Fig. 14-3).

The pregnant uterus may be palpated above the level of the symphysis pubis in the midline (see Fig. 14–3). The ovaries are located in the RLQ and LLQ and are normally palpated only during a bimanual examination of the internal genitalia.

Hollow Viscera

The stomach is a distensible, flasklike organ located in the LUQ, just below the diaphragm and in between the liver and spleen. The stomach is not usually palpable (see Fig. 14–2).

The gallbladder, a muscular sac approximately 10 cm long, is not normally palpated because it is difficult to distinguish between the gallbladder and the liver (see Fig. 14–2).

The small intestine is actually the longest portion of the digestive tract (approximately 7.0 m long). The small intestine, which lies coiled in all four quadrants of the abdomen, is not normally palpated (see Fig. 14–2).

The colon, or large intestine, has a wider diameter than the small intestine (approximately 6.0 cm) and is approximately 1.4 m long. The colon is composed of three major sections: ascending, transverse, and descending.

The sigmoid colon is often felt as a firm structure on palpation, whereas the cecum and ascending colon may feel softer. The transverse and descending colon may also be felt on palpation (see Fig. 14–2).

The urinary bladder is a distensible muscular sac located behind the pubic bone in the midline of the abdomen. A bladder filled with urine may be palpated in the abdomen above the symphysis pubis (see Fig. 14–3).

Vascular Structures

The abdominal organs are supplied with arterial blood by the abdominal aorta and its major branches. Pulsations of the aorta are frequently visible and palpable midline in the upper abdomen (see Fig. 14–3).

Equipment Needed

- Stethoscope (warm)
- Small ruler

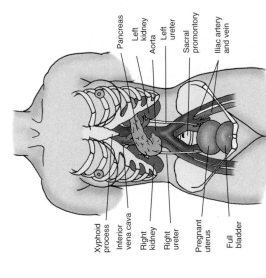

Xyphoid
process

Inferior
vena cava

Right
kidney

Right
ureter

Pregnant
uterus

Full
bladder

Pancreas

Left
kidney

Aorta

Left
ureter

Sacral
promontory

Iliac artery
and vein

FIGURE 14–3 Abdominal viscera and vascular structures (aorta and iliac artery and vein).

- Marking pencil
- Small pillows

Subjective Data: Focus Questions

Indigestion? Nausea? Vomiting? Precipitating/relieving factors? Change in appetite? Associated weight loss? Change in bowel elimination? Describe. Constipation? Diarrhea? Associated symptoms? Any past gastrointestinal (GI) disorders (ulcers, reflux, inflammatory, obstructive bowel, pancreatitis, gallbladder or liver disease, diverticulosis, appendicitis, history of viral hepatitis)? Family history of colon, stomach, pancreatic, liver, kidney, or bladder cancer? Use of medications—aspirin, anti-inflammatory drugs, steroids? Surgeries? GI diagnostic tests? Health practices: Usual diet? Exercise? Use of alcohol? Stressors?

RISK FACTORS. Risk for hepatitis B virus (HBV) exposure related to contact in population of high HBV endemicity, sexual contact with carriers, intravenous drug abusers, heterosexuals who have had more than one sex partner in past 6 months, sexually active homosexual or bisexual males, hemodialysis patients, hemophiliac patients, international travelers in high-risk HBV areas, health care workers, long-term inmates.

Risk for colon cancer related to age over 50 years; family history of colorectal cancer, patient history of endometrial, breast, or ovarian cancer, patient history of inflammatory bowel disease, polyps, or colorectal cancer.

Objective Data: Assessment Techniques

Review Figures 14–1 through 14–3 for a diagram of landmarks of the abdomen.

Assessment of the abdomen differs from other assessments in that inspection and auscultation precede percussion and palpation. This sequence allows accurate assessment of bowel sounds and delays more uncomfortable maneuvers until last. The client is placed in the supine position, with small pillows under the head and knees. The abdomen is exposed from the breasts to the symphysis pubis.

Examiner should warm hands and have short fingernails. Stand at the client's right side and carry out assessment systematically, beginning with the LUQ and progressing clockwise through the four abdominal quadrants (see Fig. 14–1). The client's bladder should be empty.

INSPECTION

PROCEDURE	NORMAL FINDINGS	DEVIATIONS FROM NORMAL
Inspect the **skin** *for the following:* • Color	• Normally paler, with white striae	• Dark bluish striae seen in Cushing syndrome, redness seen in inflammation, pale and taut with ascites, purple flank color (Grey Turner sign) seen with bleeding within the abdominal wall
• Venous pattern	• Fine veins observable	• Engorged, prominent veins seen with cirrhosis of the liver, inferior vena cava obstruction, portal hypertension, or ascites
• Integrity	• No rashes or lesions	• Rashes, lesions
Special maneuver for prominent abdominal veins: • Compress a section of vein with two fingers next to each other, remove one finger and observe for filling; repeat procedure, removing other finger.	• Blood fills from upper to lower abdomen	• Blood fills from lower to upper abdomen (obstructed inferior vena cava)

INSPECTION (continued)

PROCEDURE	NORMAL FINDINGS	DEVIATIONS FROM NORMAL
Inspect the **umbilicus** *for the following:*		
• Position	• Sunken, centrally located	• Deviated from midline with mass, hernia, enlarged organs, or fluid; everted with abdominal distention or umbilical hernia
• Color	• Pinkish	• Inflamed, crusted; bluish color (Cullen sign) seen in intra-abdominal hemorrhage
Observe the **abdomen** *for the following:*		
• Contour	• Rounded or flat	• Generalized distention seen with air or fluid accumulation; distention below umbilicus due to full bladder, uterine enlargement, ovarian tumor or cyst; distention above the umbilicus seen with pancreatic mass or gastric dilation
• Symmetry	• Symmetrical	• Asymmetrical with organ enlargement, large masses, hernia, diastasis recti, or bowel obstruction

Abdominal Assessment

INSPECTION (continued)

PROCEDURE	NORMAL FINDINGS	DEVIATIONS FROM NORMAL
• Surface motion	• No movement or slight peristalsis visualized over aorta	• Diminished abdominal movement with peritoneal irritation; bounding peristalsis, bounding pulsations with abdominal aortic aneurysm; peristaltic, ripple waves seen with intestinal obstruction
Observe **color of stools**.	Brown to dark brown	Black, tarry (melena), bright red
Observe **color of emesis**.	Varies	Bloody (hematemesis), coffee grounds (old blood)

AUSCULTATION

Using the diaphragm of a warm stethoscope, apply light pressure to auscultate for bowel sounds for up to 5 minutes in each quadrant. Use the bell to auscultate for vascular sounds.

PROCEDURE	NORMAL FINDINGS	DEVIATIONS FROM NORMAL
Auscultate for **bowel sounds**.	High-pitched, irregular gurgles 5–35 times/min; present equally in all four quadrants	Absent with peritonitis or paralytic ileus; hypoactive in abdominal surgery or late bowel obstruction; hyperactive sounds heard in diarrhea, gastroenteritis, or

AUSCULTATION (continued)

PROCEDURE	NORMAL FINDINGS	DEVIATIONS FROM NORMAL
		early bowel obstruction; high-pitched tinkling and rushes (borborygmus) heard in bowel obstruction
Auscultate for **vascular sounds** (Fig. 14-4).	No bruits, no venous hums, no friction rubs	Bruits heard over aorta, renal arteries, or iliac arteries; venous hum auscultated over epigastric or umbilical area may indicate increased collateral circulation between portal and systemic venous systems as with cirrhosis of the liver.

Caution: If bruits are heard, do *not* palpate abdomen as part of the assessment. (Bruits may be indicative of a narrowed vessel or aneurysm.)

PERCUSSION

Percussion notes will vary from dull to tympanic, with tympany dominating over the hollow organs. The hollow organs include the stomach, intestines, bladder, aorta, and gallbladder. Dull percussion notes will be heard over the liver, spleen, pancreas, kidneys, and uterus. Percuss from areas of tympany to dullness to locate borders of these solid organs.

Abdominal Assessment

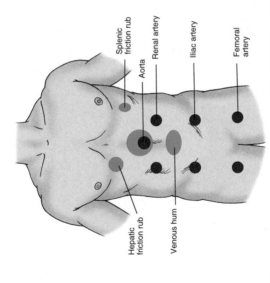

Splenic
friction rub

Aorta

Renal artery

Iliac artery

Femoral
artery

Hepatic
friction rub

Venous hum

FIGURE 14–4 Vascular sounds and friction rubs can best be heard over these areas.

Objective Data: Assessment Techniques

PROCEDURE	NORMAL FINDINGS	DEVIATIONS FROM NORMAL
Percuss **all four quadrants** for percussion tones (notes); see Figure 14–5.	Generalized tympany over bowels	Increased dullness over enlarged organs; hyperresonance over gaseous, distended abdomen
Percuss the liver for span (Fig. 14–6) as follows:		
• Percuss starting below umbilicus at client's right midclavicular line (MCL), and percuss upward until you hear dullness; mark this point. Percuss downward from lung resonance in the right MCL to dullness and mark.	• Liver span is 6–12 cm (2.5–5 inches) in the right MCL. **Note:** Span is greater in men.	• Liver span is greater than 12 cm in the right MCL with enlarged liver as seen in tumors, cirrhosis, abscess, and vascular engorgement. A liver in a lower position may be caused by emphysema, and a liver in a higher position may be caused by a mass, ascites, or paralyzed diaphragm.
• Repeat in midsternal line.	• Liver span is 4–8 cm in midsternal line.	• Liver span is greater than 8 cm in right midsternal line.
Percuss the spleen (Fig. 14–7) as follows:		
• Percuss for dullness by percussing downward in left midaxillary line, beginning with lung resonance until you hear splenic dullness. (Note: Location fluctuates with respiration.)	• Small area of dullness at sixth to tenth ribs	• Dullness extends above sixth rib or covers larger area. Enlarged spleen is seen with portal hypertension, mononucleosis, or trauma.

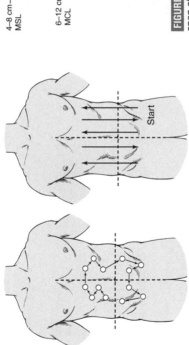

FIGURE 14-5 Abdominal percussion sequences may proceed clockwise or up and down over the abdomen.

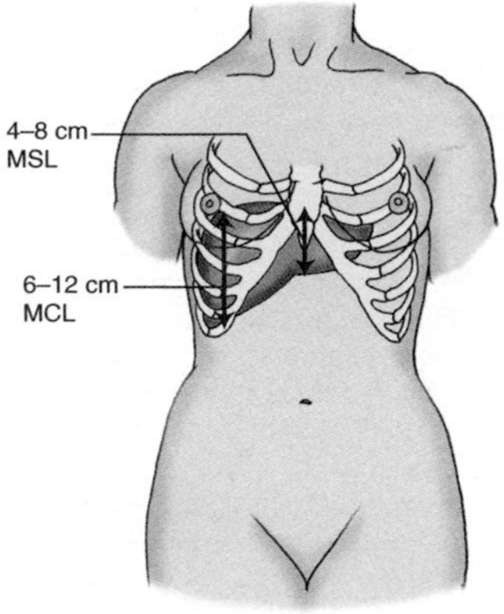

Start

FIGURE 14-6 The normal liver span at the midsternal line (MSL) is 4–8 centimeters (MCL, midclavicular line.)

4–8 cm
MSL

6–12 cm
MCL

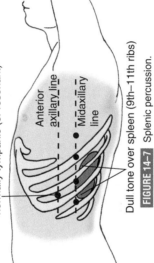

Percuss last interspace:
normally tympanic (or resonant)

Anterior
axillary line

Midaxillary
line

Dull tone over spleen (9th–11th ribs)

FIGURE 14–7 Splenic percussion.

Objective Data: Assessment Techniques (continued)

PROCEDURE	NORMAL FINDINGS	DEVIATIONS FROM NORMAL
Splenic percussion sign: Ask client to inhale deeply and hold breath; percuss lowest interspaces at left anterior axillary line.	Percussion note remains tympanic on inhalation.	Percussion note becomes dull on inhalation.

PALPATION

Light palpation precedes deep palpation to detect tenderness and superficial masses. Deep palpation is used to detect masses and size of organs.

Watch the client's facial expressions and body posture carefully to help assess pain. Examine tender areas last. Never use deep palpation over tender organs in client with polycystic kidneys, after renal transplant, or after hearing an abnormal bruit. Use deep palpation with caution.

Objective Data: Assessment Techniques (continued)

PROCEDURE	NORMAL FINDINGS	DEVIATIONS FROM NORMAL
Lightly palpate all four quadrants *for the following (also observe facial expression):*		
• Tenderness	• Nontender	• Tender, painful with infection, inflammation, pressure from gaseous distention, tumors, or enlarged organs
• Consistency	• Soft, nontender	• Rigid, boardlike
• Masses	• No masses	• Superficial masses (A superficial mass becomes more prominent against examiner's hand when client lifts head from examination table, whereas a deep abdominal mass does not.)
Deeply palpate all four quadrants *for the following:*		
• Tenderness	• Mild tenderness over midline at xiphoid, cecum, sigmoid colon	• Tenderness, severe pain seen with tumor, cyst, abscess, enlarged organ, aneurysm, or adhesions
• Guarding	• Voluntary guarding	• Involuntary guarding is seen with peritoneal irritation; right-sided guarding is seen with acute cholecystitis.

Abdominal Assessment

Objective Data: Assessment Techniques (continued)

PROCEDURE	NORMAL FINDINGS	DEVIATIONS FROM NORMAL
• Masses	• No masses; aorta; feces in colon	• Masses
*Palpate deeply for **liver border** at right costal margin (Box 14–2) for the following:*		
• Tenderness	• Nontender	• Tenderness seen in trauma or diseased liver
• Consistency	• Smooth, firm sharp edge, no masses	• Hard, firm liver may indicate cancer; nodularity may occur with tumors, metastatic cancer, late cirrhosis, or syphilis.
*Palpate deeply for **splenic border**, using bimanual technique (see Box 14–2). Check for the following:*		
• Size	• Not normally palpable	• Enlarged and palpable with trauma, mononucleosis, blood disorders, and malignancies
• Tenderness	• Nontender	• Tender

Abdominal Assessment

BOX 14–2. Guidelines for Liver and Spleen Palpation

Liver Palpation

1. Stand at client's right side and place your left hand under clients back at the 11th and 12th ribs.

2. Place right hand parallel to right costal margin.

3. Ask client to breathe deeply, and press upward with your right fingers with each inhalation.

Spleen Palpation

1. Stand at client's right side; reach across client to place your left hand under client's posterior lower ribs, and push up.

2. Place your right hand below rib margin.

3. Ask client to breathe deeply.

4. Press hands together to palpate spleen on inhalation.

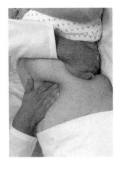

Objective Data: Assessment Techniques (continued)

PROCEDURE	NORMAL FINDINGS	DEVIATIONS FROM NORMAL
*Palpate deeply for the **kidneys** by using bimanual technique (Box 14–3). Assess for the following:*		
• Size	• Not normally palpable	• Enlarged and palpable owing to cyst, tumor, or hydronephrosis
• Tenderness	• Nontender	• Tender
• Masses	• No masses	• Masses
Special maneuvers for ascites:		
• Measure abdominal girth at same point every day.	• No increase in abdominal girth	• Increase in abdominal girth
• Fluid wave test: Place palmar surfaces of fingers and hand firmly on one side of abdomen. Tap with other hand on opposite abdominal wall side. Have assistant put lateral side of lower arm firmly on center of abdomen (Figure 14–8).	• No fluid wave transmitted	• Fluid wave palpated with ascites
• Shifting dullness: Place client in supine position and percuss from midline to flank, noting level of dullness. Then assist client to side position and percuss again for level of dullness (Fig. 14–9).	• Level of dullness does not change.	• Level of dullness is higher when client turns on side.

BOX 14-3. Guidelines for Kidney Palpation

1. Place one of your hands behind lower edge of rib cage and above iliac crest.
2. Place the other hand over corresponding anterior surface.
3. Instruct client to breathe deeply.
4. Lift up lower hand and push in with upper hand as client exhales.
5. Repeat on other side.

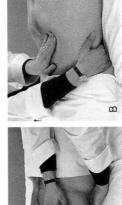
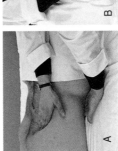

(*Note*: The kidneys are rarely palpable.)

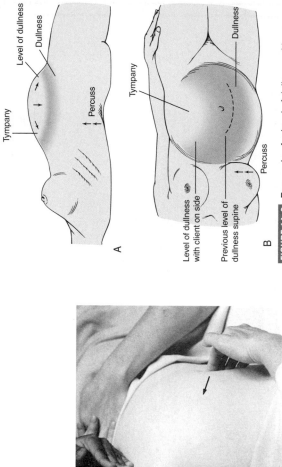

FIGURE 14-8 Performing fluid wave test.

FIGURE 14-9 Percussing for level of dullness with (A) client supine and (B) client lying on side.

Objective Data: Assessment Techniques (continued)

PROCEDURE	NORMAL FINDINGS	DEVIATIONS FROM NORMAL
Special tests for appendicitis:		
• Rebound tenderness: Palpate deeply in one of client's four abdominal quadrants, and quickly withdraw palpating hand. Do this at end of abdominal exam.	• No pain present	• Pain is present in peritoneal irritation (as in appendicitis); because of danger of rupture do not repeat if pain is present.
• Psoas sign: Ask client to lie supine and raise right leg. Place pressure on client's thigh.	• No abdominal pain present	• Right lower abdominal pain present with irritation of the iliopsoas muscle due to appendicitis
• Obturator sign: Ask client to flex right leg at hip and knee. Then rotate leg internally and externally.	• No abdominal pain present	• Lower abdominal pain present with irritation of the obturator muscle due to appendicitis
Special test for acute cholecystitis (Murphy sign):		
• Place thumb below right costal margin and ask patient to inhale deeply.	• Client has no increase in pain.	• Client has sharp increase in pain with cholecystitis.
Testing for asterixis (classic sign of hepatic coma):		
• Dorsiflex client's wrist with fingers extended.	• No tremor noted.	• Persistent, involuntary flapping tremor

Abdominal Assessment

Subjective Data: Focus Questions

Types of food, fluids, and formula? Bowel patterns? Frequent spitting up? Ability to feed self? Milk intake? Food intolerances? History of eating disorders? History of pica?

Objective Data: Assessment Techniques

INSPECTION

PROCEDURE	NORMAL VARIATIONS
Inspect **contour and size of abdomen**.	Prominent/cylindrical (protuberant) when erect, flat when supine. Superficial veins may be present in infants.
Inspect **abdominal movement** in children younger than 8 years.	Rises with inspiration in synchrony with chest; may have visible pulsations in epigastric region.

PALPATION

Palpate **liver border**.	Normal, shortened liver span on percussion. May not extend below costal margin. *Infants and young children:* Liver may be felt 1–3 cm below costal margin; may descend with inspiration.
Palpate **splenic border** (may have child roll on right side).	*Infants and young children:* Spleen may be felt 1–3 cm below costal margin.

PALPATION (continued)

PROCEDURE	NORMAL VARIATIONS
Palpate for **abdominal tenderness.**	Extremely difficult to assess in young children, who may confuse pressure of palpation with pain. Distraction is important.
Palpate **kidney borders.**	Difficult to locate except in newborns.

GERIATRIC VARIATIONS

- Decline in appetite and at risk for nutritional imbalance
- Dilated superficial capillaries visible
- Abdomen is softer and organs more easily palpated owing to a decrease in tone of abdominal musculature.
- Decreased production of saliva, decreased peristalsis, decreased enzymes, weaker gastric acid
- Gastric mucosa and parietal cell degeneration results in a loss of intrinsic factor, which decreases absorption of vitamin B_{12}.
- Bowel sounds 5 to 30 sounds/min.
- Shortened liver span on percussion due to a decrease in liver size after age 50 years
- Liver border is more easily palpated.
- Decreased nerve sensation to lower bowel contributes to constipation.

Possible Collaborative Problems

Bowel strangulation
Ascites
Metabolic acidosis/alkalosis
GI bleeding
Gastric ulcer

Intestinal obstruction
Paralytic ileus
Diverticulitis
Hepatic failure
Evisceration

Peritonitis
Malabsorption syndrome
Pancreatitis
Stromal changes
Gallbladder disease (stones and cancer)

TEACHING TIPS FOR SELECTED NURSING DIAGNOSES

Adult Client

Nursing Diagnosis: Imbalanced Nutrition: More or less than body requirements

Discuss essential components of a well-balanced diet in relation to client's level of physical development and energy expenditure (basal metabolic rate). Teach client how to keep a daily food diary in order to assess intake. Discuss with client the following:

- Decreasing calories
- Increasing carbohydrates (whole grains and vegetables)
- Decreasing saturated fats
- Decreasing refined sugars
- Decreasing intake of cholesterol to 300 mg/day and salt to 5 g/day

Provide information on support groups such as Weight Watchers, TOPS (Take Off Pounds Sensibly).

Nursing Diagnosis: Risk for Constipation

Discuss bowel habits that are "normal" for client. Caution against overuse of laxatives. Discourage overuse of mineral oil as a laxative because it decreases absorption of vitamins A, D, E, and K. Explain the effects of nutrients, bulk, fluids, and exercise on elimination. The American Cancer Society [*Cancer facts and figures*, 2003] recommends a high-fiber, low-fat diet that includes a variety of vegetables and fruits to reduce the risk of certain cancers. It also recommends limiting consumption of alcohol. Advise client to eat a varied diet, maintain a desirable weight, eliminate tobacco use and be physically active.

Pediatric Client

Nursing Diagnosis: Readiness for enhanced nutritional–metabolic pattern of child

☒ Teach parents nutritional needs of the child at various ages:
Infant: Exclusive breast-feeding is the ideal nutrition for the first 6 months. Gradually introduce iron-enriched solid food at 6 months to complement breast-feeding. When possible, continue breast-feeding for at least 1 year. Do not give cow's milk before 12 months of age. Introduce finger foods by 1 year. The American Academy of Pediatrics [1997] recommends that formula, if used, be fortified with iron. Breast-fed infants should get oral iron supplements Fluoride supplements are required only if the water supply is severely deficient in fluoride.
Toddlers: Food fads are common. Accept this as long as child gets balanced diet over period of days versus every day.

Nursing Diagnosis: Fluid Volume Deficit related to vomiting or diarrhea

☒ Teach parents to give child small amounts of clear liquids (approximately 1 oz every hour for 8 hours) until symptoms subside. May recommend Pedialyte for fluid and electrolyte replacement.

Nursing Diagnosis: Risk for Aspiration related to improper feeding and small size of stomach in newborns

☒ Explain size of infant's stomach to parents (holds 60 cc), and demonstrate proper burping technique to use after every ½ oz feeding.

Genitourinary–Reproductive Assessment

ASSESSMENT OF FEMALE GENITALIA

Equipment Needed

- Gown and drape
- Pillow
- Movable light source
- Gloves and lubricant
- Private location
- Vaginal speculum of appropriate size
- Vaginal swabs (large cotton-tipped applicators)
- pH paper
- Cotton-tipped applicators
- Mirror

Subjective Data: Focus Questions

Last menstrual period? Length of cycle? Amount of blood flow? Associated symptoms? Age of menarche? Unpleasant odor? Knowledge about toxic shock syndrome? Age of menopause if applicable? Estrogen replacement? Vaginal discharge? Pain, itching, or lumps in inguinal/groin area? Pain with intercourse? Difficulty urinating? Color or odor of urine? Difficulty controlling urine? Stress incontinence? Sexual performance? Activity? Change in libido? Fertility problems/concerns? History of gynecological problems or sexually transmitted diseases (STDs)? Pregnancies? Number of children? Chance of pregnancy now? History of family reproductive or genital cancer? Self-care: Monthly genital self-examinations? Cotton underwear? Wiping pattern after bowel movement? Douching—how often? Use of contraceptives? Number of sexual partners? Comfort level with talking with sexual partner? Fears related to sex? Tested for HIV (human immunodeficiency virus)?

RISK FACTORS. Risk for cervical cancer related to sexually active female, human papilloma virus infection, first and frequent intercourse at young age, multiple sexual partners, history of STD, multiple births, history of no prior Pap exams, lower socioeconomic status, low level of education, poor hygiene especially with uncircumcised partner.

Objective Data: Assessment Techniques

See Figure 15–1 for a diagram of the female genitalia.

INSPECTION

Have client empty bladder and lie on her back with head slightly elevated on a pillow. Knees should be bent and separated with feet resting on the bed. Light should be adjusted to provide good visualization of the genitalia.

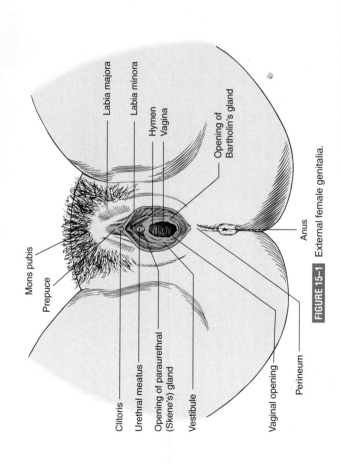

FIGURE 15-1 External female genitalia.

Labia majora
Labia minora
Hymen
Vagina
Opening of Bartholin's gland

Mons pubis
Prepuce

Anus

Clitoris
Urethral meatus
Opening of paraurethral (Skene's) gland
Vestibule

Vaginal opening
Perineum

Genitourinary–Reproductive Assessment

INSPECTION (continued)

PROCEDURE	NORMAL FINDINGS	DEVIATIONS FROM NORMAL
Inspect labia for the following:		
• Lesions, swelling, excoriation	• Equal in size, free of lesions	• Lesions seen in infectious disease; swelling and excoriation seen with scratching or self-treatment of the lesions
• Pubic hair	• Varies with age	• Nits or lice
• Skin texture	• Smooth, loose skin	• Vesicles, warts, open sores
• Color	• Pink	• Blue, visible veins, shiny
Using an examination glove, insert thumb and index or third finger between labia and separate. Inspect urinary meatus for the following:		
• Position	• Small, slitlike, anterior to vaginal orifice and in midline	• Urinary meatus not visible; located within or near anterior surface of vaginal wall
• Color	• Pink	• Red, inflamed with perineal irritation
Apply labial traction and inspect vaginal orifice for the following:		
• Hymen	• Absent; thin, elastic membrane that partially occludes orifice; varies with estrogen effects; thick in newborn and at puberty, thin in infants, prepubescent patients, and elderly	• Completely occludes orifice.

INSPECTION (continued)

PROCEDURE	NORMAL FINDINGS	DEVIATIONS FROM NORMAL
• Discharge	• Clear, milky, serosanguineous with menstrual cycle	• Any purulent, irritating, foul-smelling discharge is abnormal and should be cultured.
Have client strain down, and observe **vaginal wall** for bulging.	Slight movement	Bulging of anterior wall may be a cystocele; bulging of posterior vaginal wall may indicate a rectocele; if cervix or uterus protrudes down, the client may have a uterine prolapse; if urine is produced, stress incontinence may be present.

PALPATION

Don gloves. Using left thumb and index or third finger, gently separate labia and hold apart. Lubricate right index finger and insert into vaginal opening. Push up on anterior wall and "milk" toward opening. Push down on posterior wall and grasp tissue between thumb and index finger. Palpate tissue along entire lower half of vaginal orifice.

PROCEDURE	NORMAL FINDINGS	DEVIATIONS FROM NORMAL
Assess **Skene's glands** (see Fig. 15–1) for the following:		
• Openings	• Not visible	• Visible openings
• Discharge	• None	• Exudate from openings or urethra

PALPATION (continued)

PROCEDURE	NORMAL FINDINGS	DEVIATIONS FROM NORMAL
Assess *Bartholin's glands*		
• Palpate posterior aspect of labia majora	• Soft	• Tenderness • Pain • Swelling • Discharge
Palpate *posterior vaginal orifice* for the following:		
• Swelling	• None	• Present
• Lumps or nodules	• Smooth, soft tissue	• Hard, nonpliable tissue
Assess *internal genitalia*		
• Determine size of vaginal opening	• Size varies with age, sexual history, vaginal deliveries	
• Determine position of cervix. Insert gloved index finger into the vagina.	• Anterior or posterior • Midline • Extends into the vagina 1–3 cm	
• With index finger in vagina, ask client to squeeze around finger to check vaginal musculature.	• Able to squeeze finger	• Inability to squeeze finger indicates decreased muscle tone.
• Separate labia minora and ask client to bear down	• No bulging • No urinary discharge	• Bulging of anterior wall may indicate cystocele. • Bulging of posterior wall may indicate rectocele.

PALPATION (continued)

PROCEDURE	NORMAL FINDINGS	DEVIATIONS FROM NORMAL
Insert speculum, then inspect		
• Cervix for: color, size, position	• Surface of cervix smooth, pink, even • Pregnant clients bluish • Older women pale	• Asymmetric, reddened area, strawberry spots, white patches
• Cervical secretions	• Clear to opaque • Odorless • Nonirritating	• Discolored (gray, yellow, green) • Malodorous • Irritating • Lesions • Erosions
• Cervical os	• Small, round if nulliparous • Horizontal slit if parous	
Rotate speculum and inspect:		
• Vagina for color, surface, consistency, discharge, vaginal pH of secretions, using cotton swab on lateral or anterior (not posterior) vaginal wall. Touch swab to pH paper strip to test secretions.	• Pink, moist, smooth without lesions, irritations, or malodorous discharge • pH: 3.8–4.2	• Reddened area • Lesions • Malodorous discharge • <3.8 • >4.2–6.0: consider bacterial vaginosis, sexual intercourse (pH of semen↑) • >6.0: consider trichomoniasis

BIMANUAL EXAMINATION

Tell client you are going to perform a manual examination. Apply water-soluble lubricant to gloved middle and index fingers of your dominant hand. Stand and place nondominant hand on client's lower abdomen. Next insert index and middle fingers into the vagina.

PROCEDURE	NORMAL FINDINGS	DEVIATIONS FROM NORMAL
Apply pressure to the posterior vaginal wall; wait for relaxation of vaginal opening before palpating (Fig. 15–2).	Vaginal wall is smooth without tenderness	Tenderness, may indicate infection

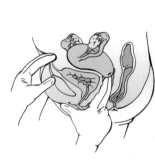

FIGURE 15–2 Hands positioned for palpating the vaginal wall.

BIMANUAL EXAMINATION (continued)

PROCEDURE	NORMAL FINDINGS	DEVIATIONS FROM NORMAL
Palpate the cervix Advance fingers to the cervix; palpate for: • Contour • Consistency • Mobility • Tenderness	• Feels firm and soft like the tip of the nose	• Hardness and immobility may indicate cancer. • Pain with movement (and chandelier sign) may indicate infection.
Palpate the uterus Move the fingers intravaginally into the opening above cervix. Apply pressure with the hand resting on the abdomen. Squeeze the uterus between the two hands. Note uterine • Size • Position • Shape • Consistency		• An enlarged uterus above the level of the pubis is abnormal. • Irregular shape may indicate abnormality.

BIMANUAL EXAMINATION (continued)

PROCEDURE	NORMAL FINDINGS	DEVIATIONS FROM NORMAL
Palpate the ovaries		
Slide your intravaginal fingers toward the left ovary in the left lateral fornix and place your abdominal hand on the left lower abdominal quadrant. Press your abdominal hand toward your intravaginal fingers and attempt to palpate the ovary.	Ovaries are approximately $3 \times 2 \times 1$ cm (or the size of a walnut) and almond shaped.	Enlarged size, masses, immobility, and extreme tenderness are abnormal and should be evaluated.
Slide your intravaginal fingers to the right lateral fornix and attempt to palpate the right ovary. Note size, shape, consistency, mobility, and tenderness.	Ovaries are firm, smooth, mobile, and somewhat tender on palpation.	Ovaries that are palpable 3 to 5 years after menopause are also abnormal.
Withdraw your intravaginal hand and inspect the glove for secretions.	A clear, minimal amount of drainage appearing on the glove from the vagina is normal.	Large amounts of colorful, frothy, or malodorous secretions are abnormal.

Genitourinary–Reproductive Assessment

BIMANUAL EXAMINATION (continued)

PROCEDURE	NORMAL FINDINGS	DEVIATIONS FROM NORMAL
Perform the Rectovaginal Examination. • Explain that you will perform a rectovaginal examination. Forewarn the client that she may feel uncomfortable as if she wants to move her bowels, but that she will not. Encourage her to relax. Change the glove on your dominant hand and lubricate your index and middle fingers (Fig. 15–3). • Ask client to bear down and insert your index finger into the vaginal orifice and your middle finger into the rectum. While pushing down on the abdominal wall with your other hand, palpate the internal reproductive structures through the anterior rectal wall. Withdraw your vaginal finger and continue with the rectal examination.	• The rectovaginal septum is normally smooth, thin, movable, and firm. The posterior uterine wall is normally smooth, firm, round, movable, and nontender.	• Masses, thickened structures, immobility, and tenderness are abnormal.

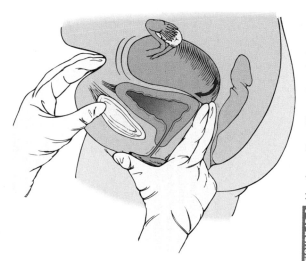

FIGURE 15–3   Hands positioned for rectovaginal examination.

ASSESSMENT OF MALE GENITALIA

Equipment Needed

- Gloves
- Private location

Subjective Data: Focus Questions

Pain in penis, scrotum, testes, or groin? Lesions in penis or genital area? Discharge from penis? Color? Odor? Lumps, masses, or swelling in scrotum, groin, or genital area? Heavy, draggy feeling in scrotum? Difficulty voiding—hesitancy, frequency, starting or maintaining stream? Change in color, odor, or amount of urine? Pain or burning when urinating? Incontinence or dribbling? Change in sexual activities? Difficulty with maintaining an erection? Problem with ejaculation? Trouble with fertility? Any bulges or pain when straining or lifting heavy objects? History of inguinal or genitalia surgery? History of STD? Self-care: Last testicular exam? Self-examination? Tested for HIV? Result? History of cancer in family? Number of sexual partners? Contraceptive form? Exposure to chemical or radiation? Fertility concerns? Comfort with communicating with sexual partner?

RISK FACTORS. Risk for HIV/AIDS (acquired immune deficiency syndrome) related to anal intercourse (especially men having sex with men), intravenous drug use, having multiple sexual partners, bisexual partners, or partner who uses intravenous drugs.

Objective Data: Assessment Techniques

See Figure 15–4 for a diagram of the male genitalia.

INSPECTION

The male genitalia should be inspected with the client in a standing position. Privacy should be ensured.

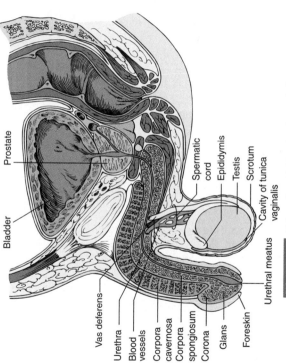

FIGURE 15–4 External and internal male genitalia.

INSPECTION (continued)

PROCEDURE	NORMAL FINDINGS	DEVIATIONS FROM NORMAL
*Observe **penis** for the following:*		
• Urinary meatus	• Located at tip of glans penis	• Displaced to ventral side (hypospadias) or dorsal side (epispadias) of penis
• Discharge	• No discharge	• Any drainage—yellow discharge is seen with gonorrhea; clear or white discharge is seen with urethritis.
• Skin texture	• Wrinkled • Hairless	• Nodules, growths, lesions • Swelling • Phimosis • Paraphimosis
*Observe **glans** for the following:*		
• Size, shape, and lesions	• Size varies; rounded, broad, or pointed; free of lesions	• Chancres (red, oval ulcerations from syphilis); pimple lesions in herpes; venereal warts
*Observe **scrotum** for the following:*		
• Size	• Left side lower than right	• Unilateral or bilateral enlargement due to presence of blood (hematocele), fluid (hydrocele), bowel (hernia), or tumor (cancer)
• Color • Texture	• Pink or normal skin color • Many skin folds	• Red, shiny, bruised • Lesions, ulcers, taut skin

PALPATION

With client standing, gently palpate shaft of penis between gloved thumb and fingers. If foreskin is present, retract from tip of penis, then replace. Grasp each testicle between thumb and fingers. Gently roll testicle so all surfaces are palpated. Client may do self-examination with instructions and report findings (Box 15-1).

PROCEDURE	NORMAL FINDINGS	DEVIATIONS FROM NORMAL
Palpate **penis** for the following:		
• Masses	• None	• Nodules, masses, or lesions anywhere on shaft or glans may indicate STDs or cancer.
• Tenderness	• Slightly tender	• Very tender or painful; hardness along central shaft may indicate cancer; tenderness is seen with infection or inflammation.
• Discharge	• None	• Clear or purulent from lesions or urinary meatus
• Foreskin	• May not be present; should retract and return easily with clean, smooth skin underneath	• Unable to retract owing to phimosis or adherence to underlying tissue; any drainage or sores under skin; discoloration of foreskin seen with scarring or infection
Palpate each **testis** for the following:		
• Location	• Each should be entirely in sac, left slightly lower than right.	• One or both are absent or cannot be palpated at inguinal border (partially descended).

BOX 15-1. Testicular Self-Examination (TSE)

Testicular self-examination (TSE) is to be performed once a month. A convenient time is often after a warm bath or shower.

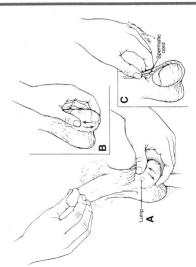

1. Use both hands to palpate the testis. The normal testicle is smooth and uniform in consistency.

2. With the index and middle fingers under the testis and the thumb on top, roll the testis gently in a horizontal plane between the thumb and fingers (A).

3. Feel for any evidence of a small lump or abnormality.

4. Follow the same procedure and palpate upward along the testis (B).

5. Locate the epididymis (C), a cordlike structure on the top and back of the testicle that stores and transports sperm.

6. Repeat the examination for the other testis. It is normal to find that one testis is larger than the other.

7. If you find any evidence of a small, pealike lump, consult your physician. It may be due to an infection or tumor growth.

PALPATION (continued)

PROCEDURE	NORMAL FINDINGS	DEVIATIONS FROM NORMAL
• Shape • Texture • Tenderness	• Oval, symmetrical • Smooth, firm • Very tender	• Enlarged, different sizes • Grainy or coarse; lumps or nodules • Pain; dull ache in lower abdomen or groin with feeling of heaviness

ASSESSMENT OF INGUINAL AREA

Objective Data: Assessment Techniques

See Figure 15–5 for a diagram of the inguinal area.

INSPECTION

Have client stand so inguinal area is visible. Have client strain down.

PROCEDURE	NORMAL FINDINGS	DEVIATIONS FROM NORMAL
Inspect **inguinal area.**	Smooth, symmetrical	Bulging on one or both sides that increases with straining indicates inguinal or femoral hernia.
Inspect **scrotum.**	Varies in size; left side of scrotal sac hangs slightly lower than the right side.	Enlarged scrotal sac is seen with presence of fluid (hydrocele), blood (hematocele), bowel (hernia), or tumor (cancer).

Genitourinary–Reproductive Assessment

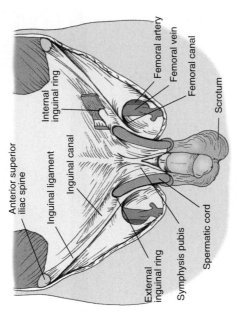

FIGURE 15-5 Inguinal area.

Anterior superior iliac spine

Inguinal ligament

Inguinal canal

Internal inguinal ring

Femoral artery

Femoral vein

Femoral canal

Scrotum

Spermatic cord

Symphysis pubis

External inguinal ring

PALPATION

Palpate inguinal area. Then have client strain down as you palpate inguinal area and scrotum (Fig. 15–6). Use right hand for right side and left hand for left side.

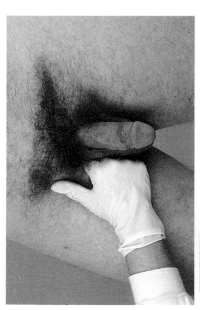

FIGURE 15-6 Palpating for an inguinal hernia (© B. Proud).

PALPATION (continued)

PROCEDURE	NORMAL FINDINGS	DEVIATIONS FROM NORMAL
Palpate for the following: • Lymph nodes • Masses	• Nonpalpable • Smooth, no masses	• Palpable, tender • Bulge of soft tissue that increases with straining indicates hernia.
• Scrotum	• No change	• Enlargement; mass felt increases with straining—bulge may disappear with scrotal hernia when client lies down; if you cannot push the mass back in, suspect an incarcerated hernia; client complains of extreme tenderness and nausea with a strangulated hernia.

ASSESSMENT OF RECTUM

Equipment Needed

• Examination gloves
• Drape
• Pillow

Subjective Data: Focus Questions

Usual bowel pattern? Changes? Diarrhea? Constipation? Color of stools? Mucus in stools? Pain? Itching? Bleeding after stools? History of rectal or anal surgery? Proctosigmoidoscopy? Family history of polyps, colon, rectal, or prostate cancer? Self-care: Use of laxatives? Engage in anal sex? Amount of roughage, fat, and water in diet? Last digital rectal exam by a physician or midlevel provider?

RISK FACTORS. Risk for colorectal cancer related to age over 40 years, history of rectal or colon polyps, inflammatory bowel disease, history of colorectal cancer, diet high in fat, protein, beef, and low in fiber; risk for prostate cancer related to dietary fat intake, age over 50 years, exposure to cadmium, high-risk occupations (eg, tire and rubber manufacturers, farmers, mechanics, sheet metal workers), lack of circumcision.

Objective Data: Assessment Techniques

See Figure 15–7 for a diagram of the anus and rectum.

INSPECTION

Have client lie on left side with right leg flexed at hip and knee. Support leg on pillow if necessary. Provide a pillow for under the head. With one hand, gently separate buttocks so rectum is exposed.

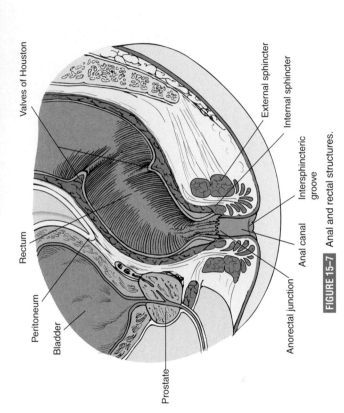

FIGURE 15–7 Anal and rectal structures.

Valves of Houston

Rectum

Peritoneum

Bladder

Prostate

External sphincter

Internal sphincter

Intersphincteric groove

Anal canal

Anorectal junction

INSPECTION (continued)

PROCEDURE	NORMAL FINDINGS	DEVIATIONS FROM NORMAL
*Palpate the **anus*** Explain to the client what you are going to do. Explain that the client may feel like his bowels will move.		
Lubricate gloved index finger and ask client to bear down. Then place the pad of your index finger on the anal opening (Fig. 15–8).	Sphincter relaxes	Sphincter tightens, preventing further examination.
Assess sphincter tone	Can close sphincter around gloved finger	Poor tone may be a result of spinal cord injury, previous surgery, trauma, prolapsed rectum, sexual abuse. Tightened sphincter may be the results of anxiety, scarring, inflammation.
Palpate for tenderness, nodules, and hardness.	Normally smooth, nontender, without nodules or hardness	Tenderness indicates hemorrhoids, fistula, fissure; nodules indicate polyps, cancer; hardness scarring, cancer.
*Palpate **rectum*** Insert finger further into rectum. Turn finger clockwise, then counterclockwise. Note tenderness irregularities, nodules, hardness.		

Genitourinary–Reproductive Assessment

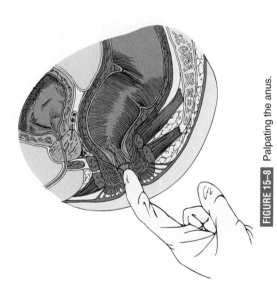

FIGURE 15–8 Palpating the anus.

INSPECTION (continued)

PROCEDURE	NORMAL FINDINGS	DEVIATIONS FROM NORMAL
Palpate the prostate On the anterior surface of the rectum, turn the hand fully counterclockwise so the pad of your index finger faces toward the client's umbilicus. Tell the client he may feel an urge to urinate but will not. Move the pad of your index finger over the prostate gland, trying to feel the sulcus between the lateral lobes (Fig. 15–9).	Prostate nontender and rubbery with two lateral lobes that are divided by a median sulcus. The lobes are normally smooth, 2.5 cm long, and heart shaped.	A swollen, tender prostate may indicate acute prostatitis. An enlarged, smooth, firm, slightly elastic prostate that may not have a median sulcus suggests benign prostatic hypertrophy (BPH). A hard area on the prostate or hard, irregular nodules on the prostate suggest cancer.
Inspect **perianal area** for color, hair, lesions, masses, or drainage.	Hairless, moist, and tightly closed with no redness, lesions, masses, or rashes	Lesions are seen in external hemorrhoids, cancer and STDs. Painful mass may be an abscess. Shiny blue skin sac suggests thrombosed hemorrhoid.
Inspect **sacrococcygeal area** for color, hair, and texture.	Smooth, free of hair and redness	Red, swollen area covered by a small tuft of hair located in the lower sacrum suggests the presence of a pilonidal cyst.

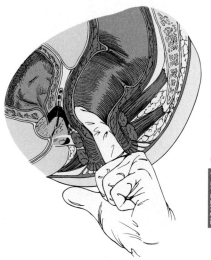

FIGURE 15-9 Palpating the prostate gland.

PEDIATRIC VARIATIONS

Subjective Data: Focus Questions

During puberty: Development of secondary sexual characteristics? Previous education on sexual development and activities? Use of contraceptives? Type?

Females: Age of menarche? Frequency of menstrual periods? Amount of flow? Pain? Irregularities? Attitude toward menstrual cycle?

Objective Data: Assessment Techniques

Inspection and palpation of external male and female genitalia constitute the *total* genitourinary assessment until puberty. Assessment of the level of sexual development of girls and boys usually begins at approximately age 11 years. This determination involves assessment of secondary characteristics associated with sexual maturity. Table 15–1 and Table 15–2 summarize the timing of sexual development for boys and girls.

CULTURAL VARIATIONS

Male and female genitalia are mutilated in pubertal rites in some cultures; for example, circumcision, removal of clitoris, or surgical incision along penile shaft and into its base for passage of urine and semen. Female pubic hair is shaved or plucked in some cultures.

GERIATRIC VARIATIONS

- Bladder capacity decreases to 250 mL owing to periurethral atrophy.
- 1 to 2 periods of nocturia

TABLE 15-1

TANNER'S SEXUAL MATURITY RATING: FEMALE PUBIC HAIR GROWTH AND BREAST DEVELOPMENT

Developmental Stage	Pubic Hair	Breast
Stage 1	Prepubertal: no pubic hair; fine vellus hair	Prepubertal: elevation of nipple only

Stage 2

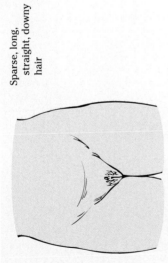

Sparse, long, straight, downy hair

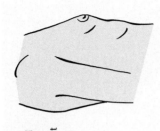

Breast bud stage; elevation of breast and nipple as small mound, enlargement of areolar diameter

(continued)

Developmental Stage	Pubic Hair	Breast
Stage 3	Darker, coarser, curly; sparse over mons pubis	Enlargement of the breasts and areola with no separation of contours

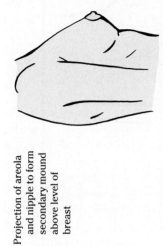

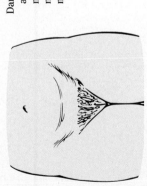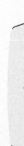

Stage 4

Dark, curly, and abundant on mons pubis; no growth on medial thighs

Projection of areola and nipple to form secondary mound above level of breast

(continued)

Developmental Stage	Pubic Hair	Breast
Stage 5	Adult pattern of inverse triangle; growth on medial thighs	Adult configuration; projection of nipple only, areola receded into contour of breast

TABLE 15–2   TANNER'S SEXUAL MATURITY RATING: MALE GENITALIA DEVELOPMENT AND PUBIC HAIR GROWTH

Developmental Stage	Genitalia	Pubic Hair
Stage 1	Prepubertal	Prepubertal: no pubic hair; fine vellus hair

(continued)

Developmental Stage	Genitalia	Pubic Hair
Stage 2	Initial enlargement of scrotum and testes with rugation and reddening of the scrotum	Sparse, long, straight, downy hair

Stage 3

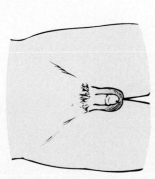

Elongation of the penis; testes and scrotum further enlarge

Darker, coarser, curly; sparse over entire pubis

(continued)

TABLE 15–2 TANNER'S SEXUAL MATURITY RATING: MALE GENITALIA DEVELOPMENT AND PUBIC HAIR GROWTH (*Continued*)

Developmental Stage	Genitalia	Pubic Hair
Stage 4	Increase in size and width of penis and the development of the glans; scrotum darkens	Dark, curly, and abundant in pubic area; no growth on thighs or up toward umbilicus

Stage 5

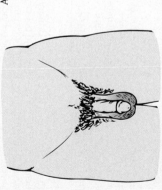

Adult configuration

Adult pattern (growth up toward
umbilicus may not be seen);
growth continues until mid 20s

GERIATRIC VARIATIONS (continued)

Female

- Decrease in size and elasticity of labia; constriction of vaginal opening
- Diminished vaginal secretions and decreased elasticity of vaginal walls
- Shortened and narrowed vaginal vault
- Cervix appears paler after menopause.

Male

- Decrease in size and firmness of testicles
- Loss of tone in musculature of scrotum
- Slowed erections and less forceful ejaculations
- Enlargement of medial lobe of prostate

Possible Collaborative Problems

Bladder perforation	Obstruction of urethra	Renal calculi
Urinary tract infection	Hemorrhage	Hypermenorrhea
Pelvic inflammatory disease	Hormonal imbalances	Polymenorrhea
Genitalia ulcers or lesions	Renal failure	

TEACHING TIPS FOR SELECTED NURSING DIAGNOSES AND COLLABORATIVE PROBLEMS

Adult Client

Nursing Diagnosis: Readiness for Enhanced Urinary Elimination and Reproductive Pattern

Teach client to drink eight glasses of fluid per day and to limit intake of alcohol, caffeine, and carbonated beverages. Teach client to avoid bubble baths and scented tissue that may irritate urethra. Teach female client to wear cotton underwear and to wipe perineum from front to back when cleansing.

Nursing Diagnosis: Readiness for Enhanced Health-Seeking Behaviors: Testicular Self-Examination

☐ Instruct client on proper method of testicular self-examination, performed once a month after a warm bath or shower. Instruct client to roll each testicle gently between thumb and fingers of both hands, feeling for lumps or nodules (see Box 15-1). Have each client demonstrate. Begin at puberty, because testicular cancer is one of the most common cancers in men 15 to 34 years old.

Nursing Diagnosis: Risk for Infection (STD) related to unprotected intercourse with multiple partners

☐ Teach early warning signs and symptoms. Discuss methods of prevention (limit to one uninfected partner and use of condoms) and modes of transmission.

Nursing Diagnosis: Ineffective Health Maintenance related to a lack of knowledge of birth control methods

☐ Teach alternate forms of birth control, proper use of methods, and advantages and disadvantages of each. Discuss the importance of increasing vitamin B_6 and folic acid in the diet because of malabsorption of these vitamins while taking birth control pills. Instruct on use of alternate birth control for 3 months after discontinuing the pill to reestablish menstrual cycle before attempting to conceive.

Nursing Diagnosis: Readiness for Enhanced Health Maintenance During Menopause

☐ Inform client that pregnancy may still occur during early menopausal years. Instruct to consume calcium 1500 mg/day along with a well-balanced diet. Explain that water-soluble lubricant may be used for vaginal dryness if intercourse is painful. Explain ways to help client cope with hot flashes (eg, use of cool clothing, fans, showers, cool drinks; avoidance of red wine, aged cheeses, and chocolate—these contain tyramine, which can trigger hot flashes). Teach male clients about the male climacteric period (during the 50s or 60s) when sexual hormones are reduced. Symptoms of hot flashes, sweating, headaches, dizziness, and heart palpitations may be experienced.

Nursing Diagnosis: Ineffective Health Maintenance related to knowledge deficit of need for colorectal and pelvic examinations and Pap smears

☐ Explain procedure. Teach relaxation. Approach sexuality as a normal part of activities of daily living. Prepare adolescent girl for first pelvic examination. The American Cancer Society [*Cancer facts and figures*, 2003] recommends that women who have been sexually active for 3 years or are 21 years old should have an annual

Pap test and pelvic examination. For a woman 30 years or older who has had three or more consecutive satisfactory and normal annual examinations, the Pap test may be performed every 2 to 3 years at the physician's discretion. Most women 70 years and older who have had recent normal Pap tests and most who have had total hysterectomies do not need continued screening. Women at high risk for endometrial cancer (major risk factors—weak immune system, estrogen replacement therapy, tamoxifen, early menarche, late menopause, never having children, and history of failure to ovulate; other risk factors—infertility, diabetes, gall bladder disease, hypertension, and obesity) should have an endometrial tissue sample at menopause and thereafter at the physician's discretion [*Cancer facts and figures*, 2003].

Men and women age 50 or older should follow one of these three examination schedules:

- A fecal occult blood test every year or a flexible sigmoidoscopy every 5 years (a combination of these two methods is preferred over either one alone)
- A colonoscopy every 10 years if normal
- A double-contrast barium enema every 5 to 10 years

A digital rectal exam should be done at the same time as sigmoidoscopy, colonoscopy, or double-contrast barium enema. People who are at moderate or high risk should talk with a doctor about a different testing schedule [*Cancer facts and figures*, 2003].

Nursing Diagnosis: Sexual Dysfunction: impotence related to unknown etiology
☐ Explore possible etiologies and alternate forms of sexual satisfaction. Refer to urologist for information on penile implants, surgery, and other alternatives.

Nursing Diagnosis: Sexual Dysfunction related to partner communication and deficient knowledge of psychological and physical health and sexual performance
☐ Teach effects and benefits of exercise. Explore communication with partner. Refer to counselor (psychiatric, sexual, marriage) as needed. Provide adequate literature on sex and health teaching for client.

Nursing Diagnosis: Sexual Dysfunction related to loss of body part or physiological limitations (eg, dyspareunia with aging)
☐ Explore prior sexual patterns. Explore alternatives. Provide resource material on self-help groups (eg, Ostomy Association, Reach for Recovery). Suggest use of foreplay and lubricants to increase secretions as necessary. Provide literature and referrals.

Pediatric Client

Nursing Diagnosis: Risk for Impaired Elimination Pattern related to parental knowledge deficit of toilet-training techniques

☐ Teach parents the importance of physiological and psychological readiness in toilet training. Explain use of "potty chairs" and that bowel control precedes bladder control. Inform parents of the benefits of positive reinforcement and that nocturnal enuresis may persist up to age 4 to 5 years.

Nursing Diagnosis: Readiness for Enhanced Sexual Function

☐ Sexual education is recommended in the early school years. Assess what child already knows and what he or she is ready to know.

Fourth to fifth grade: Interested in conception and birth

Fifth to sixth grade: Interested in their bodies and opposite sex changes. Education on birth control may be appropriate because of early experimentation. Discuss normal development of secondary sexual characteristics and the normal psychological changes associated with puberty.

Geriatric Client

Nursing Diagnosis: Impaired Urinary Elimination: functional incontinence, reflex urinary incontinence, stress incontinence

☐ Explain to family how to decrease environmental barriers (offer bedpan frequently, provide proper lighting, ensure availability and proximity of commode) for functional incontinence. Teach client cutaneous triggering mechanisms for reflex incontinence. Teach client Kegel exercises to strengthen pelvic floor muscles (ie, tightening of buttocks and practicing starting and stopping stream) for stress incontinence.

Collaborative problem: Potential complication: prostate hypertrophy

☐ Teach client about effects of normal enlargement of prostate on urination (frequency, dribbling, and nocturia). Encourage yearly rectal exams and prostate-specific antigen testing for men 50 years and older.

16

Musculoskeletal Assessment

OVERVIEW OF ANATOMY

The body's bones, muscles, and joints compose the musculoskeletal system. Two hundred and six (206) bones make up the axial skeleton (head and trunk) and the appendicular skeleton (extremities, shoulders, and hips; Fig. 16–1).

The body consists of three types of muscles: skeletal, smooth, and cardiac. The musculoskeletal system is made up of 650 skeletal (voluntary) muscles, which are under conscious control (Fig. 16–2).

The joint (or articulation) is the place where two or more bones meet. Joints provide a variety of range of motion (ROM) for the body parts. Synovial joints (eg, shoulders, wrists, hips, knees, ankles; Fig. 16–3) contain a space between the bones that is filled with synovial fluid, a lubricant that promotes a sliding movement of the ends of the bones. Bones in synovial joints are joined by ligaments, which are strong, dense bands of fibrous connective tissue. Synovial joints are enclosed by a fibrous capsule made of connective tissue and connected to the periosteum of the bone.

Equipment Needed

- Tape measure
- Goniometer (measures angles of joints)
- Marking pen

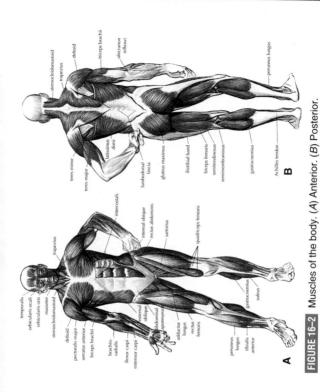

FIGURE 16–2 Muscles of the body. (A) Anterior. (B) Posterior.

FIGURE 16–1 Major bones of the skeleton.

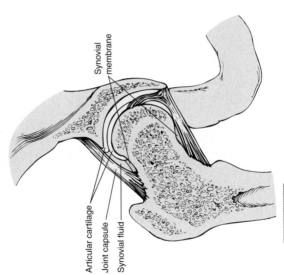

Synovial
membrane

Articular cartilage

Joint capsule

Synovial fluid

FIGURE 16-3 Components of synovial joints.

Subjective Data: Focus Questions

Pain in joints, muscles, or bones? At rest? With exercise? Changes in shape or size of an extremity? Changes in ability to carry out activities of daily living, sports, work? Stiffness? Time of day? Relation to weight bearing and exercise? Decreased, altered, or absent sensations? Redness or swelling of joints? History of past problems with bones, joints, muscles, fractures? Treatment? Orthopedic surgery? Last tetanus and polio immunizations? History of osteoporosis or osteomyelitis? Family history of rheumatoid arthritis, gout, osteoporosis? Age of menopause if applicable? Occupational and recreational history? Self-care: Exercise, weight lifting, weight reduction, diet, use of tobacco or alcohol?

RISK FACTORS. Risk for osteoporosis related to lack of exercise, low calcium intake, excessive caffeine or alcohol consumption, smoking, use of steroids, low estrogen levels in women or postmenopausal women not on estrogen replacement therapy. Risk for sports injury related to lack of wearing protective gear, poor physical fitness, lack of warm-up exercises, and overuse of joints.

Objective Data: Assessment Techniques

See Figures 16–1 and 16–2 for diagrams of the bones and muscles of the body.

Inspection and palpation are performed while client is standing, sitting, and supine. ROM can be measured by degrees, using approximation or a goniometer. (Normal trunk ROM is given as an example—pgs. 346–347) In assessing muscle weakness or swelling, size is compared bilaterally by measuring circumference with a tape measure. Joints should not be forced into painful positions. Muscle strength can be estimated using a muscle strength scale (Table 16–1).

Inspection: Observe for ROM, swelling, deformity, atrophy, condition of surrounding tissues, and pain.
Palpation: Palpate for heat, strength, tone, edema, crepitus, and nodules. (**Note:** Dominant side is normally stronger in muscle strength and tone.)

TABLE 16-1 SCALE FOR MUSCLE STRENGTH

Rating	Explanation	Strength Classification
5	Active motion against full resistance	Normal
4	Active motion against some resistance	Slight weakness
3	Active motion against gravity	Average weakness
2	Passive ROM (gravity removed and assisted by examiner)	Poor ROM
1	Slight flicker of contraction	Severe weakness
0	No muscular contraction	Paralysis

INSPECTION OF STANCE AND GAIT

Observe stance and gait as client enters and walks around the room.

Objective Data: Assessment Techniques

PROCEDURE	NORMAL FINDINGS	DEVIATIONS FROM NORMAL
Inspect the **stance** *for the following:*		
• Base of support	• Weight evenly distributed	• Uneven base, with unequal weight bearing, wide based
• Weight-bearing stability	• Able to stand on right/left heels, toes	• Weakness or inability to use either extremity
• Posture	• Erect	• Stooped
Inspect the **gait** *for the following:*		
• Position of feet	• Toes point straight ahead	• Toes point in or out
• Posture	• Erect	• Stooped
• Stride	• Equal on both sides	• Wide based, propels forward, shuffling, or limping
• Arm swing	• Swing in opposition	• No swing

INSPECTION OF THE SPINE, SHOULDER, AND POSTERIOR ILIAC CREST

With client standing, observe in the erect position and as the client bends forward to touch toes. Stabilize client at the waist, and evaluate ROM of the upper trunk.

Objective Data: Assessment Techniques

PROCEDURE	NORMAL FINDINGS	DEVIATIONS FROM NORMAL
Inspect the **spine** for the following:		
• Curves	• Cervical concave; thoracic convex: lumbar concave (Fig. 16–4)	• Kyphosis, scoliosis, lordosis (see Fig. 16–4); a flattened lumbar curve is seen with herniated lumbar disk or ankylosing spondylitis; lateral curvature of spine is seen with scoliosis; and exaggerated lumbar curve (lordosis) is seen with pregnancy or obesity.
• Posture	• Erect	• Stooped
• ROM—flexion, lateral bending, rotation, extension (Fig. 16–5)	• Full ROM	• Limited ROM with pain or crepitation

PALPATION OF THE SPINE, SHOULDER, AND POSTERIOR ILIAC CREST

With client in standing or sitting position, palpate the paravertebral muscles, using both moderate pressure and gentle sweeping motions. Ask client to shrug shoulders against resistance.

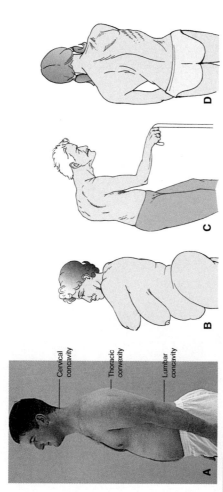

FIGURE 16–4 Normal and abnormal spinal curves. (A) Normal. (© B. Proud.) (B) Lordosis. (C) Kyphosis. (D) Scoliosis.

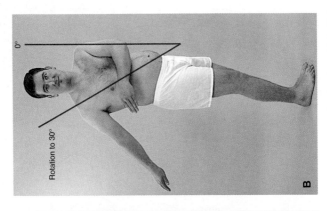

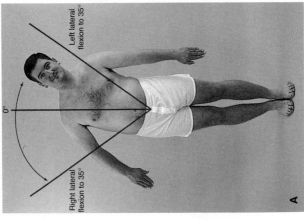

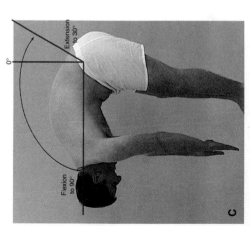

FIGURE 16-5 Range of motion of trunk. (*A*) Thoracic and lumbar spines: lateral bending. (*B*) Thoracic and lumbar spines: rotation. (*C*) Thoracic and lumbar spines: flexion. (© B. Proud.)

PALPATION OF THE SPINE, SHOULDER, AND POSTERIOR ILIAC CREST (continued)

PROCEDURE	NORMAL FINDINGS	DEVIATIONS FROM NORMAL
*Palpate the **paravertebrals** for the following:*		
• Muscle strength and tone	• Equally strong	• Weak, spasm
• Temperature	• Warm	• Hot and swollen
• Sensation	• Nontender	• Tender, painful
*Palpate the **shoulder** (trapezius muscle) for the following:*		
• Muscle strength and tone	• Able to shrug shoulders against resistance (3–5)	• Weakness with shrugging of shoulders; pain (0–2)
• Sensation	• Nontender	• Tender, painful with shoulder strains, sprains, arthritis, bursitis, and degenerative joint disease
*Palpate the **shoulder, scapula, and posterior hip** for the following:*		
• Bony prominences	• Smooth and nontender, no swelling	• Bony enlargement and tenderness, swelling, pain
• Muscle size, strength, and tone	• Equal in size bilaterally, equally strong (3–5)	• Muscle atrophy, weakness, flabbiness, or swelling (0–2)
• Temperature	• Warm to cool	• Hot

INSPECTION OF THE HEAD, THORAX, AND NECK

With client in sitting position facing you, inspect body parts. Ask client to open and close mouth to assess temporomandibular joint (TMJ) function.

PROCEDURE	NORMAL FINDINGS	DEVIATIONS FROM NORMAL
Observe the **head** *for the following:*		
• Facial structure and muscle development	• Symmetrical structure and development of muscles	• Asymmetrical structure and development of muscles
• TMJ function	• Can open mouth 2 inches	• Limited ROM; audible crepitation, click; trismus (muscle spasms), pain, tenderness, and swelling seen with TMJ syndrome
Observe the **thorax** for posture.	Erect, slight kyphosis	Stooped; abnormal spinal curves
Observe the **neck** for ROM: Flexion, extension, rotation, lateral bending (Fig. 16–6).	Full ROM; no pain	Limited ROM with crepitation or pain; nuchal rigidity; neck pain with radiation to back, shoulder, or arms seen with cervical disk degeneration. Neck pain with weakness or loss of sensation in legs is seen with cervical spine compression.

Musculoskeletal Assessment

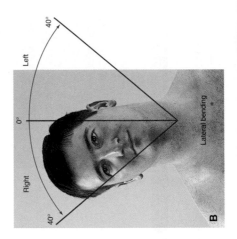

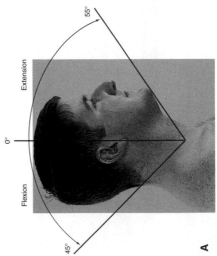

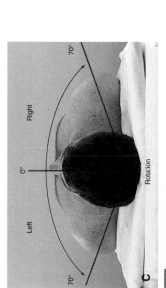

FIGURE 16-6 Normal range of motion of cervical spine. (*A*) Flexion–hyperextension. (*B*) Lateral bending. (*C*) Rotation. (© B. Proud.)

PALPATION OF THE HEAD, THORAX, AND NECK

While inspecting the TMJ, palpate it bilaterally anterior to the tragus of the ear as client opens mouth and clenches teeth. Ask client to turn head laterally against resistance.

PROCEDURE	NORMAL FINDINGS	DEVIATIONS FROM NORMAL
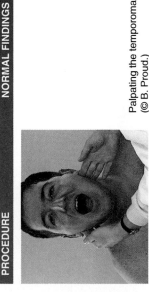	Palpating the temporomandibular joint. (© B. Proud.)	
*Palpate the **TMJ** for the following:* • Joint function	• Smooth movement bilaterally on opening, with no clicks or pain	• Palpable click, pain
• Joint contour • Temperature	• Symmetrical • Warm	• Asymmetrical • Hot and swollen
Palpate the **neck** (sternocleidomastoid) for muscle strength and tone.	Can turn head laterally against resistance without pain (3–5)	Weakness or pain when turning head against resistance (0–2)

INSPECTION OF THE UPPER EXTREMITIES

Position client in the sitting position facing you, with the upper extremities exposed. Inspect each joint and determine ROM. Both active and passive ROM may be assessed. It is easier for the client to carry out ROM if you demonstrate movements first.

PROCEDURE	NORMAL FINDINGS	DEVIATIONS FROM NORMAL
Observe the **shoulder, elbow, wrist, hand, and fingers** for bone structure, bony prominences, muscle mass, joint structure, and symmetry.	Bilaterally symmetrical	Bony deformity, muscle atrophy, swelling, deviation, contractures, nodes, tophi. Swelling of wrists, tenderness, and nodules are seen in rheumatoid arthritis; nontender, round, enlarged, swollen cysts may be ganglion of the wrists.
Observe the **shoulder, elbow, wrist, and fingers** for ROM. See Table 16–2 and Figures 16–7 through 16–10 for normal ROM.	Full ROM	Limited ROM with crepitation or pain. Catches of pain with ROM in shoulder are seen with rotator cuff tendinitis; chronic pain and limited ROM seen with calcified tendinitis; pain-limited abduction of shoulder seen with rotator cuff tear; redness and heat of elbows with bursitis; ulnar deviation of wrists and fingers with limited ROM seen in rheumatoid arthritis; inability to extend ring finger seen in Dupuytren contracture; painful extension of finger with tenosynovitis.

(text continues on p. 358)

Musculoskeletal Assessment

TABLE 16 – 2 NORMAL RANGE OF MOTION FOR JOINTS OF THE UPPER EXTREMITIES

Shoulder	Elbow	Wrist	Fingers
Flexion	Flexion	Flexion	Flexion
Extension	Extension	Hyperextension	Hyperextension
Abduction	Supination	Deviation	Abduction
Adduction	Pronation	Radial	Adduction
Rotation (internal and external)		Ulnar	Thumb away from fingers
			Thumb to base of small finger

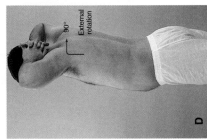

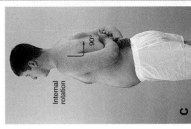

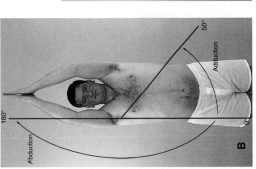

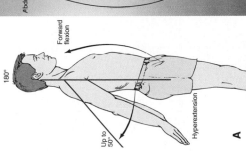

FIGURE 16-7 Normal range of motion of the shoulder. (*A*) Flexion–extension. (*B*) Adduction-abduction. (*C*) Internal rotation. (*D*) External rotation. (© B. Proud.)

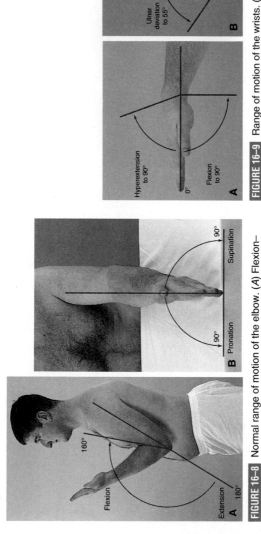

FIGURE 16–8 Normal range of motion of the elbow. (A) Flexion–extension. (B) Pronation–supination. (© B. Proud.)

FIGURE 16–9 Range of motion of the wrists. (A) Flexion–hypertension. (B) Radial–ulnar deviation. (© B. Proud.)

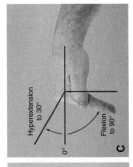

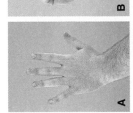

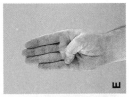

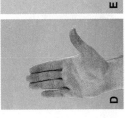

Hyperextension
to 30°

Flexion
to 90°

0°

FIGURE 16-10 Normal range of motion of the fingers. (*A*) Abduction. (*B*) Adduction. (*C*) Flexion–hyperextension. (*D*) Thumb away from fingers. (*E*) Thumb touching base of small finger. (© B. Proud.)

PALPATION OF THE UPPER EXTREMITIES

As the musculoskeletal structure of the upper extremity is going through active or passive ROM, palpate bones, muscles, tendons, and joints. Assess muscle strength and tone.

PROCEDURE	NORMAL FINDINGS	DEVIATIONS FROM NORMAL
Palpate the **arm** (biceps, triceps) for muscle strength and tone.	Can flex and extend arm against resistance (3–5)	• Weakness, paralysis (0–2)
Palpate the **hand** *for the following:* • Muscle strength, tone • Sensation	• Grip is firm and equal (3–5) • Nontender (3–5)	• Weakness, paralysis • Tenderness, pain (0–2)
Palpate the **elbow, wrist, hand, and fingers** *for the following:* • Bony landmarks • Muscle size • Joint structure	• Nontender, smooth • Regular and equal bilaterally • Symmetrical and equal	• Bony enlargement • Muscle atrophy • Loss of joint structure; joint bogginess; nodules, swelling
• Strength • Temperature • Sensation	• Equally strong (3–5) • Warm • Nontender	• Unilateral or bilateral weakness (0–2) • Hot • Tender, painful
Ask client to close eyes for 20–30 seconds with arms extended in front of body with palms up.	Arms remain up with no drifting.	Arm tends to drift downward and pronate.

INSPECTION OF THE LOWER EXTREMITIES

Position the client in standing or supine position to inspect the hips; in sitting position with legs hanging freely to inspect the knees, ankles, feet, and toes. If the client is unable to sit or stand, assessments may be made in the supine position. Both active and passive ROM may be assessed.

PROCEDURE	NORMAL FINDINGS	DEVIATIONS FROM NORMAL
Observe the **hip, knee, ankle, foot, and toes** *for the following:*		
• Bone structure and bony landmarks	• Bilaterally symmetrical and equal	• Bony deformity
• Muscle mass	• Symmetrical and equal	• Muscle atrophy
• Joint structure	• Feet maintain straight position	• Swelling, deviation, or contractures; bunion, hammer toe
• Leg length	• Bilateral leg lengths within 1 inch of each other	• Unequal lengths
Observe the **hip, knee, ankle, and toes** for ROM. See Table 16–3 and Figures 16–11 through 16–13 for normal ROM.	Full ROM	Limited ROM with crepitation or pain in joint and muscle disease. Hip pain, decreased ROM, and crepitus in hip inflammation and degenerative joint disease; tenderness and warmth with boggy consistency in synovitis; turned-in knees (genu valgum), knees turned out (genu varum); fluid bulge in knee joint effusion; pain or clicking in torn meniscus.

Musculoskeletal Assessment

TABLE 16–3   NORMAL RANGE OF MOTION FOR JOINTS OF THE LOWER EXTREMITIES

Hip	Knee	Ankle	Toes
Rotation (internal and external)	Flexion	Dorsiflexion	Flexion
Flexion	Extension	Plantar flexion	Extension
Extension		Inversion	
Abduction		Eversion	
Adduction			

PALPATION OF THE LOWER EXTREMITIES

As the musculoskeletal structure of the lower extremity is going through active or passive ROM, palpate bones, bony landmarks, muscles, and joints. Assess muscle strength and tone.

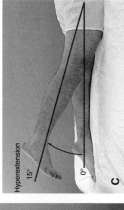

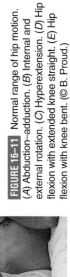

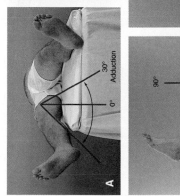

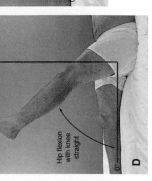

FIGURE 16–11 Normal range of hip motion. (A) Abduction–adduction. (B) Internal and external rotation. (C) Hyperextension. (D) Hip flexion with extended knee straight. (E) Hip flexion with knee bent. (© B. Proud.)

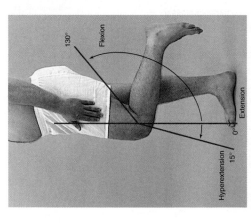

FIGURE 16–12 Normal range of motion of knee. (© B. Proud.)

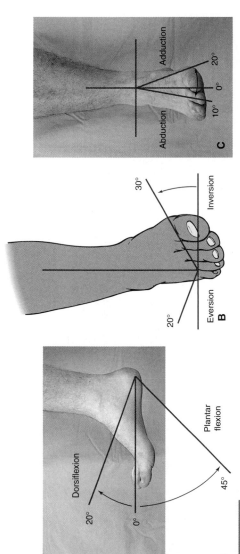

FIGURE 16-13 Normal range of motion of the feet and ankles. (*A*) Dorsiflexion–plantar flexion. (*B*) Eversion–inversion. (*C*) Abduction-adduction. (Photos © B. Proud.)

PALPATION OF THE LOWER EXTREMITIES (continued)

PROCEDURE	NORMAL FINDINGS	DEVIATIONS FROM NORMAL
Palpate the **hip** *(quadriceps, gastrocnemius) for the following:*		
• Bony landmarks	• Bilaterally symmetrical and equal	• Bony enlargement
• Muscle size and strength	• Smooth, regular, strong (3–5)	• Muscle atrophy and weakness (0–2)
• Joint structure	• Bilaterally symmetrical; strong	• Loss of joint structure; joint bogginess
• Temperature	• Warm	• Hot and swollen
• Sensation	• Nontender	• Tenderness, pain

PEDIATRIC VARIATIONS

Subjective Data: Focus Questions

Birth injuries? Alignment of hips? Trauma? Participation in sports or outdoor activities? Frequent pain in joints?

Objective Data: Assessment Techniques

PROCEDURE	NORMAL VARIATIONS
Infant: Inspect lower extremities.	A distinct bowlegged growth pattern persists and begins to disappear at 18 months. At 2 years, a knock-kneed pattern is common (Fig. 16–14), persisting until age 6–10, when legs straighten. A greater ROM in joints is present in infants. Legs are wide set until the child begins walking; weight is borne on the inside of the feet.

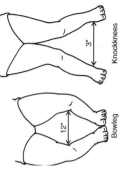

Bowleg   Knockknees

FIGURE 16–14 Normal pediatric variations of the lower extremities.

Objective Data: Assessment Techniques (continued)

PROCEDURE	NORMAL VARIATIONS
Perform Ortolani maneuver to test for congenital hip dysplasia. With the infant supine, flex the knees while holding your thumbs on mid thigh and your fingers over the greater trochanters; abduct the legs, moving the knees outward and down toward the table (Fig. 16–15, A).	Positive Ortolani sign: A click heard along with feeling the head of the femur slip in or out of the hip.
Perform Barlow maneuver. With the infant supine, flex the knees while holding your thumbs on mid thigh and your fingers over the greater trochanters; adduct legs until thumbs touch (Fig. 16–15, B).	Positive Barlow sign: A feeling of the head of the femur slipping out of the hip socket (acetabulum).
Over age 2 years: Inspect gait.	Wide-based gait common until age 2 years
3–7 years of age: Measure distance between knees with ankles together.	Less than 2 inches
3–7 years of age: Measure distance between ankles with knees together. Longitudinal arch of foot is often obscured by adipose until age 3 years, and infant appears flatfooted.	Less than 3 inches
4–13 years of age: See also Appendix 2 for developmental milestones.	

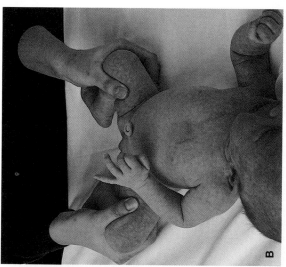

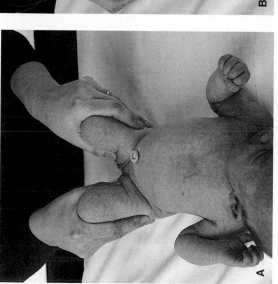

FIGURE 16–15 (A) Ortolani maneuver. (B) Barlow maneuver.

Objective Data: Assessment Techniques (continued)

PROCEDURE	NORMAL VARIATIONS
Inspect curvature of spine: • Stand behind erect child and note asymmetry of shoulders and hips. • Have child bend forward at waist until back is parallel to floor; observe from side, looking for asymmetry or prominence of rib cage.	• Shoulders symmetrical, parallel with hips • Shoulders, scapulae iliac crests symmetrical

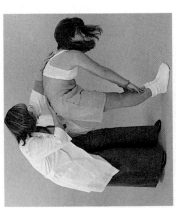

Assessing spinal curvature for scoliosis.
(© B. Proud.)

GERIATRIC VARIATIONS

- Decrease in total bone mass due to decreased activity level, change in hormones, and bone resorption; this results in weaker, softer bones.
- Slower gait with wide-based stance and smaller arm swing
- Accentuated dorsal spinal curve (kyphosis)
- Loss of muscle bulk and tone
- Decreased ROM of spine, neck, extremities
- Decrease in height (1.2 cm of height lost every 20 years)
- Shoulder width decreases; chest and pelvis width increase.
- May have bowlegged appearance due to decreased muscle control

CULTURAL VARIATIONS

- Some variation in muscle size and mass and in bone length and density are seen in different racial/ethnic group. Overfield (1995) noted that the peroneus tertius in foot or palmaris longus muscles in wrist may be absent in some groups; the number of vertebrae may differ (black women may have 23, Eskimo and Native American man, 25). A large gluteal prominence in some blacks may be mistaken as lordosis, and the ulna and radius may have unequal lengths (eg, Swedes and Chinese). Bone density (and osteoporosis) vary, with men having denser bones, blacks denser than whites, and most East Asians (except Polynesian woman) less dense than Caucasians (Overfield, 1995).
- Blacks tend to be advanced in and Asians tend to fall behind in the growth and development norms established for U.S. whites.

Possible Collaborative Problems

Bone fractures   Osteoporosis   Osteoarthritis

Sprains   Dislocation of joints   Rheumatoid arthritis

Contractures of joints   Compartment syndrome

TEACHING TIPS FOR SELECTED NURSING DIAGNOSES

Adult Client

Nursing Diagnosis: Readiness for Enhanced Mobility

☐ Teach client the importance of maintaining an ideal weight. Explain the importance of doing weight-bearing and muscle-toning exercises at least three times per week. Encourage client to wear seat belts in vehicles, to wear low well-fitted shoes, and to use walking aids (eg, cane) as needed to prevent injury.

Nursing Diagnosis: Chronic Pain (muscles and joints)

☐ Discuss independent pain management measures the client may find useful (eg, massage, relaxation, distraction). Weight loss may also reduce discomfort if obesity is straining the bones, muscles, and joints. Explain use and side effects of pain medications.

Nursing Diagnosis: Risk for Injury related to excessive exercise/improper body mechanics

☐ Caution the client against the dangerous effects of excessive exercise. Teach proper body mechanics and correct posture.

Pediatric Client

Nursing Diagnosis: Risk for Injury related to premature physical developmental level

☐ Caution parents on home safety precautions (eg, gates at stairways, removal of objects that may cause unnecessary falls, avoiding leaving child near water alone) based on child's level of musculoskeletal development. Develop home safety checklist with parents. Teach normal milestones of musculoskeletal development, and advise parent to encourage these skills as appropriate.

Geriatric Client

Nursing Diagnosis: Risk for Injury related to decalcification of bones secondary to sedentary lifestyle and post-menopausal state

☐ Discuss importance of calcium supplements in diet for postmenopausal women. Explain effects of exercise on decreasing bone decalcification.

Nursing Diagnosis: Risk for Injury related to unstable gait secondary to aging process

☐ Explain correct use of aids (eg, crutches, canes, walkers) and other prostheses. Use referrals as necessary. Instruct client on measures to prevent falls (eg, adequate lighting, avoidance of loose board ends and scatter rugs on floor). Discourage use of sleeping pills and suggest alternate methods of promoting sleep (eg, watching TV, reading, warm bath, music, warm milk).

Nursing Diagnosis: Impaired Physical Mobility related to decreased activity secondary to aging process

☐ Instruct client on the hazards of immobility and methods to prevent complications (eg, turning, coughing, deep breathing, repositioning, ROM, adequate diet, plentiful fluid intake, and diversional activities). Encourage mild exercise to loosen joint stiffness.

Nursing Diagnosis: Self-Care Deficit (specify) related to decreased mobility and/or weakness

☐ Assess safe level of activity with client, and teach methods to increase activity gradually to that level. Explore alternate self-help methods of maintaining self-care (eg, feeding aids, wheelchairs, crutches, hygienic aids). Assist client with identifying and utilizing services and groups to assist with activities of daily living (eg, Meals on Wheels). Support and teach family caregivers.

17 Neurologic Assessment

ANATOMY OVERVIEW

The very complex neurologic system is responsible for coordinating and regulating all body functions. It consists of two structural components: the central nervous system (CNS) and the peripheral nervous system.

Central Nervous System

The CNS encompasses the brain and spinal cord. Located in the cranial cavity, the brain has four major divisions: the cerebrum, the diencephalon, the brainstem, and the cerebellum.

The cerebrum is divided into the right and left cerebral hemispheres, which are joined by the corpus callosum. The diencephalon lies beneath the cerebral hemispheres and consists of the thalamus and hypothalamus. Located between the cerebral cortex and the spinal cord, the brainstem consists of the midbrain, pons, and medulla oblongata. The cerebellum, located behind the brainstem and under the cerebrum, also has two hemispheres.

The spinal cord (Fig. 17–2) is located in the vertebral canal and extends from the medulla oblongata to the first lumbar vertebra.

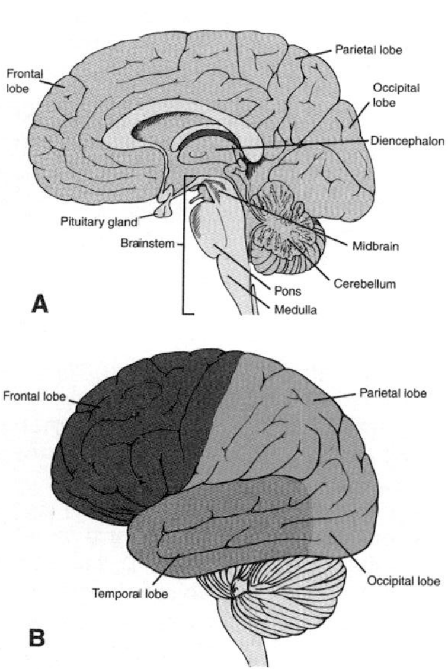

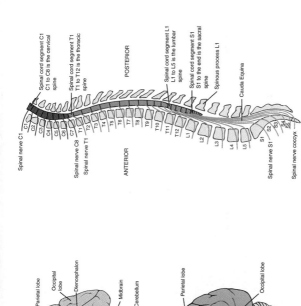

FIGURE 17-1 (A) Structures of the brain. (B) Lobes of the brain.

FIGURE 17-2 Spinal cord.

Peripheral Nervous System

Carrying information to and from the CNS, the peripheral nervous system consists of 12 pairs of cranial nerves and 31 pairs of spinal nerves. The cranial nerves evolve from the brain or brainstem (Table 17–1).

Comprising 8 cervical, 12 thoracic, 5 lumbar, 5 sacral, and 1 coccygeal nerve, the 31 pairs of spinal nerves are named after the vertebrae below each one's exit point along the spinal cord (see Fig. 17–2). Each nerve is attached to the spinal cord by two nerve roots. The sensory (afferent) fiber enters through the dorsal (posterior) roots of the cord, whereas the motor (efferent) fiber exits through the ventral (anterior) roots of the cord. The sensory root of each spinal nerve innervates an area of the skin called a dermatome (Fig. 17–3).

The neurologic assessment is performed last because several of its components may have been integrated into previous parts of the examination. For example, the eighth cranial nerve (CN VIII) may have been tested during the ear examination and therefore will not need to be tested again.

The neurologic assessment consists of six parts: (1) mental status, (2) cranial nerves, (3) sensory function, (4) motor function, (5) cerebellar function, and (6) reflexes.

Equipment Needed

- Penlight
- Tuning fork
- Reflex hammer
- Cotton wisp
- Paper clip (for detection of sharp/dull sensations)
- Salt
- Sugar
- Cotton-tipped applicators
- Glass of water
- Tongue blade
- Ophthalmoscope

Subjective Data: Focus Questions

Numbness? Paralysis? Tingling? Neuralgia? (Timing, duration, associated factors?) Seizures? Auras? Medications taken for seizures? Wear Medicalert identification? Tremors? Headaches? (Frequency, duration, character, precipitating/relieving factors?) Loss of consciousness? Dizziness? Fainting? Confusion? Visual loss, blurring, pain? Facial pain,

TABLE 17-1   CRANIAL NERVES: TYPE AND FUNCTION

Cranial Nerve (Name)	Type of Impulse	Function
I (olfactory)	Sensory	Carries smell impulses from nasal mucous membrane to brain
II (optic)	Sensory	Carries visual impulses from eye to brain
III (oculomotor)	Motor	Contracts eye muscles to control eye movements (inferior lateral, medial, and superior), constricts pupils, and elevates eyelids
IV (trochlear)	Motor	Contracts one eye muscle to control inferomedial eye movement
V (trigeminal)	Sensory	Carries sensory impulses of pain, touch, and temperature from the face to the brain
	Motor	Influences clenching and lateral jaw movements (biting, chewing)
VI (abducens)	Motor	Controls lateral eye movements
VII (facial)	Sensory	Contains sensory fibers for taste on anterior two thirds of tongue and stimulates secretions from salivary glands (submaxillary and sublingual) and tears from lacrimal glands
	Motor	Supplies the facial muscles and affects facial expressions (smiling, frowning, closing eyes)
VIII (acoustic, vestibulocochlear)	Sensory	Contains sensory fibers for hearing and balance

(continued)

Neurologic Assessment

TABLE 17-1 CRANIAL NERVES: TYPE AND FUNCTION (*continued*)

Cranial Nerve (Name)	Type of Impulse	Function
IX (glossopharyngeal)	Sensory	Contains sensory fibers for taste on posterior third of tongue and sensory fibers of the pharynx that result in the "gag reflex" when stimulated
	Motor	Provides secretory fibers to the parotid salivary glands; promotes swallowing movements
X (vagus)	Sensory	Carries sensations from the throat, larynx, heart, lungs, bronchi, gastrointestinal tract, and abdominal viscera
	Motor	Promotes swallowing, talking, and production of digestive juices
XI (spinal accessory)	Motor	Innervates neck muscles (sternocleidomastoid and trapezius) that promote movement of the shoulders and head rotation. Also promotes some movement of the larynx
XII (hypoglossal)	Motor	Innervates tongue muscles that promote the movement of food and talking

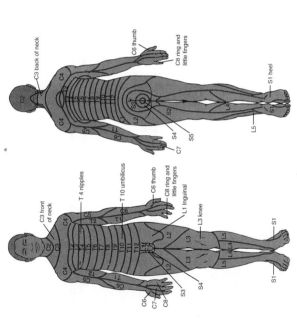

FIGURE 17-3 Anterior (*left*) and posterior (*right*) dermatomes (areas of the skin innervated by spinal nerves).

weakness, twitching? Speech problems (aphasia—expressive/receptive)? Swallowing problems? Drooling? Neck weakness, spasms? Any muscle weakness or loss of bowel or urinary control? History of head injury? Meningitis? Encephalitis? Treatment? Family history of high blood pressure, stroke, Alzheimer disease, epilepsy, brain cancer, or Huntington chorea?

Self-care: Use of medications? Alcohol intake? Use of drugs such as marijuana, tranquilizers, barbiturates, or cocaine? Smoking? Use of seat belt, head gear for sports? Daily diet and exercise? Prolonged exposure to lead, insecticides, pollutants, or other chemicals?

RISK FACTORS. Risk for cerebrovascular accident (stroke) related to hypertension, smoking, chronic alcohol intake, history of cardiovascular disease, high levels of fibrinogen, diabetes mellitus, drug abuse, oral contraceptives, high estrogen levels, postmenopausal woman not taking estrogen replacement, older adult, African American, and newly industrializing environment.

MENTAL STATUS ASSESSMENT

Assessment of mental status is performed by observing the client and asking questions. Much of this information may have already been assessed during the initial interview and general survey.

Objective Data: Assessment Techniques

See Figure 17–1 for a diagram of the brain.

PROCEDURE	NORMAL FINDINGS	DEVIATIONS FROM NORMAL
Observe level of consciousness • Response to calling the client's name. If the client does not respond, call the name louder. If	• Alert and awake with eyes open and looking at examiner; client responds appropriately	• Lethargy: Opens eyes, answers questions, and falls back asleep.

Objective Data: Assessment Techniques (continued)

PROCEDURE	NORMAL FINDINGS	DEVIATIONS FROM NORMAL
necessary, shake the client gently. If the client still does not respond, apply a painful stimulus.		• Obtunded: Opens eyes to loud voice, responds slowly with confusion, seems unaware of environment.
		• Stupor: Awakens to vigorous shake or painful stimuli, but returns to unresponsive sleep.
		• Coma: Remains unresponsive to all stimuli; eyes stay closed. Client with lesions of the corticospinal tract draws hands up to chest (*decorticate* or abnormal flexor posture) when stimulated.
		• Client with lesions of the diencephalon, midbrain, or pons extends arms and legs, arches neck and rotates hands and arms internally (*decerebrate* or abnormal extensor posture) when stimulated.
*Observe **appearance and movement.***		
• Posture	• Relaxed, with shoulders back and both feet stable	• Tense, rigid, slumped, asymmetrical posture. Slumped posture is seen with depression or organic brain disease.

Neurologic Assessment

Objective Data: Assessment Techniques (continued)

PROCEDURE	NORMAL FINDINGS	DEVIATIONS FROM NORMAL
• Gait	• Smooth, coordinated movements; client alters position occasionally	• Uncoordinated—staggering, shuffling, stumbling
• Motor movements	• Same as above	• Jerky, uncoordinated; tremors, tics, fast or slow movements. Bizarre movements are seen with schizophrenia; tense, fidgety, and restless behavior in anxious patients.
• Dress	• Clothes fit and are appropriate for occasion and weather	• Clothes extra large or small and inappropriate for occasion. Inappropriate dress is seen with depression, dementia, Alzheimer disease, and schizophrenia.
• Hygiene	• Skin clean, nails clean and trimmed	• Dirty, unshaven; dirty nails; foul odors. Poor hygiene is seen with depression, dementia, Alzheimer disease, and schizophrenia; meticulous, finicky grooming in obsessive–compulsive disorder.
• Facial expression	• Good eye contact, smiles/frowns appropriately	• Poor eye contact is seen in apathy or depression; mask-like expression in Parkinson disease; extreme anger or happiness in anxious clients.

Objective Data: Assessment Techniques (continued)

PROCEDURE	NORMAL FINDINGS	DEVIATIONS FROM NORMAL
• Speech	• Clear with moderate pace	• High pitched; monotonal; hoarse; very soft or weak. Slow, repetitive speech is present in depression or Parkinson disease; loud and rapid in manic phases; irregular, uncoordinated speech in multiple sclerosis; dysphonia in impairment of CN X; dysarthria in Parkinson or cerebellar disease; aphasia in lesions of dominant hemisphere.
*Observe **mood*** by asking, "How are you feeling?" or "What are your plans for the future?"		
• Feelings (varies from joy to anger)	• Responds appropriately to topic discussed; expresses feelings appropriate to situation	• Expresses feelings inappropriate to situation (eg, extreme anger or euphoria)
• Expressions	• Expresses good feelings about self, others, and life; verbalizes positive coping mechanisms (talking, support systems, counseling, exercise, etc)	• Expresses dissatisfaction with self, others, and life in general; verbalizes negative coping mechanisms (use of alcohol, drugs, etc); prolonged negative feelings seen with depression; elation and high energy seen with manic phases; exces-

Objective Data: Assessment Techniques (continued)

PROCEDURE	NORMAL FINDINGS	DEVIATIONS FROM NORMAL
Observe **thought process and perceptions** by stating, "Tell me your understanding of your current health situation."		sive worry seen in obsessive–compulsive disorders; eccentric moods not relevant to situation are seen in schizophrenia.
• Clarity and content	• Expresses full and free-flowing thoughts during interview	• Expressed thoughts are jumbled, confusing, and not reality oriented. Repetition and expression of illogical thoughts are seen with schizophrenia; rapid flight of ideas with manic phases; irrational fears with phobias; delusions seen with psychotic disorders, delirium, and dementia; illusions seen with acute grief, stress reactions, schizophrenia, and delirium; hallucinations with organic brain disease or psychotic illness.
• Perceptions	• Follows directions accurately; perceptions realistic and consistent with yours and others.	• Is unable to follow through with directives; perceptions unrealistic and inconsistent with yours and others.

Objective Data: Assessment Techniques (continued)

PROCEDURE	NORMAL FINDINGS	DEVIATIONS FROM NORMAL
• Judgment	• Answers to questions are based on sound rationale.	Impaired judgment may be seen in organic brain syndrome, emotional disturbances, mental retardation, or schizophrenia.
*Observe **cognitive abilities.***		
• Orientation—Ask client name, hour, date, season, where he lives now.	• Aware of self, others, place, time, have address	• Unable to express where he or she is, time, and who others are; does not follow instructions. Reduced level of orientation is seen with organic brain disorders.
• Length of concentration	• Listens to you and responds with full thoughts	• Fidgets; does not listen attentively to you; expresses incomplete thoughts. Distraction and inability to focus are noted with anxiety, fatigue, attention deficit disorders, and altered states due to drug or alcohol intoxication.
• Memory—Ask client "What did you eat today?" (recent) "When is your birthday?" (past)	• Correctly answers questions about current day's activities; recalls significant past events	• Unable to recall any recent events with delirium, dementia, depression, and anxiety; unable to recall past events with cerebral cortex disorders
• Abstract reasoning—Ask client to explain a proverb, eg, "A stitch in time saves nine."	• Explains proverb accurately	• Unable to give abstract meaning of proverb with schizophrenia, mental retardation, delirium, or dementia

Objective Data: Assessment Techniques (continued)

PROCEDURE	NORMAL FINDINGS	DEVIATIONS FROM NORMAL
• Ability to make sound judgments—Ask client question such as "Why did you come to the hospital?" or "What do you do when you have pain?"	• Answers to questions based on sound rationale	• Answers to questions are not based on sound rationale in organic brain syndrome, emotional disturbances, mental retardation, or schizophrenia.
• Ability to identify similarities—Ask client questions such as "How are birds and bees alike?"	• Identifies similarity	• Unable to identify similarity with schizophrenia, mental retardation, delirium, or dementia
• Sensory perception and coordination—Ask client to write name and draw the face of a clock or copy simple figures such as:	• Writes name, draws clock and/or simple figures	• Does not write name or draw clock/figures accurately with mental retardation, dementia, parietal lobe dysfunction

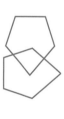

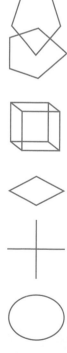

Figures to be drawn by client.

The Glasgow Coma Scale

Use the Glasgow Coma Scale (GCS) for clients who are at high risk for rapid deterioration of the nervous system (Table 17–2). A GCS score of 14 points indicates an optimal level of consciousness. A GCS score of less than 14 points indicates some impairment in the level of consciousness. A score of 3 points, the lowest possible score, indicates deep coma.

Mini-Mental State Examination

Perform the Mini-Mental State Examination if time is limited and a quick standard measure is needed to evaluate or reevaluate cognitive function (Box 17–1).

Scores from 24 to 30 points are normal. Scores lower than 21 points may be seen in organic brain disease (delirium or dementia) or affective disorders. Scores of 21 to 24 points are questionable with regard to disease and require further evaluation.

Note that potential harm from labeling or identifying clients with possible dementia must be weighed against benefits of assessment.

PEDIATRIC VARIATIONS

Subjective Data: Focus Questions

Excessive difficulty in relationships with siblings, peers, parents, and teachers? Sudden changes in activities such as play or school activities? Excessive fears? Change in attention span?

NORMAL VARIATIONS

- Abstract reasoning is not possible before ages 10 to 12 years. Judgment ability varies with level of development.
- From birth to 11 years, knowledge of normal development is most important in evaluating cognition. Cues for evaluating cognition in infants and young children are primarily *not* valid. Awareness, attention to mother, and a parent's report on

(text continues on p. 391)

TABLE 17–2 GLASGOW COMA SCALE

Response	Score	
Eye-opening response	Spontaneous opening	4
	To verbal stimuli	3
	To pain	2
	None	1
Most appropriate verbal response	Oriented	5
	Confused	4
	Inappropriate words	3
	Incoherent	2
	None	1
Most integral motor response (arm)	Obeys commands	5
	Localizes pain	4
	Flexion to pain	3
	Extension to pain	2
	None	1
TOTAL SCORE		3–15

The GCS is useful for rating one's response to stimuli. The client who scores 10 points or lower needs emergency attention. The client with a score of 7 points or lower is generally considered to be in a coma. Teasdale, G., & Jennelt, B. (1974). Assessment of coma and impaired consciousness: A practical scale. *Lancet, 2,* 81.

BOX 17–1. Annotated Mini-Mental State Examination

NAME OF SUBJECT _____   Age _____

NAME OF EXAMINER _____   Years of School Completed _____

                                          Date of Examination _____

Approach the patient with respect and encouragement

Ask: Do you have any trouble with your memory?   ☐ Yes   ☐ No

May I ask you some questions about your memory?   ☐ Yes   ☐ No

SCORE   ITEM

5 ( )   Time orientation

Ask:

What is the year _____ (1), season _____ (1).

month of the year _____ (1), date _____ (1).

day of the week _____ (1)?

5 ( )   Place orientation

Ask:

Where are we now? What is the state _____ (1), city _____ (1),

part of the city _____ (1), building _____ (1), city _____ (1) floor of the building _____ (1)?

3 ( )   Registration of three words

Say: Listen carefully. I am going to say three words. You say them back after I stop. Ready? Here they are . . . PONY (wait 1 second), QUARTER (wait 1 second), ORANGE (wait one second). What were those words?

_____ (1)

_____ (1)

_____ (1)

Give 1 point for each correct answer, then repeat them until the patient learns all three.

Neurologic Assessment

BOX 17–1. *(continued)*

5 ( ) **Serial 7s as a test of attention and calculation**

Ask: Subtract 7 from 100 and continue to subtract 7 from each subsequent remainder until I tell you to stop.

What is 100 take away 7? ———— (1)

Say:

Keep Going. ———— (1), ———— (1).

———— (1), ———— (1).

3 ( ) **Recall of three words**

Ask:

What were those three words I asked you to remember?

Give one point for each correct answer ———— (1).

———— (1), ———— (1).

2 ( ) **Naming**

Ask:

What is this? (show pencil) ———— (1). What is this? (show watch) ———— (1).

1 ( ) **Repetition**

Say:

Now I am going to ask you to repeat what I say. Ready? No ifs ands or buts.

Now you say that ———— (1)

3 ( ) **Comprehension**

Say:

Listen carefully because I am going to ask you to do something:

Take this paper in your left hand (1), fold it in half (1), and put it on the floor. (1)

1 ( ) Reading

Say:

Please read the following and do what it says, but do not say it aloud. (1)

Close your eyes

1 ( ) Writing

Say:

Please write a sentence. If patient does not respond say: Write about the weather. (1)

1 ( ) Drawing

Say: Please copy this design.

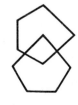

TOTAL SCORE _____ Assess level of consciousness along a continuum

Alert	Drowsy	Stupor	Coma

BOX 17–1. (*continued*)

	YES	NO		YES	NO
Cooperative	☐	☐	Deterioration from previous level of functioning	☐	☐
Depressed	☐	☐	Family history of dementia	☐	☐
Anxious	☐	☐	Head trauma	☐	☐
Poor vision	☐	☐	Stroke	☐	☐
Poor hearing	☐	☐	Alcohol abuse	☐	☐
Native language			Thyroid disease	☐	☐

FUNCTION BY PROXY

Please record date when patient was last able to perform the following tasks.

Ask caregiver if patient independently handles.

	YES	NO	DATE
Money bills	☐	☐	—
Medication	☐	☐	—
Transportation	☐	☐	—
Telephone	☐	☐	—

Used with permission from Folstein, M. F., Folstein, S. E., & McHugh, P. R. (1975). Mini-Mental State: A practical method for grading the cognitive state of patients for the clinician. *Journal of Psychiatric Research, 12*(3), 189–198.

the infant's attentiveness are also important. Play activities or games can be used to elicit many desired responses. For example, a young child can be asked to recall three to four numbers in sequence as a test of memory.

● From birth to 6 years, objective findings can be determined using the Denver Developmental Screening Test.

CULTURAL VARIATIONS

The stroke rate, although decreasing in industrialized countries, remains high in African Americans, and across the U.S. "Stroke belt" of southern states, Indiana, and Washington, D.C. [National Stroke Association, 2000]. A changing pattern is expected with decreasing incidence in Alabama and Mississippi and increases in Oregon, Washington, and Arkansas. Stroke rates are also expected to continue to decrease in New York and Florida (Howard et al., 2001).

GERIATRIC VARIATIONS

● May seem confused in a new or acute care setting owing to slowed thought processes and slowed responses to questions; however, is oriented to person, time, and place
● Decreased ability to recall directions
● Slight decline in short-term memory
● Use the GDS-5/15 Geriatric Depression Scale to screen older adults for depression (Box 17-2).
● Slowed reaction time
● Likes to reminisce and tends to wander from topic at hand
● May have hesitation with short-term memory
● Clients over 80 years should be able to recall 2 to 4 words after a 5-minute time period.

Possible Collaborative Problems

Depression	Suicide attempt
Alcohol abuse	Drug abuse

BOX 17-2. The GDS-5/15 Geriatric Depression Scale

Directions: If the patient scores 0 or 1 point on the GDS-5, the patient is classified as "not depressed" and no further questions are asked. If the patient scores 2 points or more on the GDS-5, the screener continues asking the remaining 10 questions and classifies the patient as "suggesting depressed" or "not depressed" according to the GDS guidelines. Those classified as "suggesting depressed" on the full GDS-5/15 need to be referred for further clinical investigation for symptoms of depression.

1. Are you basically satisfied with your life?[1,2,3]	Yes	No*
2. Do you often get bored?[3]	Yes*	No
3. Do you often feel helpless?[3]	Yes*	No[3]
4. Do you prefer to stay home rather than going out and doing new things?[2,3]	Yes*	No
5. Do you feel pretty worthless the way you are now?[3]	Yes*	No

Score GDS-5 = _____

Score of 2 or more on GDS-5? Please continue with the remaining 10 questions:

6. Have you dropped many of your activities and interests?[2]	Yes*	No
7. Do you feel that your life is empty?[1]	Yes*	No
8. Are you in good spirits most of the time?	Yes	No*
9. Are you afraid that something bad is going to happen to you?[1]	Yes*	No
10. Do you feel happy most of the time?[1,2]	Yes	No*

11. Do you feel you have more problems with memory than most?	Yes*	No
12. Do you think it is wonderful to be alive now?	Yes	No*
13. Do you feel full of energy?	Yes	No*
14. Do you feel your situation is hopeless?	Yes*	No
15. Do you think that most people are better off than you are?	Yes*	No

Score GDS-15=_____

Circle each answer. Each answer indicated by * counts as 1 point.

Note.
[1] = Included on 4-Item, D'Ath.
[2] = Included on 4-Item, van Marwijk.
[3] = Included on 5-Item, Hoyl.

GDS-5 score of 2 or more indicates possible depression (Hoyl et al., 1999); ask remaining 10 questions.
GDS-15 score of 5–9 indicates possible depression; scores above 9 usually indicate depression (Sheikh & Yesavage, 1986).
Used with permission from Weeks, S. K., McGarin, P. E. Michaels. T. K., & Pennius, B. W. J. H. (2003). Comparing various short-form geriatric depression scales leads to the GDS-5/15. *Journal of Nursing Scholarship 35(2)* 133–137. © Sigma Theta Tau International.

TEACHING TIPS FOR SELECTED NURSING DIAGNOSES

Adult Client

Nursing Diagnosis: Disturbed Thought Processes related to neurological changes (aging, head injury, stroke, etc)

☐ Inform client of the purpose and benefits of community agencies that offer support. Refer client as necessary. Assist family in coping, and explain how to communicate accurately using short sentences.

Nursing Diagnosis: Ineffective Individual Coping related to inadequate opportunity to prepare for stressor

☐ Teach client the use of appropriate stress-reducing measures (eg, relaxation techniques, biofeedback, exercise, hobbies). Inform client of beneficial effects of decreasing coffee, sugar, and salt in diet and maintaining adequate B and C vitamins in diet for adequate functioning of the endocrine and nervous systems. Refer client to community agencies and support groups as necessary.

Nursing Diagnosis: Impaired Memory

☐ Teach client memory-enhancing techniques.

Nursing Diagnosis: Readiness for enhanced critical thinking

☐ Teach client critical-thinking skills. Assist client to obtain resources to enhance critical thought processes.

Pediatric Client

Nursing Diagnosis: Compromised Family Coping: Compromised related to family developmental crisis adjusting to infant

☐ Discuss social development of the child. Infant's "stranger anxiety" is normal. Teach parents ways to assist infant to warm up to strangers. Encourage verbalization, reassurance, and cuddling. Help parent assess child's readiness to begin school and to verbalize any school problems with child.

CRANIAL NERVE ASSESSMENT

Various techniques are used to assess cranial nerve (CN) functioning.

Objective Data: Assessment Techniques

Assess CN I through XII.

PROCEDURE	NORMAL FINDINGS	DEVIATIONS FROM NORMAL
CN I—Olfactory: Hold scent (eg, coffee, orange) under one nostril with other occluded while client closes eyes. Repeat with other nostril.	Identifies scent correctly with each nostril	Unable to identify correct odor
CN II—Optic: Assess vision. Assess visual fields. Do funduscopic examination for direct visualization of optic nerve.	See Chapter 8, Eye Assessment.	See Chapter 8, Eye Assessment.
CN III—Oculomotor **CN IV—Trochlear** **CN VI—Abducens:** Assess extraocular movements. Assess PERRLA (pupils equal, round, and reactive to light and accommodation).	See Chapter 8, Eye Assessment.	See Chapter 8, Eye Assessment.

Neurologic Assessment

Objective Data: Assessment Techniques (continued)

PROCEDURE	NORMAL FINDINGS	DEVIATIONS FROM NORMAL
CN V—Trigeminal: Assess sensory function by: • Touching cornea lightly with wisp of cotton (Fig. 17–4) • Testing client's ability to feel light touch, dull, and sharp facial sensations on both sides of face at the forehead, cheek, and chin areas (with client's eyes closed; Fig. 17–5)	• Eyelids blink bilaterally • Identifies light touch, dull, and sharp sensations to forehead, cheeks, and chin	• Absent blink of eyelids with lesion of CN V (trigeminal) or lesions of the motor part of CN VII (facial) • Unable to identify or feel facial sensations with lesions of CN V, spinothalamic tract, or posterior columns

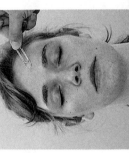

FIGURE 17-5 Testing sensory function of cranial nerve V: dull stimulus using a paper clip. (© B. Proud.)

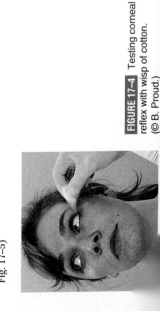

FIGURE 17-4 Testing corneal reflex with wisp of cotton. (© B. Proud.)

Neurologic Assessment

Objective Data: Assessment Techniques (continued)

PROCEDURE	NORMAL FINDINGS	DEVIATIONS FROM NORMAL
Assess motor function by palpating masseter and temporal muscles as client clenches teeth (Fig. 17–6).	Muscles contract bilaterally.	Asymmetrical or no muscle contractions; irregular facial movements; pain or bilateral muscle weakness is seen with peripheral or CNS dysfunction. Unilateral weakness is seen with lesion of CN V.
CN VII—Facial: Assess sensory function by asking client to identify sugar, lemon, salt on anterior two thirds of tongue, with eyes closed and tongue protruded.	Identifies taste correctly	Unable to taste or to identify taste correctly with impaired CN VII.

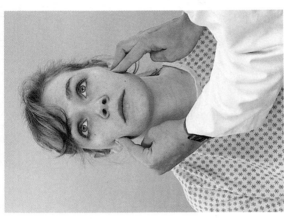

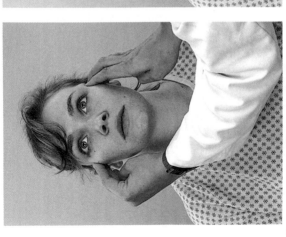

FIGURE 17-6 Testing motor function of cranial nerve V: (*left*) palpating temporal muscles; (*right*) palpating masseter muscles. (© B. Proud.)

Objective Data: Assessment Techniques (continued)

PROCEDURE	NORMAL FINDINGS	DEVIATIONS FROM NORMAL
Assess motor function by asking client to do the following: • Smile • Frown • Show teeth • Blow out cheeks • Raise eyebrows and tightly close eyes	• Smiles • Frowns • Shows teeth • Blows out cheeks • Raises eyebrows and closes eyes tightly as instructed; facial movements are symmetrical	• Unable to perform facial movements as instructed, or movements asymmetrical on one side of face. Unable to do facial movements along with paralysis of the lower part of the face seen in Bell palsy; paralysis of lower part of face on opposite side is seen with central lesion affecting upper motor neurons from cerebrovascular accident.
CN VIII—Acoustic: Assess hearing.	See Chapter 9, Ear Assessment.	See Chapter 9, Ear Assessment.
CN IX—Glossopharyngeal Assess taste and gag reflex	See CN VII for taste and CN X for gag reflex.	See CN VII (taste) and CN IX (gag reflex).
Ask client to identify lemon juice and salt on posterior one third of tongue with eyes closed.	• Identifies taste and gag reflex present	Unable to identify correct taste with lesion of CN IX

Neurologic Assessment

Objective Data: Assessment Techniques (continued)

PROCEDURE	NORMAL FINDINGS	DEVIATIONS FROM NORMAL
CN X—Vagus: Ask client to open mouth and say "ah."	Bilateral, symmetrical rise of soft palate and uvula	Unequal or absent rise of soft palate and uvula with lesions of CN X
Touch back of tongue or soft palate with tongue blade (Fig. 17–7).	Gag reflex present	Gag reflex absent with lesions of CN IX or X
CN XI—Spinal Accessory: Palpate strength of trapezius muscles by asking client to shrug shoulders against your hands (Fig. 17–8).	Symmetrical, strong contraction of trapezius muscles	Asymmetrical, weak, or absent contraction of trapezius muscles seen with paralysis or muscle weakness
Palpate strength of sternocleidomastoid muscles by asking client to turn head against your hand (Fig. 17–9).	Strong contraction of sternocleidomastoid muscle on opposite side that head is turned	Weak or absent contraction of sternocleidomastoid muscle on opposite side that head is turned seen with peripheral nerve disease
CN XII—Hypoglossal: Ask client to protrude tongue and move it to each side against tongue blade.	Symmetrical tongue with smooth outward movement and bilateral strength	Asymmetrical tongue; deviation to one side seen with unilateral lesion; fasciculations and atrophy of tongue seen with peripheral nerve disease; unequal or no strength

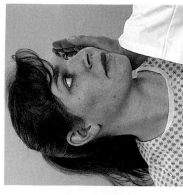

FIGURE 17-9   Testing cranial nerve XI: assessing strength of sternocleidomastoid muscle. (© B. Proud.)

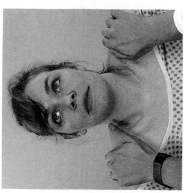

FIGURE 17-8   Testing cranial nerve XI: assessing strength of the trapezius muscle. (© B. Proud.)

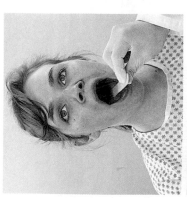

FIGURE 17-7   Testing cranial nerves IX and X: checking uvula rise and gag reflex. (© B. Proud.)

Neurologic Assessment

GERIATRIC VARIATIONS

● Decreased ability to see, hear, taste, and smell

Possible Collaborative Problems

Cranial nerve impairment
Corneal ulceration
Increased intraocular pressure

TEACHING TIPS FOR SELECTED NURSING DIAGNOSES

Adult Client

Nursing Diagnosis: Sensory/Perceptual Alterations (specify) related to injury or aging

Explain to family the use and benefits of sensory therapy. Refer for hearing/visual aids as necessary. Teach client slowly and concisely. Speak clearly and demonstrate instructions from client's best side for hearing and seeing. Teach client how to prevent thermal injuries.

SENSORY NERVE ASSESSMENT

To test the client's ability to perceive various sensations over the extremities and abdomen, stimuli must be scattered to cover all dermatomes. The client is asked to close his or her eyes and identify the type of sensation perceived and the body area where it was felt. If a perceptual deficit is identified, the area is mapped out to determine the extent of impaired sensation.

Objective Data: Assessment Techniques

PROCEDURE	NORMAL FINDINGS	DEVIATIONS FROM NORMAL
Test for *primary sensations* with client's eyes closed by touching client with the following:		
• Piece of cotton	• Identifies area of light touch	• Unable to identify location or light touch sensation
• Alternately with sharp tip and dull tip of paper clip	• Identifies area touched and differentiates between sharp and dull sensations	• Unable to identify location or differentiate touch sensations
• Vibrating tuning fork on major distal bony prominences of wrist, sternum	• Identifies vibratory sensation	• Unable to identify vibratory sensation
Test for *cortical and discriminatory sensation* with client's eyes closed by asking client to identify the following:		
• The number of points touching him or her while you touch client with two points simultaneously (two-point discrimination; Fig. 17–10)	• Identifies two points on: forearm at 40 mm apart; back at 40–70 mm apart; dorsal hands at 20–30 mm apart; fingertips at 2–5 mm apart	• Unable to identify two points at normal ranges with lesions of the sensory cortex

Objective Data: Assessment Techniques (continued)

PROCEDURE	NORMAL FINDINGS	DEVIATIONS FROM NORMAL
• The object (eg, a coin) you place in client's hand (stereognosis)	• Identifies correct object	• Unable to identify object with lesions of the sensory cortex
• A number you write on client's palm with a tongue blade (graphesthesia)	• Identifies correct number	• Unable to identify number with lesions of the sensory cortex
• The direction you move a part of client's body (eg, move fingers or toes up or down with eyes closed; kinesthesia; Fig. 17–11)	• Identifies correct direction body part is moved	• Unable to identify direction in which body part is moved with lesions of the sensory cortex

GERIATRIC VARIATIONS

- Touch sensations may diminish normally with aging due to atrophy of peripheral nerve endings
- Decreased light touch and pain perception
- Vibratory sensation at ankles often decreased after age 70 years

Possible Collaborative Problems

Peripheral nerve impairment

Neuropathies

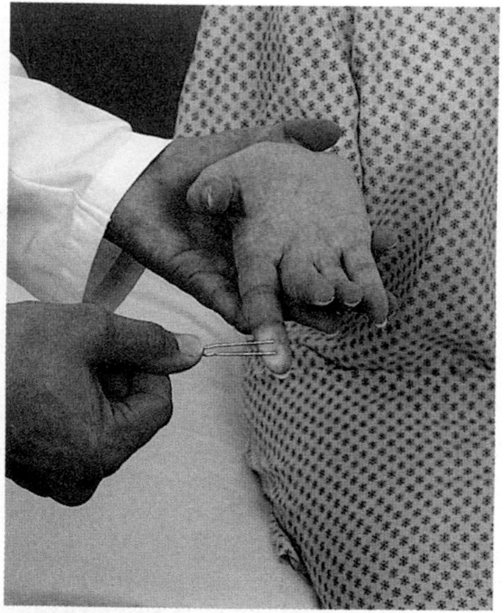

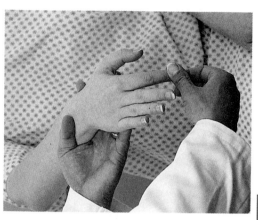

FIGURE 17-11 Testing position sense (kinesthesia). (© B. Proud.)

FIGURE 17-10 Two-point discrimination. (© B. Proud.)

TEACHING TIPS FOR SELECTED NURSING DIAGNOSES

Adult Client

Nursing Diagnosis: Risk for Injury related to decreased tactile sensations

Instruct on proper inspection and protective care of extremities. Caution client on dangers of exposure to extreme hot and cold temperatures, contact with sharp objects, and wearing tight-fitting shoes or garments.

MOTOR ASSESSMENT

Assess muscle size, tone, movement, voluntary movements, and strength. See Chapter 16, Musculoskeletal Assessment.

CEREBELLAR ASSESSMENT

Ask the client to perform the following actions, after you demonstrate them, in order to assess coordination.

Objective Data: Assessment Techniques

Ask client to do the following:

PROCEDURE	NORMAL FINDINGS	DEVIATIONS FROM NORMAL
Close eyes, and hold arms over head and straight out in front.	Holds arms over head and straight out steadily for 20 seconds	Downward drift; a flexion of one or both arms
With arms extended to the sides, touch each forefinger alternately to nose, first with eyes open and then with eyes closed (Fig. 17–12).	Smooth accurate movements while touching finger to nose	Uncoordinated jerky movements; inability to touch nose seen with cerebellar disease

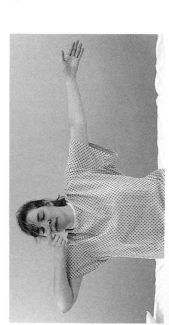

FIGURE 17–12 Testing coordination: finger-to-nose test. (© B. Proud.)

Objective Data: Assessment Techniques (continued)

PROCEDURE	NORMAL FINDINGS	DEVIATIONS FROM NORMAL
Put the palms of both hands down on both legs, then turn the palms up, then turn the palms down again. Ask client to increase speed (Fig. 17–13).	Rapidly turns palms up and down	Uncoordinated movements or tremors are seen with cerebellar disease.
Button and unbutton coat/shirt.	Buttons and unbuttons clothes smoothly	Clumsy attempts to button and unbutton clothes
Run each heel down opposite shin one at a time (Fig. 17–14).	Runs each heel smoothly down each shin	Unable to place heel on shin and move it down with coordination with cerebellar disease
Stand erect with feet together and arms at sides, first with eyes open and then with eyes closed. (Put your arms around client to prevent client falls—Romberg test.)	Stands straight with minimal swaying	Sways, moves feet out to prevent fall with disease of posterior column, vestibular dysfunction, or cerebellar disorders
Walk naturally.	Steady gait with opposite arm swing	Unsteady gait, uncoordinated arm swing; uses wide foot stance; shuffles or drags feet; lifts feet high off ground; crosses feet when walking. Gait is affected by disorders of the motor, sensory, vestibular, and cerebellar systems.

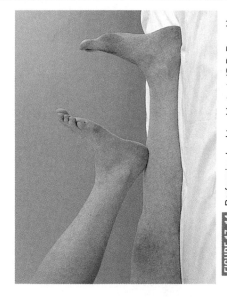

FIGURE 17-14 Performing heel-to-shin test. (© B. Proud.)

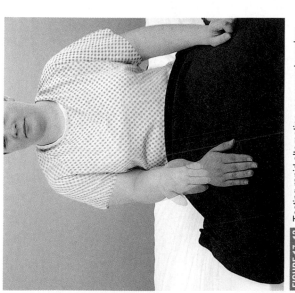

FIGURE 17-13 Testing rapid alternating movements: palms. (© B. Proud.)

Objective Data: Assessment Techniques (continued)

PROCEDURE	NORMAL FINDINGS	DEVIATIONS FROM NORMAL
Walk in a heel-to-toe fashion (tandem walk, Fig. 17–15).	Maintains balance with tandem walk	Unsteady tandem walk; unable to walk tandem style.
Stand on each foot (one at a time).	Stands on one foot at a time	Unable to stand on one foot at a time
Hop on each foot (one at a time). (Fig. 17–16)	Hops on each foot without losing balance	Inadequate strength or balance to hop on each foot with muscle weakness or disease of the cerebellum
Walk on heels, then toes	Walks on heels, then toes	Unable to walk on heels or toes

GERIATRIC VARIATIONS

- Slowed coordination and voluntary movements
- Decreased fine motor coordination
- May see tremors of the hand or head, or repetitive movements of the lips, jaw, or tongue
- May have slower and less certain gait; tandem walking may be very difficult for older client.
- Hopping on one foot is often impossible because of decreased flexibility and strength; it is best to avoid this test with the older client because of risk for injury.

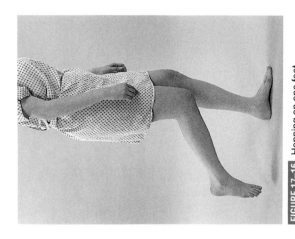

FIGURE 17-15 Testing balance: tandem walking. (© B. Proud.)

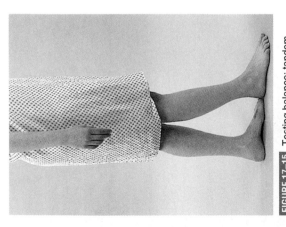

FIGURE 17-16 Hopping on one foot. (© B. Proud.)

REFLEX ASSESSMENT

Objective Data: Assessment Techniques

The reflex (or percussion) hammer is used to elicit deep tendon reflexes. Proceed as follows to elicit a deep tendon reflex:

1. Encourage the client to relax and position the client properly.

2. Hold the handle of the reflex hammer between your thumb and index finger so it swings freely.

3. Palpate the tendon and use a rapid wrist movement to strike the tendon briskly. Observe the response.

4. Compare the response of one side with the other.

5. For arm reflexes, ask the client to clench his or her jaw or to squeeze one thigh with the opposite hand, then immediately strike the tendon. For leg reflexes, ask the client to lock the fingers of both hands and pull them against each other, then immediately strike the tendon.

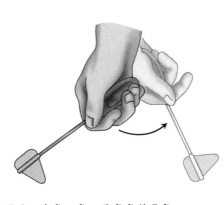

6. Rate and document reflexes using the following scale and figure:
- Grade 4+ Hyperactive, very brisk, rhythmic oscillations (clonus); abnormal and indicative of disorder
- Grade 3+ More brisk or active than normal, but not indicative of a disorder
- Grade 2+ Normal, usual response
- Grade 1+ Decreased, less active than normal
- Grade 0 No response

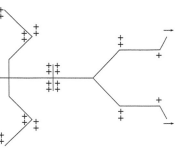

(text continues on p. 414)

REFLEX ASSESSMENT (continued)

To elicit superficial reflexes, lightly stroke the skin with a moderately sharp instrument (eg, key, tongue blade). Finally, certain maneuvers are performed to elicit any pathologic reflexes.

PROCEDURE	NORMAL FINDINGS	DEVIATIONS FROM NORMAL
Elicit deep tendon reflexes as follows:		
• Biceps reflex: With reflex hammer, tap your thumb placed over biceps tendon with client's arm flexed (tests nerve roots C5, C6; Fig. 17–17).	• Biceps contract (1+, 2+, 3+ biceps reflex).	• Absent or hyperactive contraction of biceps (0, 4+ biceps reflex).
• Brachioradialis reflex: Tap brachioradialis tendon just above wrist on radial side with client's arm resting midway between supination and pronation (tests nerve roots C5, C6; Fig. 17–18).	• Elbow flexes with pronation of forearm (1+, 2+, 3+ brachioradialis reflex).	• Absent or hyperactive flexion of elbow and forearm pronation (0+, 4+ brachioradialis reflex).
• Triceps reflex: Tap triceps tendon (just above elbow) with client's arm abducted and forearm hanging freely (tests nerve roots C6, C7, C8; Fig. 17–19).	• Elbow extends (1+, 2+, 3+ triceps reflex).	• Absent or hyperactive elbow extension (0, 4+ triceps reflex).

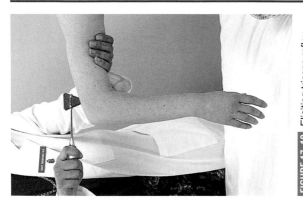

FIGURE 17-17 Eliciting biceps reflex. (© B. Proud.)

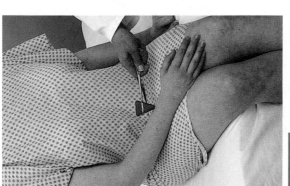

FIGURE 17-18 Eliciting brachioradialis reflex. (© B. Proud.)

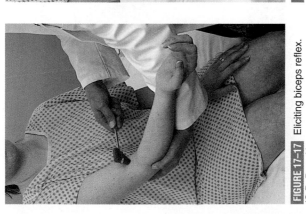

FIGURE 17-19 Eliciting triceps reflex. (© B. Proud.)

Objective Data: Assessment Techniques (continued)

PROCEDURE	NORMAL FINDINGS	DEVIATIONS FROM NORMAL
• Patellar reflex: Tap patellar tendon with client's knee flexed and thigh stabilized (tests nerve roots L2, L3; Fig. 17–20).	• Extension of knee (1+, 2+, 3+ patellar reflex)	• Absent or hyperactive extension of knee (0, 4+ patellar reflex)

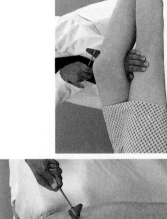 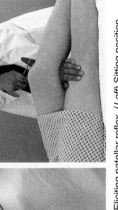

FIGURE 17–20 Eliciting patellar reflex. (*Left*) Sitting position. (*Right*) Supine position. (© B. Proud.)

Objective Data: Assessment Techniques (continued)

PROCEDURE	NORMAL FINDINGS	DEVIATIONS FROM NORMAL
• Achilles reflex: Tap Achilles tendon with client's foot slightly dorsiflexed and stabilized (tests nerve roots S1, S2; Fig. 17–21).	• Plantar flexion of foot (1+, 2+, 3+ Achilles reflex)	• Absent or hyperactive plantar flexion of foot (0, 4+ plantar flexion)

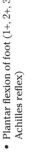
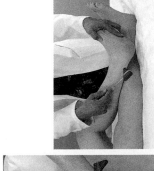
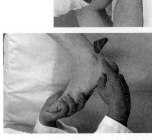

FIGURE 17–21 Eliciting Achilles reflex. (*Left*) Sitting position. (*Right*) Supine position. (© B. Proud.)

Objective Data: Assessment Techniques (continued)

PROCEDURE	NORMAL FINDINGS	DEVIATIONS FROM NORMAL
Elicit **superficial reflexes** *as follows:* • Lightly stroke each side of abdomen above and below umbilicus (umbilicus reflexes; Fig. 17–22). • Stroke gluteal area. • Stroke inner upper thigh of males.	• Bilateral upward and downward movements of umbilicus toward stroke; abdomen contracts. • Anal sphincter contracts. • Scrotum elevates on side stimulated.	• Absent or unilateral movement of umbilicus; no abdominal contraction • Absent contraction of gluteal reflex • No elevation of scrotum

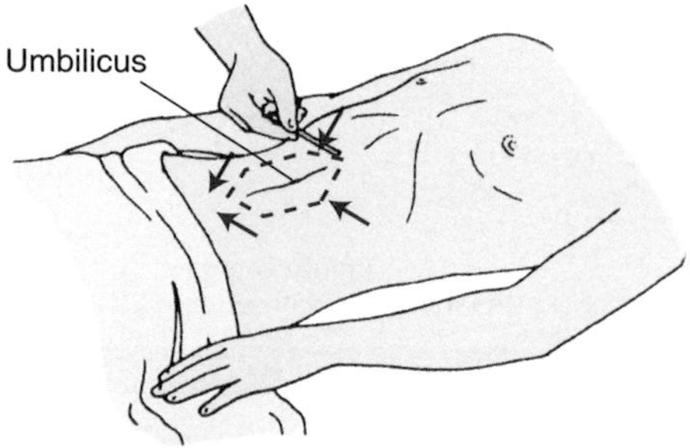

Umbilicus

FIGURE 17–22 Umbilicus reflex.

Objective Data: Assessment Techniques (continued)

PROCEDURE	NORMAL FINDINGS	DEVIATIONS FROM NORMAL
Assess for **pathologic reflexes** *as follows:* • Plantar reflex: Use end of reflex hammer to stroke lateral aspect of sole from heel to ball of foot (Fig. 17–23).	• Flexion of all toes (plantar response) seen in adults (see Fig. 17–23)	• Except in infancy, extension (dorsiflexion) of the big toe and fanning of all toes (positive plantar reflex; Babinski response) are seen with lesions of upper motor neurons. Unconscious states resulting from drug and alcohol intoxication or subsequent to an epileptic seizure may also cause it.

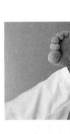

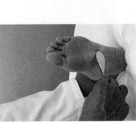

FIGURE 17–23 Eliciting plantar reflex (*left*). Normal plantar response (*right*). (© B. Proud.)

Objective Data: Assessment Techniques (continued)

PROCEDURE	NORMAL FINDINGS	DEVIATIONS FROM NORMAL
• Ankle clonus: Sharply dorsiflex foot with knee supported and partially flexed, and hold this way (Fig. 17–24).	• Foot stays dorsiflexed with no movement.	• Foot oscillates between dorsiflexion and plantar flexion.
• Brudzinski sign: Ask client to flex the neck; watch the hips and knees in reaction to the maneuver.	• Hips and knees remain relaxed and motionless.	• Flexion of the hips and knees is a positive Brudzinski sign and suggests meningeal inflammation.
• Kernig sign: Flex the client's leg at both the hip and the knee, then straighten the knee.	• No pain felt. Discomfort behind the knee during full extension occurs in many normal people.	• Pain and increased resistance to extending the knee are a positive Kernig sign. When Kernig sign is bilateral, the examiner suspects meningeal irritation.

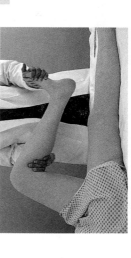

FIGURE 17–24 Testing for ankle clonus. (© B. Proud.)

PEDIATRIC VARIATIONS: BIRTH TO 1 YEAR

See Appendix 2 for developmental milestones for ages 1 to 3 years.

Objective Data: Assessment Techniques

REFLEXES	NORMAL VARIATIONS
Cough	No cough reflex until 1–2 days of age; after 1–2 days, cough should be strong and present even during sleep throughout infancy.
Rooting: Infant turns head toward side of face stroked.	Disappears at about age 3–12 months
Extension: When tongue is pressed or touched, infant forces tongue outward.	Disappears at about age 4 months
Grasp: Touch to palm of hand or soles of feet causes flexion of hands/toes.	Palmar grasp should disappear at about age 3 months.
Plantar reflex: Stroking outer sole of foot from heel to toe causes big toe to rise (dorsiflexion) and other toes to fan out.	Disappears after 1 year
Moro: Sudden jarring or change in equilibrium causes sudden extension and abduction of extremities, with thumb forming "C" shape; crying.	Disappears at about age 3–4 months
Startle: Sudden noise causes abduction of arms, clenched hands.	Disappears at about age 4 months

Neurologic Assessment

Objective Data: Assessment Techniques (continued)

REFLEXES	NORMAL VARIATIONS
Crawling: Infant on abdomen will make crawling movements with arms and legs.	Disappears at about age 6 weeks
Dance: Infant held so soles of feet touching table will simulate walking movements.	Disappears at about age 3–4 weeks
Neck righting: In supine infant, if head is turned to one side, shoulder and trunk will turn to that side.	Disappears around age 10 months
Asymmetrical tonic neck: Infant's head quickly turns to one side, arm and leg on that side will extend, opposite leg and arm will flex.	Disappears at about age 3–4 months

GERIATRIC VARIATIONS

- Generalized decreased deep tendon reflexes and slowed reflexes
- Decrease in transmission of impulses along with a delay in reaction time

Possible Collaborative Problems

Increased intracranial pressure Spinal cord compression
Meningitis Seizures
Paralysis

TEACHING TIPS FOR SELECTED NURSING DIAGNOSIS

Adult Client

Nursing Diagnosis: **Risk for Injury** related to seizure activity

☑ Teach appropriate precautions and care, including the following:

- Use of padded tongue blade, wallet, or cloth to maintain airway
- Protection of client from harm during seizures
- Positioning on side after seizure
- Significance of drug maintenance

Nursing Diagnosis: **Risk for Adult Failure to Thrive**

☑ Teach client and family or caregivers to assess behavior patterns that suggest anorexia, fatigue, dehydration, onset of incontinence (bowel or bladder), increase in chronic health problems such as pneumonia and urinary tract infections, cognitive decline, self-neglect, apathy, sadness. Teach client and caregivers to seek appropriate referrals if pattern is detected.

18

Nutritional Assessment

Equipment Needed

- Beam balance scale
- Metric measuring tape
- Skinfold calipers

Subjective Data: Focus Questions

Describe your appetite and nutritional status. Have you had anything to eat or drink during the past 3 days? Do you consider your usual dietary intake to be healthy? What are your food preferences and intolerances? Are you allergic to any foods? Explain. Do you have any food preferences related to your religious or cultural practices? Explain. Who usually shops for food and prepares food for you? Have you ever used particular health foods, vitamins, or diets? Explain. What are your usual activities during a day? Have you had any recent weight loss or gain?

Objective Data: Assessment Techniques

Assessment of the client's nutritional status consists of an overall inspection of muscle mass, distribution of fat, and skeleton. The examiner must determine if abnormalities found during assessment of the skin, thyroid, mouth, lungs, abdomen, and nervous system are related to alterations in nutrition. (Refer to Chapters 5, 6, 7, 10, 11, 14, and 17.)

GENERAL INSPECTION

PROCEDURE	NORMAL FINDINGS	DEVIATIONS FROM NORMAL
Observe the **muscle mass** *over temporal areas, dorsum of hands, and spine for:*		
• Tone	• Firm, developed	• Flaccid, wasted, underdeveloped
• Strength with voluntary movement	• Strength equal bilaterally	• Weak, sluggish, or unequal
Observe **body fat** for distribution over waist, thighs, and triceps.	Equal distribution; some fat under skin	Lack of fat under skin, increased bony prominences, emaciated, cachectic, abundant fatty tissue, abdominal ascites (due to fluid shift in protein)
Observe **posture.**	Erect, no malformations, smooth and coordinated gait	Poor posture, difficulty walking, bowlegged, knock-kneed
Observe **energy level.**	Energetic	Fatigued, irritable
Observe **skin** for color and texture.	Pink, smooth, turgor present	Pale, rough, dry, flaky, petechiae, lacks subcutaneous fat, loss of turgor
Observe **nails** for color and texture.	Nails firm; skin under nails pink	Pale, brittle, opaque, spoon shaped, ridged
Observe **hair** for texture.	Lustrous and shiny	Brittle, dry

GENERAL INSPECTION (continued)

PROCEDURE	NORMAL FINDINGS	DEVIATIONS FROM NORMAL
Observe **lips** for color and texture.	Pink, smooth, moist	Swollen, puffy, lesions, fissures at corners of mouth
Observe **tongue** for color and texture.	Deep red with papillae	Beefy red, smooth, swollen, atrophy or hypertrophy; dry tongue seen with dehydration
Observe **teeth** for position and condition.	Straight with no cavities	Missing, malpositioned, cavities
Observe **gums** for condition and color.	Smooth, firm, pink	Inflamed, spongy, swollen, red, bleed easily
Observe **eyes** for moisture, lesions.	Clear, moist surfaces, transparent cornea	Pale or red eye; membranes dry, increased vascularity, dull appearance of cornea; sunken eyeballs seen with dehydration
Observe **reflexes.**	Reflexes normal	Loss of or decreased ankle and knee reflexes
Observe **pulse and blood pressure.**	Normal heart rate and blood pressure for age	Tachycardia, hypertension, irregular pulse; blood pressure that drops 20 mm Hg from lying to standing position may indicate fluid volume deficit.

ANTHROPOMETRIC MEASUREMENTS

PROCEDURE	NORMAL FINDINGS	DEVIATIONS FROM NORMAL
Measure **height:** Have client stand erect against wall without shoes. Record height in centimeters and inches.	Compare findings for normal adult height and weight.	Extreme shortness seen with Achondroplastic dwarfism and Turner syndrome. Extreme heights are seen with Marfan syndrome, gigantism, and with excessive secretion of growth hormone.
Measure **weight** on a balance beam scale. Ask client to remove shoes and heavy outer clothing and to stand on the scale. Record weight (1 lb = 2.2 kg). If you are weighing a client at home, you may have to use a scale with an automatically adjusting true zero. Determine **ideal body weight** (IBW) and **percentage of IBW**	Desirable weights for men and women are listed in Table 18–1.	Weight does not fall within range of desirable weights for women and men.
Use this formula to calculate the client's IBW: *Female:* 100 lb for 5 ft + 5 lb for each inch over 5 ft ± 10% for small or large frame	Body weight is within 10% of ideal range.	A current weight that is 80–90% of IBW indicates a lean client and possibly mild malnutrition. Weight that is 70–80% indicates moderate malnutrition; less than 70% may indicate severe malnutrition possi-

TABLE 18-1 HEIGHT AND WEIGHT TABLE: WEIGHTS FOR PERSONS 25 TO 59 YEARS ACCORDING TO BUILD*

Men

Height		Small Frame	Medium Frame	Large Frame
Feet	Inches			
5	2	128–134	131–141	138–150
5	3	130–136	133–143	140–153
5	4	132–138	135–145	142–156
5	5	134–140	137–148	144–160
5	6	136–142	139–151	146–164
5	7	138–145	142–154	149–168
5	8	140–148	145–157	152–172
5	9	142–151	148–160	155–176
5	10	144–154	151–163	158–180
5	11	146–157	154–166	161–184
6	0	149–160	157–170	164–188
6	1	152–164	160–174	168–192
6	2	155–168	164–178	172–197
6	3	158–172	167–182	176–202
6	4	162–176	171–187	181–207

Women

Height†		Small Frame	Medium Frame	Large Frame
Feet	Inches			
4	10	102–111	109–121	118–131
4	11	103–113	111–123	120–134
5	0	104–115	113–125	122–137
5	1	106–118	115–129	125–140
5	2	108–121	118–132	128–143
5	3	111–124	121–135	131–147
5	4	114–127	124–138	134–151
5	5	117–130	127–141	137–155
5	6	120–133	130–144	140–159
5	7	123–136	133–147	143–163
5	8	126–139	136–150	146–167
5	9	129–142	139–153	149–170
5	10	132–145	142–156	152–173
5	11	135–148	145–159	155–176
6	0	138–151	148–162	158–179

Courtesy Metropolitan Life Insurance Company (2000). *Statistical bulletin.*
*Indoor clothing weighing 5 lb for men and 3 lb for women.
†Shoes with 1-inch heels.

ANTHROPOMETRIC MEASUREMENTS (continued)

PROCEDURE	NORMAL FINDINGS	DEVIATIONS FROM NORMAL
Make: 106 lb for 5 ft + 6 lb for each inch over 5 ft ± 10% for small or large frame. Calculate the client's percentage of IBW by the following formula: $$actual\ weight \times 100 = \%\ IBW.$$ Measure **body mass index** (BMI) Determine BMI using one of these formulas: $$\frac{Weight\ in\ kilograms}{Height\ in\ meters^2} = BMI$$ or $$\frac{Weight\ in\ pounds}{Height\ in\ inches^2} \times 705 = BMI$$	BMI between 20 and 25	bly from systemic disease, eating disorders, cancer therapies, and other problems. Weight exceeding 10% of the IBW range is called overweight; weight exceeding 20% of IBW is called obesity. BMI < 20 is associated with health problems in some people. BMI between 25 and 27 may lead to health problems in some people. BMI > 27 indicates increased risk of developing health problems.

ANTHROPOMETRIC MEASUREMENTS (continued)

PROCEDURE	NORMAL FINDINGS	DEVIATIONS FROM NORMAL
Determine **waist-to-hip ratio.** Have the client stand. Measure the waist. Then measure the hips midway between the iliac crest and the greater trochanter. Use this formula to calculate the waist-to-hip ratio: $$\text{Waist-to-hip ratio} = \frac{\text{waist circumference}}{\text{hip circumference}}$$	*Females:* Waist 20% smaller than hips or waist-to-hip ratio less than or equal to 0.80 *Males:* Waist-to-hip ratio less than or equal to 1.0	Females with a waist-to-hip ratio greater than 0.80 and males with a waist-to-hip ratio greater than 1.0 have a three to five times greater risk for having a heart attack or stroke.
Measure **mid-arm circumference** (MAC; Fig. 18–1). The MAC measurement evaluates skeletal muscle mass and fat stores. Have the client dangle the nondominant arm freely next to the body. Locate the arm's midpoint (halfway between the top of the acromion process and the olecranon process). Mark the midpoint and measure the MAC, holding the tape measure firmly around, but not pinching, the arm.	Compare the client's current MAC to prior measurements and compare to standard MAC measurements for the client's age and sex.	Measurements that are significantly higher or lower than the 50th percentile on the standard reference charts indicate that further assessment of the client's nutritional status is needed. The MAC may increase with obesity to the upper percentiles and decrease to the lower percentiles in malnutrition (see Table 18–2).

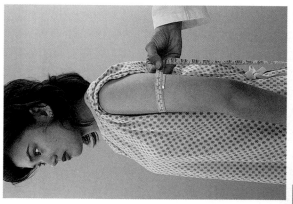

FIGURE 18–1 Measuring mid-arm circumference. (© B. Proud.)

ANTHROPOMETRIC MEASUREMENTS (continued)

PROCEDURE	NORMAL FINDINGS	DEVIATIONS FROM NORMAL
Measure **triceps skinfold thickness** (TSF; Fig. 18–2). Take the TSF measurement to evaluate the degree of fat stores. Instruct the client to stand and hang the nondominant arm freely. Grasp the skinfold and subcutaneous fat between the thumb and forefinger 1 cm above the midpoint mark. Pull the skin away from the muscle (ask client to flex arm—if you feel a contraction with this maneuver, you still have the muscle) and apply the calipers. Repeat three times and average the three measurements.	Compare the client's current measurement to past measurements and to standard TSF measurements for the client's age and sex.	Fat stores decrease in malnutrition and increase in obesity.
Calculate **mid-arm muscle circumference** (MAMC). The MAMC calculation determines skeletal muscle reserves from	Compare the client's current MAMC to past measurements and to data	The MAMC decreases to the lower percentiles with malnutrition and in obesity

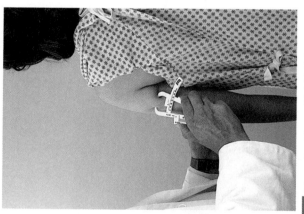

FIGURE 18–2 Measuring triceps skinfold thickness. (© B. Proud.)

TABLE 18–2 DETERMINING DEGREE OF OBESITY BY BODY MASS INDEX

BMI	Weight Classification
25.0–29.9	Overweight (preobese)
30.0–34.9	Class 1 obesity
35.0–39.9	Class 2 obesity
≥40	Class 3 obesity

ANTHROPOMETRIC MEASUREMENTS (continued)

PROCEDURE	NORMAL FINDINGS	DEVIATIONS FROM NORMAL
MAC and TSF measurements by this formula: MAMC (cm) = MAC (cm) − (0.314 × TSF)	for MAMCs for the client's age and sex.	if TSF is high. If the MAMC is in a lower percentile and the TSF is in a higher percentile, the client may benefit from muscle-building exercises that increase muscle mass and decrease fat.
Calculate **mid-arm muscle area** (MAMA). To determine skeletal muscle reserves and evaluate malnourishment in clients, calculate the MAMA. MAMA is more sensitive than MAMC for malnutrition, particularly for growing children and clients with long-term malnutrition. MAMA is derived from MAC and MAMC by the following formula: $$\frac{(\text{MAC} - \text{MAMC})^2}{4\pi(12.56)} = \text{MAMA}$$	Compare with normal values.	Malnutrition Mild—MAMA of 90% Moderate—MAMA 60–90% Severe—MAMA < 60%

DIETARY ASSESSMENT

Assess client's dietary requirements and intake by asking client to keep 3-day diary of food and fluid intake. May also use Box 18–1, Speedy Checklist for Nutritional Health.

PROCEDURE	NORMAL FINDINGS	DEVIATIONS FROM NORMAL
Calculate client's daily caloric requirements with following formula:	Meets caloric requirements	Consumes more or less than caloric requirements for age, height, body build, and weight
Multiply IBW in lb × cal/lb of IBW based on sex and activity level found in Table 18–3. Compare daily caloric requirements with client's daily consumption.		
Compare client's intake with USDA-recommended food guidelines (Fig. 18–3).	Consumes 2–3 dairy products, 2–3 meats, 2–4 fruits, 3–5 vegetables, and 6–11 grains per day. Compare with Figure 18–3 Asian and Latin American pyramids.	Consumes more or less than 2–3 dairy products, 2–3 meats, 2–4 fruits, 3–5 vegetables, and 6–11 grains per day Compare with Figure 18–3 Asian and Latin American pyramids.

PEDIATRIC VARIATIONS

Physiologic Growth Patterns

● See Appendix 5 for height/weight parameters.
● Growth is most rapid during the first year of life.

BOX 18–1. Speedy Checklist for Nutritional Health

Some warning signs of poor nutritional health are noted in this checklist. Use it to find out if your client is at nutritional risk. Read the statements below. Circle the number in the yes column for those that apply to the client. For each yes answer, score the number in the box. Total the nutrition score.

	YES
Illness or condition that made client change the kind and/or amount of food eaten	2
Eats fewer than two meals per day	3
Eats few fruits or vegetables, or milk products	2
Has three or more drinks of beer, liquor, or wine almost every day	2
Tooth or mouth problems that make it hard to eat	2
Does not always have enough money to buy the food needed	4
Eats alone most of the time	1
Takes three or more different prescribed or over-the-counter drugs a day	1
Without wanting to, has lost or gained 10 lb in the last 6 months	2
Not physically able to shop, cook, and/or feed self	2

TOTAL

Total the nutritional score.
0–2   Good. Recheck the score in 6 months.
3–5   Moderate nutritional risk. See what can be done to improve eating habits and lifestyle. Recheck score in 3 months.
6 or more   High nutritional risk. Consult with physician, dietitian, or other qualified health or social service professional.
Note: Remember that warning signs suggest risk but do not represent diagnosis of any condition.

Nutritional Assessment

TABLE 18-3	USDA GUIDELINES FOR CALCULATING DAILY CALORIE REQUIREMENTS (CAL/LB IBW)	
Activity Level	**Male**	**Female**
Sedentary	16	14
Moderate	21	18
Heavy	28	22

Based on activity level, multiply IBW in pounds by appropriate number of calories/pound according to sex.

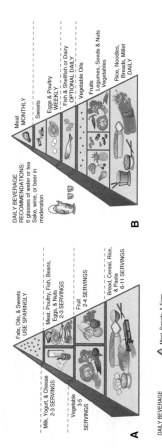

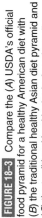

DAILY BEVERAGE
RECOMMENDATIONS:
6 glasses of water or tea
Sake, wine, or beer in
moderation

Meat
MONTHLY

Sweets

Eggs & Poultry
WEEKLY

Fish & Shellfish or Dairy
OPTIONAL DAILY

Vegetable Oils

Fruits
Legumes, Seeds & Nuts
Vegetables

Rice, Noodles,
Breads, Millet
DAILY

B

Fats, Oils, & Sweets
USE SPARINGLY

Milk, Yogurt, & Cheese
2-3 SERVINGS

Meat, Poultry, Fish, Beans,
Eggs, & Nuts
2-3 SERVINGS

Vegetable
3-5
SERVINGS

Fruit
2-4 SERVINGS

Bread, Cereal, Rice,
& Pasta
6-11 SERVINGS

A

DAILY BEVERAGE
RECOMMENDATIONS:
6 glasses of water
Alcohol in moderation

Meat, Sweets, & Eggs
WEEKLY

Fish & Shellfish
Plant Oils & Dairy
Poultry
DAILY

Fruits
Whole Grains, Tubers,
Beans, & Nuts
Vegetables
AT EVERY MEAL

DAILY PHYSICAL EXERCISE

C

FIGURE 18-3 Compare the (A) USDA's official
food pyramid for a healthy American diet with
(B) the traditional healthy Asian diet pyramid and
(C) the traditional healthy Latin American diet
pyramid.

- Birth weight doubles at age 4 to 6 months and triples by 1 year.
- Length increases 50% the first year of life.
- Teeth erupt first year of life.
- Growth decreases from ages 1 to 6 years, but biting, chewing, and swallowing abilities increase.
- Muscle mass and bone density increase from ages 1 to 6 years.
- There is a latent uneven period of growth from ages 1 to 12 years.
- Permanent teeth erupt at ages 6 to 12 years.
- School-age children tolerate larger, less frequent meals.
- Nutritional needs increase during growth spurts (ages 10–15 years for girls and ages 12–19 years for boys).

Dietary Requirements

- Allow 1000 calories plus 100 more per each year of age (eg, a 5-year-old needs 1500 calories per day).
- Children need three milks, two meats, four fruits or vegetables, and four grains per day.
- Adolescents need four milks, two meats, four fruits or vegetables, and four grains per day.
- The American Academy of Pediatrics (1997) recommends infants be breast-fed the first year of life. Solid foods should not be introduced before age 6 months, and they should be iron enriched.

Assessment Techniques

- *Infants:* Use pediatric pan scale. Obtain weight, length, and head circumference. Identify type of feeding and iron source.
- *Children and adolescents:* Weigh child and obtain height. Identify adequacy of meals and snacks and sources of iron, calories, and protein.

GERIATRIC VARIATIONS

- Elderly clients may have atrophy on dorsum of hands even with good nutrition.
- Assess for poor-fitting dentures and decreased ability to taste.

- Body weight may decrease with aging because of a loss of muscle or lean body tissue.
- Elderly tend to consume less food and eat more irregularly as they get older. This tends to increase with social isolation.
- Elderly have decreased peristalsis and nerve sensation, which may lead to constipation. Encourage fluids and dietary bulk to avoid laxative abuse.
- Caloric requirements decrease in response to a decreased basal metabolic rate, decreased activity, and change in body composition. A 10% decrease in calories is recommended for people ages 51 to 75 years and a 20 to 25% decrease in calories for people older than 75 years.
- A decrease in mobility and vision may impair the ability to purchase and prepare food. Sensory taste losses may lead to anorexia.
- Fifty percent of elderly are thought to be economically deprived, which may affect nutrition when meats and milks are omitted from diet to save money.
- Dietary recall may be difficult for the elderly.
- Skinfold measurements are often inaccurate owing to changes in subcutaneous fat.

CULTURAL VARIATIONS

- Great variations may be seen in nutritional preferences, eating habits, and patterns of various groups [Andrews & Boyle, 2002; Giger & Davidhizar, 2003].
- Foods, beverages, and medications are classified as hot/cold by many Asians and Hispanics (eg, yin/yang by Chinese); it is very important to these clients to seek a balanced consumption based on these theories.
- Many people, especially of non-northern European descent, have some degree of lactose intolerance.*

---

*Clients with lactose intolerance may be able to consume yogurt, buttermilk, fermented cheese, and acidophilus milk, or they may use products such as chewable tablets or liquid drops to act in place of the lactose enzyme.

- Classifications of "food" and "nonfood" items vary in cultures.
- Cultural or religious dietary rules or laws are of great importance to some groups (eg, Orthodox Jews).
- Some groups may have diseases precipitated by certain foods or medications (eg, glucose-6-phosphate dehydrogenase [G-6-PD] deficiency, lactose deficiency).
- Some cultural food preferences are contraindicated in specific disease states (eg, Japanese client with hypertension who consumes high-sodium soy sauce).

Possible Collaborative Problems

Hypoglycemia
Hyperglycemia
Electrolyte imbalance
Anemia

TEACHING TIPS FOR SELECTED NURSING DIAGNOSES

Adult Client

Nursing Diagnosis: **Readiness for enhanced nutritional–metabolic pattern**
Encourage proper oral hygiene. Teach nutritional guidelines:

- Eat a variety of foods.
- Balance the food you eat with physical activity—maintain or improve your weight.
- Choose a diet with plenty of grain products, vegetables, and fruits.
- Choose a diet low in fat, saturated fat, and cholesterol.
- Choose a diet moderate in sugar.
- Choose a diet moderate in salt and sodium.
- If you drink alcoholic beverages, do so in moderation.

(Recommended by U.S. Department of Agriculture, U.S. Department of Health and Human Services [2000]. Nutrition and your health: Dietary guidelines for Americans.)

Teach client how to get the most for his or her food dollar, how to read food labels, and ways to maintain nutrients in foods:

- Buy frozen vegetables and ripe produce.
- Encourage proper food storage and preparation to retain nutritional value.
- Prepare low-fat foods—suggest substituting applesauce or yogurt for butter when baking. Use bouillon or tomato juice instead of oil for sautéing. Use herbs and spices to replace the fat with flavor.

Nursing Diagnosis: Imbalanced Nutrition: more than body requirements

Provide client with information on social support groups. Teach client self-assessment and rewarding techniques when proper nutrition is followed. Teach client how to calculate caloric intake and caloric expenditure and how to explore forms of exercise that meet client's needs. Assist client to replace frequent unhealthy snacking with nutritious snacks. Teach dietary guidelines and food choices for Americans recommended by the U.S. Department of Health and Human Services.

Pediatric Client

Nursing Diagnosis: Imbalanced Nutrition: risk for more than body requirements

Teach parents to avoid overfeeding infants. Encourage proper formula dilution. Teach avoidance of empty caloric foods. Discourage use of food for rewarding behavior.

Nursing Diagnosis: Imbalanced Nutrition: risk for less than body requirements

Teach parents to avoid restricting normal intake of fat. Teach that low-fat diets are dangerous to growing infants because fat is essential to metabolism of some vitamins and other substances and to hormone production associated with growth and development.

CHAPTER 19

Maternal Physical Assessment

The body experiences many anatomical/physiologic changes during pregnancy. Findings in a physical assessment that would be considered abnormal in the nonpregnant client may be a result of pregnancy and not an abnormal state. In this chapter, the physical changes that occur in a woman as a result of pregnancy are identified as *normal variations*. Changes that are not a result of pregnancy or that represent an abnormal state during pregnancy are identified as *deviations from normal*.

For the sake of brevity, those systems described previously will not be repeated. Only variations of pregnancy will be noted. For procedures, the reader is referred to sections describing assessment of specific body systems.

During pregnancy, physical assessment should be performed every month for the first 27 weeks, every 2 weeks from week 28 to week 36, and then every week. More frequent examinations may be indicated for pregnancies at risk.

This chapter is divided into four sections: Prenatal Maternal Assessment, Prenatal Fetal Assessment, Intrapartum Maternal Assessment, and Postpartum Maternal Assessment.

PRENATAL MATERNAL ASSESSMENT

Equipment Needed

See Chapters 4 through 14 for the specific body system to be assessed.

Subjective Data: Focus Questions

Past pregnancies: Outcome of each? Number of living children? Complications? Length of labor? Years since last pregnancy?

Current pregnancy: Estimated due date? Confirmed by ultrasound? Planned pregnancy? Problems during pregnancy? Cramping or bleeding? Planned pregnancy? Date of first prenatal visit? Prenatal education?

Concurrent disease? Medications?

Objective Data: Assessment Techniques

Review of Systems

Perform a general physical survey.

PROCEDURE	NORMAL FINDINGS	DEVIATIONS FROM NORMAL
Assess the following:		
• Age	• Ideal childbearing years: 16–35	• Younger than 16 or older than 35; advanced maternal age increases risk of genetic abnormalities such as Down syndrome; increased risk to mother and baby with age extremes.

Maternal Physical Assessment

Objective Data: Assessment Techniques (continued)

PROCEDURE	NORMAL FINDINGS	DEVIATIONS FROM NORMAL
• Weight	• Average total weight gain: 25–35 lb (Fig. 19–1). *First trimester:* 2–4 lb *Second trimester:* 11 lb (1 lb/wk) *Third trimester:* 11 lb (1 lb/wk)	• Prepregnant weight <100 or >200 lb; sudden gain of more than 2 lb/wk may be seen in pregnancy-induced hypertension (PIH); weight loss or failure to gain weight.
• Blood pressure	• Range of 90–139/60–89 mm Hg; falls during second trimester, prepregnant level first and third trimesters	• ≥140/90 mm Hg or increase of 30 mm Hg above baseline systolic or 15 mm Hg above baseline diastolic taken with client in side-lying position; increased levels are seen with PIH.
• Pulse	• 60–90 bpm; may increase 10–15 bpm higher than prepregnant levels	• Irregularities; persistently <60 or >100 bpm at rest
• Behavior	• *First trimester:* Tired, ambivalent *Second trimester:* Introspective, energetic *Third trimester:* Restless, preparing for baby, labile moods (The father may experience some of these same behaviors)	• Denial of pregnancy, withdrawal, depression, psychosis

Maternal Physical Assessment

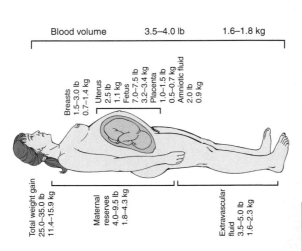

Total weight gain
25.0–35.0 lb
11.4–15.9 kg

Maternal reserves
4.0–9.5 lb
1.8–4.3 kg

Extravascular fluid
3.5–5.0 lb
1.6–2.3 kg

Blood volume   3.5–4.0 lb   1.6–1.8 kg

Breasts
1.5–3.0 lb
0.7–1.4 kg

Uterus
2.5 lb
1.1 kg

Fetus
7.0–7.5 lb
3.2–3.4 kg

Placenta
1.0–1.5 lb
0.5–0.7 kg

Amniotic fluid
2.0 lb
0.9 kg

FIGURE 19–1 Distribution of weight gain during pregnancy.

Objective Data: Assessment Techniques (continued)

PROCEDURE	NORMAL FINDINGS	DEVIATIONS FROM NORMAL
Observe **skin color.**	Linea nigra (Fig. 19–2), striae gravidarum (see Fig. 19–2); chloasma (Fig. 19–3); spider nevi	Pale, yellowing changes of the skin as seen with liver diseases

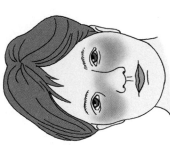

FIGURE 19–3 Marked chloasma of pregnancy.

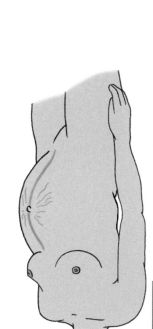

FIGURE 19–2 Pregnancy pigmentation: abdominal midline (linea nigra) and striae gravidarum. Dark-haired, brown-skinned women are more prone to pregnancy pigmentation.

Maternal Physical Assessment

Objective Data: Assessment Techniques (continued)

PROCEDURE	NORMAL FINDINGS	DEVIATIONS FROM NORMAL
Assess *head and neck.*		Facial edema, headache
• Nose	• Nasal stuffiness, nosebleeds	
• Eyes		• Blurred vision and visual spots are symptoms of PIH.
• Neck	• Slight enlargement of thyroid	• Nodules or marked enlargement, asymmetry of thyroid gland as seen with thyroid disease
Assess *cardiovascular system.*		
• Heart	• Short systolic blowing murmurs	• Progressive dyspnea, palpitations, markedly decreased activity tolerance may be seen with cardiac diseases.
• Blood volume	• Increases throughout pregnancy; peaks at 32–34 weeks, reaching 30–50% above prepregnancy levels	
Assess **peripheral vascular system.**	Late pregnancy: dependent edema, varicose veins, supine hypotension	Perineal varicosities; calf pain may be related to deep vein thrombosis; generalized edema; diminished pedal pulses.

Objective Data: Assessment Techniques (continued)

PROCEDURE	NORMAL FINDINGS	DEVIATIONS FROM NORMAL
Assess **respiratory system.**	Increased anteroposterior diameter, thoracic breathing, slight hyperventilation, shortness of breath in late pregnancy	Dyspnea may be seen in patients with cardiac disease and/or lung diseases such as asthma.
Assess **breasts.**	Increased size and nodularity, tenderness, prominent vascularization, darkening of nipples and areola, colostrum in third trimester (Fig. 19–4)	Localized redness; localized pain and warmth; erythemic streaks are commonly seen with mastitis; inverted nipples may cause difficulty for breast-feeding infants.
Assess **gastrointestinal system.**	Nausea and vomiting, increased saliva, heartburn, bloating, constipation	Severe epigastric pain is seen with PIH; severe nausea and vomiting may be seen during the first trimester with hyperemesis gravidarum.
Assess **genitourinary–reproductive systems.**	Urinary frequency in first and third trimesters, increased pigmentation of vulva and vagina, increased vaginal discharge	Flank pain, dysuria, oliguria, proteinuria, purulent vaginal discharge, vaginal bleeding
Assess **musculoskeletal system.**	Relaxation of pelvic joints: "waddling" gait; increased lumbar curve, backache, diastasis recti, leg cramps	
Assess **neurologic system.**		Hyperactive reflexes, positive clonus seen with PIH

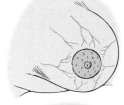

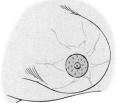
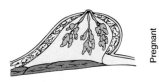
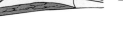
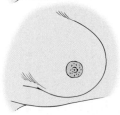

FIGURE 19–4 Breast changes during pregnancy.

Lactating

Pregnant

Non-pregnant

PRENATAL FETAL ASSESSMENT

Equipment Needed

- Bed or examination table
- Drape
- Pillow
- Paper centimeter tape measure
- Fetoscope or Doppler

Subjective Data: Focus Questions

Note date of initial fetal movement felt.
Has the fetus been active?

Objective Data: Assessment Techniques

Inspection

With client supine and head slightly elevated on a pillow, inspect abdomen for shape and contour of fetus. (Time spent in the supine position should be minimal. This position puts the weight of the fetus and uterus on the aorta and obstructs blood flow.)

Palpation

Using both hands, gently palpate the outline of the fetus and the top of the uterus (fundus). Using the centimeter tape, measure from the top of the symphysis pubis to the top of the uterine fundus (Fig. 19–5).

PROCEDURE

Measure fundal height and multiply by 8/7 (this equals weeks of gestation; Fig. 19–6).

NORMAL FINDINGS

Accurate within 2 weeks until 36 weeks. Obesity or extremes in height may alter findings.

DEVIATIONS FROM NORMAL

Lag in progression may indicate problems with fetal development and/or oligohydramnios commonly seen with congenital abnormalities. Sudden increase in fundal height size may also indicate fetal abnormalities such as congenital anomalies.

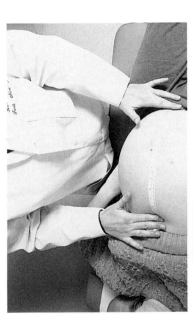

FIGURE 19–5 Measuring the fundal height.

Maternal Physical Assessment

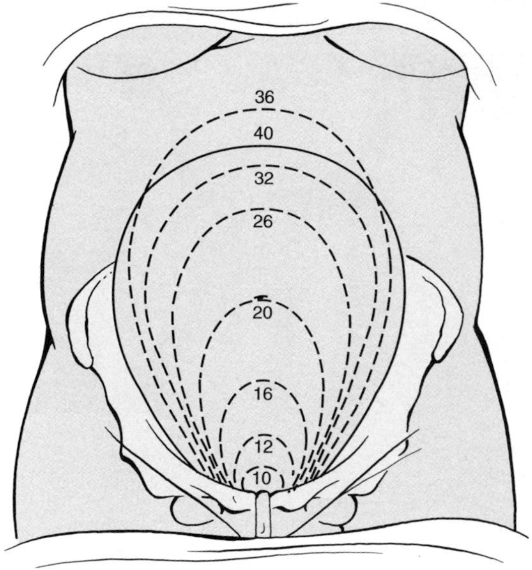

FIGURE 19-6 Approximate height of fundus at various weeks of gestation.

Auscultation

With Doppler or fetoscope, listen for fetal heartbeat. Locate fundus; begin listening halfway between the fundus and the pubis. Work outward in widening circles until a beating sound is heard. Compare with the maternal pulse. If different, count fetal heart rate for 1 full minute.

PROCEDURE	NORMAL FINDINGS	DEVIATIONS FROM NORMAL
Auscultate *fetal heart rate (FHR)* for the following:		
• Presence	• Audible at 10–12 weeks gestation with fetal Doppler; audible at 15–20 weeks gestation with fetoscope	• Absence of fetal heart tones after the 20th week of gestation indicates intra-uterine fetal demise.
• Rate	• Very rapid initially; gradually slows to 120–160 bpm at term; increased rate with fetal movement; during fetal sleep cycle, FHR may be in the 110–120 range.	• <120 bpm; no change or decrease in FHR with movement may indicate fetal distress.
• Rhythm	• Regular	• A marked variance or variance of < 5 beats/min may indicate fetal distress.

Maternal Physical Assessment

CULTURAL VARIATIONS

- Rh-negative blood is rare in nonwhite groups
- Dizygote twinning is higher in blacks than whites or Asians

Possible Collaborative Problems

Bleeding disorder of pregnancy
Spontaneous abortion
Placenta previa
Abruptio placentae
Pregnancy-induced hypertension
Dehydration
Gestational diabetes
Preeclampsia

Hyperemesis gravidarum
Ectopic pregnancy
Preexisting medical conditions
Hyperglycemia/hypoglycemia
Hypertension
Renal malfunctioning
Cardiac conditions

TEACHING TIPS FOR SELECTED NURSING DIAGNOSES

Nursing Diagnosis: Risk for Ineffective Therapeutic Regimen Management during pregnancy

Inform client of normal variations during the prenatal period. Also inform client of those abnormal symptoms to be reported immediately. Encourage client to write down questions; provide time to discuss them. Instruct client on methods to cope with normal variations (eg, nausea and vomiting). Encourage attendance at prenatal classes and appropriate reading material.

Nursing Diagnosis: Risk for Imbalanced Nutrition: Less Than Body Requirements related to increased metabolism and fetal demands

Diet should be selected from basic five food groups, with an additional 300 calories per day over recommended daily allowances. A balanced diet should provide all essential nutrients during pregnancy except folic acid and iron. These should be supplemented throughout pregnancy, because adequate amounts are closely related to fetal well-being and pregnancy outcome.

Nursing Diagnosis: Disturbed Body Image related to effects of physical changes during pregnancy

An exercise program started early in pregnancy and continued throughout will help maintain muscle tone and facilitate a return to prepregnant size after delivery. Exercise has the added benefit of creating a feeling of well-being and satisfaction. Exercise programs should be approved by the obstetrician prior to initiation. In general, those activities practiced prior to pregnancy can be continued unless they have a potential of causing physical harm to mother and baby.

Allow client to express her feelings about body changes, and reassure her that most changes are reversible or minimized after delivery. Emphasize positive changes.

Nursing Diagnosis: Readiness for Enhanced Parenting

Beginning education on growth and development of fetus and infant early in pregnancy can provide an opportunity for prospective parents to anticipate and understand development and expected patterns of developmental skill mastery.

Nursing Diagnosis: Readiness for Enhanced Infant Nutrition

The decision to breast- or bottle-feed the infant is usually made prior to or during pregnancy. Providing factual information with an opportunity for questions and answers early in pregnancy will facilitate a decision best suited to the client's needs and lifestyle.

INTRAPARTUM MATERNAL ASSESSMENT

During the intrapartum period, an initial physical assessment should be done on admission to the labor room, and findings should be compared with those of the prenatal period. The order of the assessment will vary based on presenting signs of labor.

Maternal Physical Assessment

Equipment Needed

- Bed with pillow
- Sterile examination glove
- Lubricant
- Electronic fetal monitor or Doppler
- Nitrazine paper
- Reflex hammer

Subjective Data: Focus Questions

History of prenatal care? Gravida? Para? Age? Estimated date of confinement (EDC)? When did contractions begin? Rupture of membranes? Color of vaginal fluid? Vaginal bleeding and amount? Frequency and duration of contractions? Problems with this pregnancy? Duration and outcome of previous labors? Childbirth preparation? Blood type and Rh status? Concurrent disease?

Objective Data: Assessment Techniques

Abdominal Assessment

INSPECTION

Have client completely undress except for gown. Place in a supine position with head slightly elevated. Knees and hips should be flexed with feet resting on mattress. Examination with the client in this position should be performed as rapidly as possible to prevent supine hypotension or fetal compromise.

PROCEDURE	NORMAL FINDINGS	DEVIATIONS FROM NORMAL
*Inspect **abdomen** for the following:*		
• Uterine size (see Fig. 19–5)	• Large variation; fundus just below xiphoid process	• Uterus small or large for gestational age may indicate fetal malformations.
• Uterine shape	• Fetal outline longitudinal	• Fetal outline horizontal indicates the presentation of the baby may be transverse or breech.

PALPATION

With client on back and head slightly elevated, place fingertips on fundus. During a contraction, the fundus becomes firm. Client should relate when she feels a contraction begin and when it ends. Time seconds from beginning to end of contractions (duration). Calculate elapsed time from beginning of one contraction to beginning of another (frequency). Do this for several contractions in sequence to determine regularity. During contraction, gently push in on uterus with fingertips and note degree to which uterus indents (intensity). A large amount of subcutaneous tissue over the uterus may interfere with accurate assessment of intensity. Palpate several contractions in a row. To palpate bladder, gently push in on abdomen directly above symphysis pubis and release. Note degree of resistance met.

PROCEDURE	NORMAL FINDINGS	DEVIATIONS FROM NORMAL
Palpate uterus for the following:		
• Frequency of contractions	• As labor progresses, contractions gradually get closer together, in a regular pattern progressing to every 2–3 minutes; may be less frequent during second stage.	• Irregular pattern; more frequent than every 2 minutes may cause placental insufficiency for the fetus to get sufficient oxygenation during labor.

Maternal Physical Assessment

Objective Data: Assessment Techniques (continued)

PROCEDURE	NORMAL FINDINGS	DEVIATIONS FROM NORMAL
• Duration of contractions	• Gradually increases to 60–90 seconds as labor progresses	• No increase; duration > 90 seconds may deplete fetal oxygenation reserves.
• Intensity of contractions	• Gradually become stronger, uterus feels firm (rocklike); internal pressure monitor 40–60 mm Hg.	• No increase; pressure > 60 mm Hg is seen with hypertonic contractions.
Note: Contraction frequency and duration may be monitored with an electronic fetal monitor tocodynamometer. Initial assessment of contraction frequency and duration may be performed by palpation. Accurate intensity can only be determined, however, with an intrauterine pressure catheter.		
Palpate above symphysis pubis for the bladder.	Soft, spongy	Bouncy, full, distended is seen with over-distention of the bladder.

AUSCULTATION
Locate FHR (see Prenatal section) and apply external fetal monitor ultrasound transducer or Doppler. FHR must be monitored every 5 minutes during the second stage of labor. High-risk pregnancies with ruptured amniotic fluid membranes should be monitored with internal electrodes to assess fetal well-being accurately.

PROCEDURE	NORMAL FINDINGS	DEVIATIONS FROM NORMAL
Monitor FHR for the following:		
• Baseline rate (must be determined by a 10-minute strip)	• 120–160 bpm	• < 120 or > 160 bpm for a 10-minute period may indicate fetal distress.
• Baseline variability (measurable only with internal fetal electrode)	• 5–25 bpm	• < 5 bpm for longer than 20 minutes and not associated with maternal medication
• Periodic changes	• Periodic acceleration (increased FHR with fetal movement, stimulation, or contractions); early-onset deceleration (mirrors contraction and occurs in late first stage and second stage of labor)	• Periodic deceleration; decreased FHR occurs with contractions; repetitive variable decelerations are seen with cord compression; late decelerations are seen in fetal distress; prolonged or slow return to baseline and associated loss of variability may be seen in fetal distress

Perineal Assessment
INSPECTION
With client supine, have her rest her feet on the bed with knees and hips flexed. Instruct client to relax and separate knees.
If discharge is noted, obtain specimen to assess for ruptured membranes with Nitrazine paper.

Maternal Physical Assessment

PROCEDURE	NORMAL FINDINGS	DEVIATIONS FROM NORMAL
Observe **perineum** *for the following:*		
• Lesions	• None	• Vesicles could indicate genital herpes; genital warts, open sores may be seen with sexually transmitted infections.
• Discharge	• Bloody mucus; clear or milky fluid; amniotic fluid will turn Nitrazine paper blue	• Bright red blood is seen with placenta previa; purulent fluid; green or brown fluid may indicate meconium stool in utero, which puts the fetus at risk for meconium aspiration at delivery. Lubricant or blood may give a false-positive result with Nitrazine paper.
• Swelling	• May be present in second stage of labor	• Present before second stage of labor
Observe **perineal area** *for the following:*		
• Shape	• As fetal head descends, perineum flattens and bulges.	
• Fetal parts	• Occiput becomes visible during second stage of labor.	• Fetal hand or foot may indicate breech presentation; loop of umbilical cord visible on the perineum puts the fetus at high risk and requires immediate cesarean section

PALPATION

Have client separate knees, and instruct her to relax perineum. Put on sterile examination glove, and lubricate index and middle fingers. Gently insert fingers into vagina and palpate cervix and fetal presenting part. Insert finger between cervix and presenting part, and rotate entire circumference of cervix. This examination should be performed on admission and thereafter only when behavior and contraction pattern indicate progression of labor.

PROCEDURE	NORMAL FINDINGS	DEVIATIONS FROM NORMAL
Palpate **cervix** *for the following:*		
• Position	• In early labor, cervix may be in posterior vaginal vault; it becomes more anterior as labor progresses.	
• Effacement	• *Primipara:* Effacement before dilatation *Multipara:* Effacement and dilatation simultaneous	• Swelling of part or all of cervix occurs when the patient begins pushing before the cervix is completely dilated.
• Dilatation (in cm)	• *Primipara:* Average 1 cm/hr; may be slower in early phase *Multipara:* Average 1.5 cm/hr	• Failure to progress with active labor longer than 24 hours; complete dilatation in < 3 hours of labor
Palpate **presenting part of the fetus** *for the following:*		
• Amniotic membrane	• If intact, can be felt over presenting part; may rupture prior to or during labor	

Objective Data: Assessment Techniques (continued)

PROCEDURE	NORMAL FINDINGS	DEVIATIONS FROM NORMAL
• Presentation	• Cephalic; should feel skull, suture lines, and one or both fontanelles (Fig. 19–7); caput succedaneum may mask landmarks.	• Breech: soft tissue, anus, or testicles; other small parts such as hands, feet seen in breech presentation
• Position	• Cephalic; posterior fontanelle felt in anterior position, anterior fontanelle in posterior position	• Anterior fontanelle in anterior position; fontanelles in transverse position
• Station (Fig. 19–8)	• *Primipara:* 0 station; gradually descends during second stage *Multipara:* May be –1 station or higher at onset of labor	• Failure to descend to 0 station during first stage of labor; failure to descend during second stage with pushing longer than 2 hours is seen in failure to progress, which requires cesarean section
• Umbilical cord	• Not palpable	• May feel loop or pulsations in the umbilical cord, which requires immediate cesarean section
Note: If painless, bright red vaginal bleeding occurs, vaginal examination should be omitted. If fetal gestational age is less than 34 weeks and membranes have ruptured with no evidence of labor, vaginal examination should be omitted.		

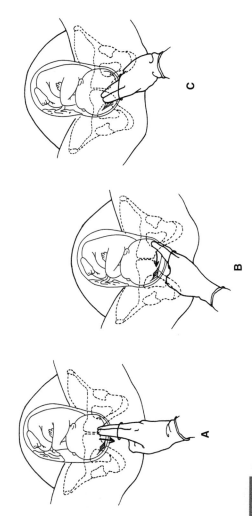

FIGURE 19-7 Assessment of fetal position and station. (*A*) Palpate the sagittal suture and assess station. (*B*) Identify posterior fontanelle. (*C*) Identify anterior fontanelle.

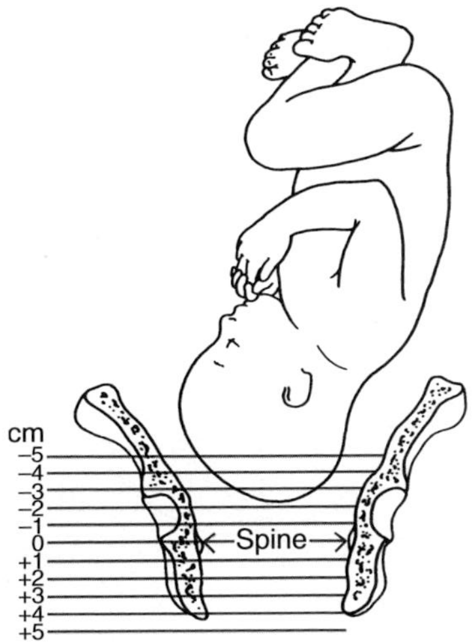

FIGURE 19-8 Measuring station of the fetal head while it is descending.

Peripheral Vascular Assessment

INSPECTION

With client in semi-Fowler position, observe face, hands, legs, and feet.

PROCEDURE	NORMAL FINDINGS	DEVIATIONS FROM NORMAL
Observe **face** *for the following:*		
• Color	• Pink	• Red, pale
• Edema	• None	• Periorbital edema
Observe **extremities** *for the following:*		
• Color	• Pink	• Pale, blue seen with cyanosis
• Swelling	• Dependent in ankles	• Swelling in the tibia or hands, not relieved by elevating

AUSCULTATION

With client in a sidelying position, auscultate blood pressure (BP) between contractions.

PROCEDURE	NORMAL FINDINGS	DEVIATIONS FROM NORMAL
Auscultate BP every hour or more often as indicated.	BP < 140/90 mm Hg. May see BP increase during contractions	BP ≥ 140/90 mm Hg or increase of 30 mm Hg systolic or 15 mm Hg diastolic over prenatal baseline seen in PIH

Maternal Physical Assessment

PERCUSSION

PROCEDURE	NORMAL FINDINGS	DEVIATIONS FROM NORMAL
Percuss extremities for reflexes and clonus.	See Chapter 17 for normal findings.	Hyperreflexia or clonus seen in PIH

Behavioral Assessment

PROCEDURE	NORMAL FINDINGS	DEVIATIONS FROM NORMAL
Observe for behavior changes: • Early labor (1–4 cm) • Active labor (4–7 cm) • Transition (7–10 cm)	• Excited, happy • Cooperative; increased dependence on support person • Irritable, inner focused, hopeless	• Irrational • Uncooperative, psychotic • Confused

Possible Collaborative Problems

Preeclampsia/eclampsia   Hypertension
Bleeding disorders   Fetal distress
Placenta previa   Labor dystocia
Abruptio placentae   Cephalopelvic disproportion
Uterine rupture   Premature labor
Fetal malpresentation   Fetal malposition

TEACHING TIPS FOR SELECTED NURSING DIAGNOSES

Nursing Diagnosis: Acute pain related to uterine contractions

Instruct and demonstrate relaxation techniques. Provide feedback on muscle relaxation. Offer encouragement and support. Provide comfort measures such as gentle massage; temperature control; clean, dry, and wrinkle-free linens; ice chips or lip lubricant. The laboring woman should be encouraged to assume varying positions of comfort and to ambulate unless complications contraindicate this. Provide analgesics as needed.

Nursing Diagnosis: Fear related to unfamiliar environment, pain, and concern for fetal well-being

Orient to surroundings. Provide short and simple explanation for all procedures and encourage questions. Provide evidence of fetal well-being (monitor data). Encourage support person to stay with client. Client should not be left alone during active labor.

Nursing Diagnosis: Risk for Fluid Volume Deficit related to increased muscle activity, increased respiratory rate, nausea and vomiting, and decreased gastric motility or absorption

Offer small amounts of fluids such as ice chips or popsicles. Avoid solid foods, which are difficult to digest and often promote vomiting. Consider antiemetics for persistent vomiting. Monitor for dehydration or decreased placental perfusion. Administer intravenous fluids as indicated.

POSTPARTUM MATERNAL ASSESSMENT

The postpartum period begins with the delivery of the placenta and lasts an average of 6 weeks, during which time all body systems return to prepregnant levels. Some changes are rapid and others occur over time. During the first 24 hours many changes occur and frequent assessment is essential.

Changes occurring as an expected part of postpartum recovery are identified as *normal findings*. The reader is referred to Chapter 3 for a more detailed description of technique for assessing various body systems.

Subjective Data: Focus Questions

Problems during pregnancy? Labor—induction, augmentation, length of labor? Gravida, para? Method of delivery? Size of baby? Anesthesia/analgesia? Concurrent disease?

Objective Data: Assessment Techniques

PROCEDURE	NORMAL FINDINGS	DEVIATIONS FROM NORMAL
Monitor the following:		
• Temperature	• 100.4°F (38°C) in first 24 hours	• Higher than 100.4°F (38°C) in first 24 hours or 100.4°F (38°C) and above on any 2 of the first 10 days postpartum seen in puerperal infection
• Blood pressure	• No change from prepregnant levels	• PIH can occur up to 48 hours postpartum; persistent elevation of blood pressure from PIH beyond 48 hours
• Pulse	• Bradycardia (50–70 bpm) for 6–10 days	• Tachycardia; preexisting hypertension may be difficult to control; postural hypotension may occur when assuming the upright position after delivery.
• Weight	• Initial 10- to 12-lb loss; 10- to 20-lb loss in next 6–8 weeks	
• Behavior	*First 2–3 days postpartum:* Preoccupied with food and sleep; passive and dependent	• Psychosis is noted when patient is unable to care for herself and newborn.

Objective Data: Assessment Techniques (continued)

PROCEDURE	NORMAL FINDINGS	DEVIATIONS FROM NORMAL
	After 2–3 days postpartum: Increased interest in control of body functions, mothering skills; gradually includes others in social circle; transient depression, let down feeling, cries easily	• Failure to assume maternal role; prolonged depression; unrealistic expectations of newborn

Breast Assessment

INSPECTION
With client in supine or semi-Fowler position, inspect breasts.

PROCEDURE	NORMAL FINDINGS	DEVIATIONS FROM NORMAL
*Inspect the following in **nonnursing mother:***		
• Size	• May be enlarged initially; will gradually return to prepregnant size	• Full, engorged breasts
• Shape	• May sag	

Maternal Physical Assessment

Objective Data: Assessment Techniques (continued)

PROCEDURE	NORMAL FINDINGS	DEVIATIONS FROM NORMAL
• Color	• May have striae	• Localized redness, tenderness may be seen with mastitis.
*Inspect the following in **nursing mother:***		
• Size	• Enlarged	• Heat, localized pain
• Texture	• Increased nodularity	• Blisters, cracked, bleeding
• Nipples	• Everted, tender	• Purulent, bloody discharge may indicate infection.
• Discharge	• Colostrum, thin milk, may leak between feedings	

PALPATION
Gently palpate all quadrants of each breast.

PROCEDURE	NORMAL FINDINGS	DEVIATIONS FROM NORMAL
*Palpate **nonnursing mother** for:*		
• Tenderness	• Soft	• Full, tender
• Texture	• Nodular	• Lumps, masses may be seen with clogged breast ducts

Objective Data: Assessment Techniques (continued)

PROCEDURE	NORMAL FINDINGS	DEVIATIONS FROM NORMAL
*Palpate in **nursing mother** for:*		
• Tenderness	• Full, slightly tender	• Painful breasts are seen with mastitis.
• Texture	• Small lumps	• Hardened area, most often in upper, outer quadrant, indicates clogged milk ducts and/or mastitis.

Abdominal Assessment

INSPECTION

Place client in a supine position with knees extended and head slightly elevated on a pillow.

PROCEDURE	NORMAL FINDINGS	DEVIATIONS FROM NORMAL
Inspect abdomen for the following:		
• Size	• Uterus visible, outlined unless obese; gradually recedes to prepregnant size with exercise	• Distention seen when patient is unable to void and bladder becomes distended
• Color	• Striae dark red or purple; recede to silvery or white and become smaller	• Yellow, pale
• Texture	• Loose and flabby	• Dry, cracked

PALPATION

Have client empty bladder and assume supine position. Place one hand over lower abdomen above symphysis pubis to support uterus. With the fingertips of the other hand, locate the fundus. Start in the midline, slightly above the umbilicus, and press in and down. Work fingers gradually down toward the symphysis pubis until the fundus of the uterus is located. It should feel like a firm, round ball, similar to a grapefruit. Measure the distance above or below the umbilicus in finger breadths (Figs. 19–9 and 19–10). If the uterus is not firm, gently massage until firm, then gently push down on fundus and observe for expression of clots from the vagina.

PROCEDURE	NORMAL FINDINGS	DEVIATIONS FROM NORMAL
Palpate fundus for the following:		
• Location	• Midline	• Deviated to left or right could indicate a distended bladder
• Consistency	• Firm; boggy to firm with massage; smooth surface	• Boggy; does not stay firm after massage may indicate uterine atony and/or retained placental fragments
• Height	• Halfway between umbilicus and symphysis immediately after delivery; within 12 hours, at the umbilicus or 1 cm above; descends 1 cm/day	• More than 1 cm above umbilicus; failure to descend
• Expression of clots	• Small clots or increased flow with massage	• Large clots; continuous trickle of blood with firm fundus indicates an unrepaired laceration.

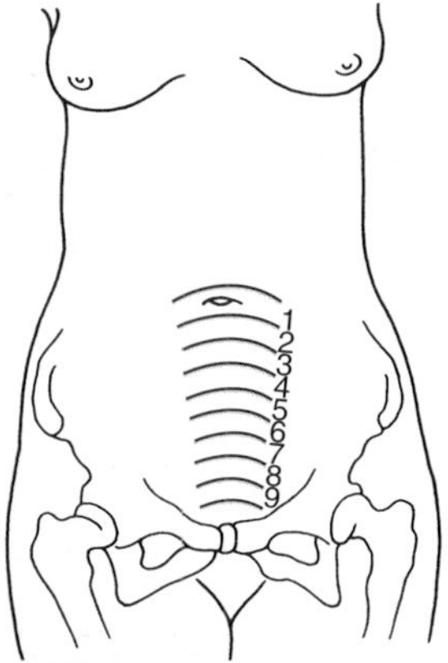

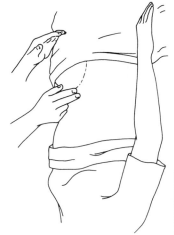

FIGURE 19–10 Measurement of the descent of the fundus. The fundus is located two finger breadths below the umbilicus.

FIGURE 19–9 Involution of the uterus. The height of the fundus decreases about one finger breadth (approximately 1 cm) each day.

Face and Extremities Assessment

INSPECTION

To inspect the face and extremities, the supine position is preferred. Adequate light must be available.

PROCEDURE	NORMAL FINDINGS	DEVIATIONS FROM NORMAL
*Inspect **face** for the following:*		
• Color	• Petechiae after prolonged second stage of labor	• Paleness may be seen with anemia.
• Edema	• None	• Periorbital
*Inspect **extremities** for the following:*		
• Color	• Pink; red tones visible under dark pigmentation	• Dusky, mottled color indicates decreased oxygenation.
• Edema	• Slight pedal edema	• Pitting edema, edema of hands seen with PIH

PALPATION

With legs extended, gently palpate calves. Place one hand on knee, and gently dorsiflex each foot.

PROCEDURE	NORMAL FINDINGS	DEVIATIONS FROM NORMAL
*Palpate **calves** for the following:*		
• Tenderness	• Calves may have generalized muscle tenderness	• Calf with localized tenderness or pain seen with deep vein thrombosis

Objective Data: Assessment Techniques (continued)

PROCEDURE	NORMAL FINDINGS	DEVIATIONS FROM NORMAL
• Texture	• Smooth	• Knots or lumps in calf
• Homans sign	• Negative (no pain)	• Positive (pain in calf) may indicate deep vein thrombosis.

PERCUSSION

Pregnancy-related seizures can occur for up to 48 hours postpartum. Reflexes should be assessed for hyperreflexia and clonus during this time. See Chapter 17 for technique.

Bladder Assessment

INSPECTION

Have client void within 4 hours after delivery or sooner if there are bleeding problems during the immediate postpartum period.

PROCEDURE	NORMAL FINDINGS	DEVIATIONS FROM NORMAL
Inspect voiding for the following:		
• Amount	• 200 mL or more each voiding; diuresis of greater than 2000 mL in first 24 hours	• Less than 100 mL per voiding; unable to void
• Color	• Yellow, clear; may be mixed with lochia	• Dark, cloudy, bloody urine may indicate urinary tract infection.

PALPATION

Have client empty bladder and assume supine position. Palpate for bladder above the symphysis pubis. If unable to void within 4 hours after delivery or if bladder is full, empty bladder with a catheter.

PROCEDURE	NORMAL FINDINGS	DEVIATIONS FROM NORMAL
Palpate bladder.	Nonpalpable	Spongy mass in lower abdomen

Perineum Assessment

INSPECTION

Have client turn to side and flex upper leg. Place one hand on upper buttock and gently separate so perineum is visible.

PROCEDURE	NORMAL FINDINGS	DEVIATIONS FROM NORMAL
Inspect perineum for the following: • Approximation of episiotomy • Color • Swelling • Lochia	• Skin edges meet. • Pink to red • Generalized swelling for 12–24 hours • *Color: days 1–3:* rubra (dark red); small clots may also be expelled. *Days 4–10:* Serosa (pinkish red) *Days 11–20:* Alba (creamy yellow) *Amount: days 1–10:* Vaginal discharge requires 6–10 pads per day (moderate flow).	• Skin edges gape. • Purple, mottled • Localized swelling with increased pain indicates hematoma. • More than 8 peri pads per day or saturated peri pad in 1 hour seen in postpartum hemorrhage; purulent; large clots; return to dark red after several days

Objective Data: Assessment Techniques (continued)

PROCEDURE	NORMAL FINDINGS	DEVIATIONS FROM NORMAL
	Days 11–20: Decreased amount of vaginal discharge still requires pad change (less than 6–8 pads per day).	
• Odor	• None; musky scent	• Foul odor with bacterial infections
• Hemorrhoids	• Small; nontender	• Swollen, painful

Possible Collaborative Problems

Urinary retention — Retained placenta
Breast engorgement/abscess — Infections
Preeclampsia/eclampsia — Exacerbation of preexisting medical conditions
Hemorrhage — Heart conditions
Uterine atony — Hypertension
Hematoma — Hyperglycemia
Cervical/vaginal lacerations — Hypoglycemia

TEACHING TIPS FOR SELECTED NURSING DIAGNOSES

Nursing Diagnosis: Disturbed Sleep Pattern related to fatigue and increased need for sleep

All teaching sessions should be brief and reinforced with written information about infant care and self-care (eg, care of breasts). Encourage mother to sleep when baby sleeps. Advise mother to avoid strenuous activities until 6-week postpartum physical examination. Enlist help of other family members.

Maternal Physical Assessment

Nursing Diagnosis: Readiness for Enhanced Infant Care and Self-Care

☐ Demonstrate infant care and allow time for mother to practice. A follow-up phone call or home visit can assist in evaluation and reinforcement of information taught. Include father whenever possible.

Nursing Diagnosis: Readiness for Enhanced Family Coping related to addition of family member and role changes

☐ Discuss plans for incorporating new member into family. Offer suggestions to decrease sibling jealousy. Explore plans for infant care, division of labor, and changes in activities of daily living.

Nursing Diagnosis: Risk for Impaired Parent/Infant Attachment related to unrealistic expectations of self

☐ Discuss normal growth and development of infant; emphasize things infant can do. Provide early and continued contact of infant and parents to maximize bonding. Teach parents skills needed to meet infant's physical and psychological needs.

Nursing Diagnosis: Impaired Parenting related to inadequate skills, unrealistic expectation of infant, stress, lack of adequate support

☐ Be aware of risk factors for child abuse/neglect that may be evident during postpartal period. Explore resources available to parents, and make appropriate referrals for follow-up or support groups.

Nursing Diagnosis: Ineffective Breast-feeding related to lack of knowledge

☐ Clarify misconceptions, and provide instructions or proper technique. Assist with first feedings and problems such as soreness or difficulty latching on to breasts, etc.

Nursing Diagnosis: Ineffective Infant Feeding Pattern

May use nipple with larger hole. Hold infant in upright position during feeding. Burp infant often (after every ½ oz). Needs frequent feedings with careful monitoring of intake and weight gain. May need to teach parents gavage feedings. If so, infant will attempt to nurse at each feeding and be gavage-fed remaining formula/breast milk.

Nursing Diagnosis: Interrupted Breast-feeding related to change in daily routine lifestyle

To continue breast milk supply, mother should pump breasts at intervals similar to infant feeding patterns. Milk letdown is optimal immediately after infant contact. Mother should be relaxed and have privacy. If possible, both breasts should be emptied at each feeding. Increased fluid consumption is needed for milk production. To terminate breast-feeding, mother should avoid any stimulation of breasts. Encourage use of good support bra. Painful engorgement may be alleviated with analgesics and intermittent ice packs to breasts.

20

Initial Newborn Physical Assessment

Equipment Needed

- Gloves
- Stethoscope
- Tape measure

Subjective Data: Focus Questions

Prenatal history: Gravida? Para? Estimated date of confinement (EDC)? Gestational age? Maternal history? Risk factors? Prenatal exposure to drugs? Complications? Blood type? Maternal testing?

Labor and delivery history: Date, time, type of delivery? Prolonged labor? Narcotics? Time of rupture of membranes? Intrapartum complications? Shoulder dystocia?

Delivery history: Apgar scores? Respiratory effort? Resuscitation efforts? Medications? Procedures performed? Evidence of injury? Void? Stool?

Social history: Parent interaction? Significant others? Cultural variations? Type of infant feeding? Male circumcision requested?

Objective Data: Assessment Techniques

Immediately after delivery the general state of the newborn should be evaluated while the infant is supine under a radiant warmer with the temperature probe attached to the abdomen. Apgar scores (Table 20–1) are assigned at 1 and 5 minutes after delivery.

APGAR SCORE ASSESSMENT

PROCEDURE	NORMAL FINDINGS	DEVIATIONS FROM NORMAL
Auscultate apical pulse.	>100 bpm	<100 bpm indicates bradycardia; absent heart beat indicates fetal demise.
Inspect chest and abdomen for respiratory effort.	Crying	Absent, slow, irregular respirations
Stroke back or soles of feet.	Crying	Delayed neurological function may be seen in grimace, no response.
Inspect muscle tone by extending legs and arms. Observe degree of flexion and resistance in extremities.	Extremities flexed, active movement	Moderate degree of flexion, limp may indicate neurological deficits.
Inspect body and extremities for skin color.	Full body pink, acrocyanosis	Cyanosis, pale
Determine total Apgar score at 1 and 5 minutes after birth (see Table 20–1).	8–10 points	<8 points may indicate poor transition from intrauterine into extrauterine life.

TABLE 20–1 APGAR SCORE

	Scores 0	Scores 1	Scores 2
Heart rate	Absent	<100 bpm	>100 bpm
Respiratory rate	Absent	Slow, irregular	Good lusty cry
Reflex irritability	No response	Grimace, some motion	Cry, cough
Muscle tone	Flaccid, limp	Flexion of extremities	Active flexion
Color	Cyanotic, pale	Pink body, acrocyanosis	Pink body, pink extremities

ASSESSMENT OF VITAL SIGNS AND MEASUREMENTS

After the Apgar score has been assigned, a thorough assessment including vital signs, measurements, and gestational age assessment is performed.

PROCEDURE	NORMAL FINDINGS	DEVIATIONS FROM NORMAL
Monitor axillary temperature.	97.5–99°F (36.4–37.2°C)	<97.5°F (<36.4°C): hypothermia, which may indicate sepsis >99°F (>37.2°C): hyperthermia (Consider infection or improper monitoring of temperature probe.)
Inspect and auscultate lung sounds.	Easy, nonlabored, clear lungs bilaterally	Labored breathing, nasal flaring, rhonchi, rales, retractions, grunting
Monitor respiratory rate.	Rate: 30–60 breaths/min	Rate <30 or >60 breaths/min is seen with respiratory distress.
Auscultate apical pulse.	Regular 120–160 bpm (100 sleeping, 180 crying)	Irregular <100 or >180 bpm may indicate cardiac abnormalities.
Weigh newborn unclothed using a newborn scale (Fig. 20–1).	2500–4000 g	<2500 g >4000 g
Measure length.	44–55 cm	<44 cm >55 cm

Initial Newborn Physical Assessment

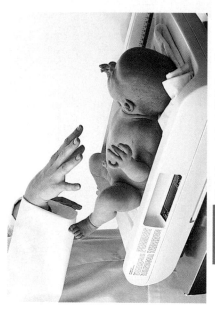

FIGURE 20-1 Weighing an infant. (© B. Proud.)

ASSESSMENT OF VITAL SIGNS AND MEASUREMENTS (continued)

PROCEDURE	NORMAL FINDINGS	DEVIATIONS FROM NORMAL
Measure head circumference (see Fig. 4–4).	33–35.5 cm	<33 cm >35.5 cm
Measure chest circumference.	30–33 cm (1–2 cm < head)	<29 cm >34 cm

ASSESSMENT OF GESTATIONAL AGE

The newborn's gestational age is examined within 4 hours after birth to identify any potential age-related problems that may occur within the next few hours. The newborn's neuromuscular and physical maturity are examined. After examination, boxes on the New Ballard Scale (Fig. 20–2 and Fig. 20–3) that most closely describe and depict the newborn's neuromuscular and physical maturity are marked, and scores are assigned to assess gestational age.

PROCEDURE	NORMAL FINDINGS	DEVIATIONS FROM NORMAL
Assess *neuromuscular maturity* (see Fig. 20–2) by performing each of the following with the newborn in the supine position: • Posture (with newborn undisturbed)	• Arms and legs flexed	• Arms and legs limp, extended away from body seen with premature infants

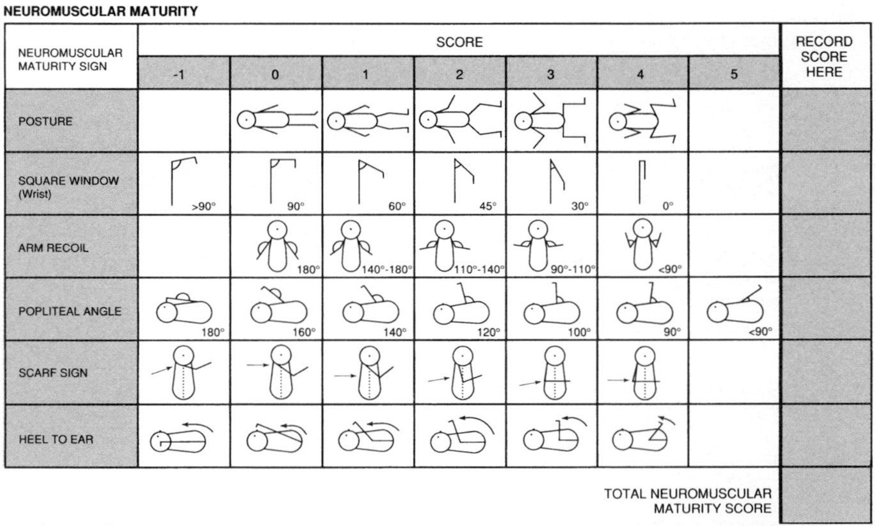

NEUROMUSCULAR MATURITY

FIGURE 20-2 Neuromuscular maturity for the maturational assessment of gestational age (New Ballard Scale).

PHYSICAL MATURITY

PHYSICAL MATURITY SIGN	-1	0	1	2	3	4	5	RECORD SCORE HERE
SKIN	sticky friable transparent	gelatinous red translucent	smooth pink visible veins	superficial peeling &/or rash, few veins	cracking pale areas rare veins	parchment deep cracking no vessels	leathery cracked wrinkled	
LANUGO	none	sparse	abundant	thinning	bald areas	mostly bald		
PLANTAR SURFACE	heel-toe 40-50 mm:-1 <40 mm:-2	>50 mm no crease	faint red marks	anterior transverse crease only	creases ant. 2/3	creases over entire sole		
BREAST	imperceptible	barely perceptible	flat areola no bud	stippled areola 1-2 mm bud	raised areola 3-4 mm bud	full areola 5-10 mm bud		
EYE/EAR	lids fused loosely: -1 tightly: -2	lids open pinna flat stays folded	sl. curved pinna; soft; slow recoil	well-curved pinna; soft but ready recoil	formed & firm instant recoil	thick cartilage ear stiff		
GENITALS (Male)	scrotum flat, smooth	scrotum empty faint rugae	testes in upper canal rare rugae	testes descending few rugae	testes down good rugae	testes pendulous deep rugae		
GENITALS (Female)	clitoris prominent & labia flat	prominent clitoris & small labia minora	prominent clitoris & enlarging minora	majora & minora equally prominent	majora large minora small	majora cover clitoris & minora		

SCORE: Neuromuscular _____ Physical _____ Total _____

TOTAL PHYSICAL MATURITY SCORE

MATURITY RATING

score	weeks
-10	20
-5	22
0	24
5	26
10	28
15	30
20	32
25	34
30	36
35	38
40	40
45	42
50	44

GESTATIONAL AGE (weeks)

By dates _____
By ultrasound _____
By exam _____

Initial Newborn Physical Assessment

FIGURE 20-3 Physical maturity and maturity rating scale for the maturational assessment of gestational age (New Ballard Scale).

ASSESSMENT OF GESTATIONAL AGE (continued)

PROCEDURE	NORMAL FINDINGS	DEVIATIONS FROM NORMAL
• Square window: bend wrist toward ventral forearm until resistance is met. Measure angle (see Fig. 20–4).	• 0–30°	• Premature infants may have square window measurement of >30°

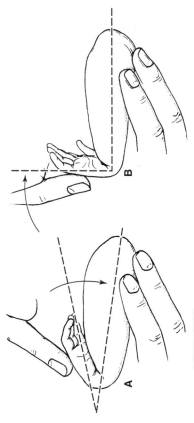

FIGURE 20–4 Square window sign. (*A*) Term infant. (*B*) Preterm infant.

ASSESSMENT OF GESTATIONAL AGE (continued)

PROCEDURE	NORMAL FINDINGS	DEVIATIONS FROM NORMAL
• Arm recoil: bilaterally flex elbows up with hands next to shoulders and hold approximately 5 seconds; extend arms down next to side, release; observe elbow angle and recoil.	• Elbow angle <90°, rapid recoil to flexed state	• Elbow angle >110°, delayed recoil seen in premature infants
• Popliteal angle: flex thigh on top of abdomen; push behind ankle and extend lower leg up toward head until resistance is met; measure angle behind knee.	• <100°	• >100°
• Scarf sign: Lift arm across chest toward opposite shoulder until resistance is met; note location of elbow in relation to middle of chest (Fig. 20–5).	• Elbow position less than midline of chest	• Elbow position midline of chest or greater, toward opposite shoulder seen in premature infants

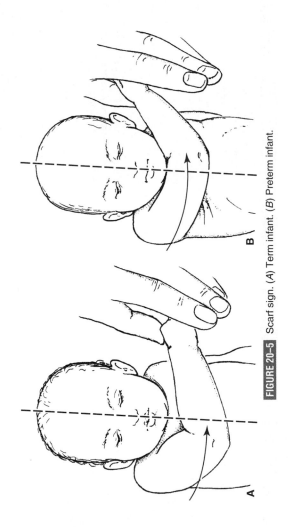

FIGURE 20–5 Scarf sign. (*A*) Term infant. (*B*) Preterm infant.

ASSESSMENT OF GESTATIONAL AGE (continued)

PROCEDURE	NORMAL FINDINGS	DEVIATIONS FROM NORMAL
• Heel to ear: pull leg toward ear on same side, keeping buttocks flat on bed; inspect popliteal angle and proximity of heel to ear.	• Popliteal angle <90°, heel distal from ear	• Popliteal angle >90°, heel proximal to ear seen in premature infants
*Assess **physical maturity** (see Fig. 20–3) by performing the following:*		
• Observe skin.	• Parchment, few or no vessels on abdomen, cracking in ankle area especially	• Translucent, visible veins; rash; leathery, wrinkled skin seen in postmature infants
• Inspect for lanugo.	• Thinning, balding on back, shoulders, knees	• Abundant amount of fine hair on face seen in premature infants
• Inspect plantar surface of feet for creases.	• Creases on anterior two thirds or entire sole	• Anterior transverse crease on sole only, no creases; fewer creases indicate prematurity.
• Inspect and palpate breast bud tissue with middle finger and forefinger; measure bud in millimeters.	• Raised areola, full areola	• Absence of bud tissue, bud <3 mm seen in premature infants
• Observe ear cartilage in upper pinna for curving. Fold pinna down toward side of head and release; observe recoil of ear.	• Pinna well curved, cartilage formed, instant recoil	• Pinna slightly curved, slow recoil seen in premature infants

Initial Newborn Physical Assessment

ASSESSMENT OF GESTATIONAL AGE (continued)

PROCEDURE	NORMAL FINDINGS	DEVIATIONS FROM NORMAL
• Inspect genitals. *Male:* Observe scrotum for rugae and palpate position of testes. *Female:* Observe labia majora, labia minora, and clitoris.	• *Male:* Deep rugae; testes positioned down in scrotal sac *Female:* Labia majora cover labia minora and clitoris.	• *Male:* Decreased presence of rugae; testes positioned down inguinal canal *Female:* Labia majora and labia minora equally prominent, clitoris prominent seen with premature infants
Determine **score rating:** On Figure 20–2 and Figure 20–3, mark the boxes that most closely represent each observation.		
• Add the total scores from both tables.	• Total score: 35–45 points	• Total score: <35 points or >45 points
• Using Figure 20–2, plot total score in column on right-hand side of page; this score corresponds to the number in weeks on the maturity rating scale; circle the number of weeks.	• Gestational age: 38–42 weeks	• Gestational age: <38 or >42 weeks
• Using gestational weeks assessed, plot weight, length, and head circumference on Figures 20–6 through 20–9.	• 10th through 90th percentile is appropriate for gestational age (AGA).	• Less than the 10th percentile (small for gestational age), greater than the 90th percentile (large for gestational age)

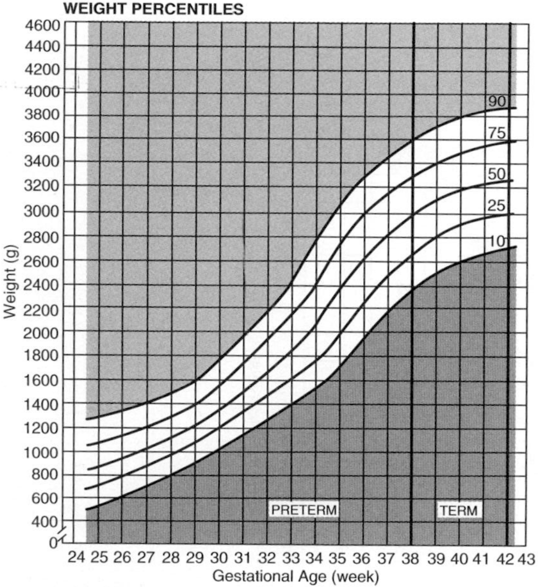

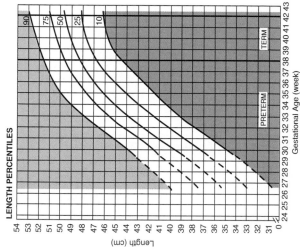

WEIGHT PERCENTILES

FIGURE 20-6 Weight percentiles for newborn infants.

LENGTH PERCENTILES

FIGURE 20-7 Length percentiles for newborn infants.

Initial Newborn Physical Assessment

HEAD CIRCUMFERENCE PERCENTILES

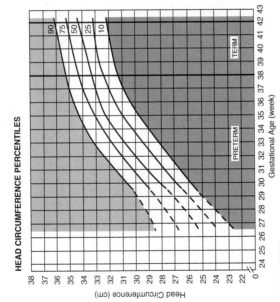

FIGURE 20–8 Head circumference percentiles for newborn infants.

CLASSIFICATION OF INFANT*	Weight	Length	Head Circ.
Large for Gestational Age (LGA) (>90th percentile)			
Appropriate for Gestational Age (AGA) (10th to 90th percentile)			
Small for Gestational Age (SGA) (<10th percentile)			

*Place an "X" in the appropriate box (LGA, AGA or SGA) for weight, for length and for head circumference.

FIGURE 20–9 Classification of infant for gestational age.

PHYSICAL ASSESSMENT

In addition to the Apgar assessment and the gestational age assessment, the nurse also performs a thorough head-to-toe physical assessment. The head-to-toe assessment is reviewed at the end of each chapter under Pediatric Variations.

PROCEDURE	NORMAL FINDINGS	DEVIATIONS FROM NORMAL
Assess **respiratory system.**	30–60 breaths/min. Unlabored, chest/abdominal movement synchronized, lung sounds clear bilaterally, transient rales, nose appears normal with patent nares bilaterally, nose breathers.	<30 or >60 breaths/min. Retractions, nasal flaring, grunting, tachypnea, see-saw movement of chest, apnea, decreased breath sounds indicate respiratory distress.
Assess **cardiovascular system.**	120–160 bpm: regular rhythm; color pink, acrocyanosis; capillary refill <2 seconds; brachial/femoral pulses present, equal bilaterally	<110 or >180 bpm. Weak pulse, tachycardia, bradycardia, persistent murmur, cyanosis indicates congenital heart defects. Unequal pulses may be seen with coarctation of the aorta.
Assess **neurological system.**	Alert when awake; normal, lusty cry Reflexes: see Neurologic Assessment, Chapter 17.	Asymmetrical, weak, or absent response to stimulation seen with neurological deficits
Assess *sensory system.* • Ears	• Symmetrical, well formed, parallel to outer canthus of eye, infant responds to sound.	• Preauricle dimple or tag, low-set ears often seen in infants with Down syndrome

PHYSICAL ASSESSMENT (continued)

PROCEDURE	NORMAL FINDINGS	DEVIATIONS FROM NORMAL
• Eyes	• Symmetrical, alert, clear sclera; iris slate gray or brown, infant follows objects to midline; eyelids have transient edema, absence of tears.	• Unequal pupils, purulent discharge seen with sexually transmitted infections (gonorrhea, *Chlamydia*)
Assess musculoskeletal system.	Tone flexed, extremities resist when extended and return to flexed state when released	Limp, flaccid, poor tone may be seen in infants with neurological deficits.
• Head	• Anterior fontanelle (Fig. 20–10) has diamond shape, 3–4 cm × 2–3 cm, soft, flat. Posterior fontanelle (Fig. 20–11) has triangular shape, 1–2 cm. Head is round with mild to moderate molding. Sutures are palpable, overriding. A common variation is *caput succedaneum* (Fig. 20–12, A). Face is symmetrical.	• Cephalhematoma (Fig. 20–12B). Hydrocephalus may be caused by metabolic disturbances or by intrauterine infections. Bulging fontanelle represents increased cranial pressure. Microcephaly may be seen in newborns who have been exposed to congenital infections.

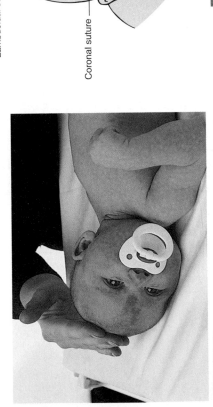

FIGURE 20–10 Palpating the anterior fontanelle. (© B. Proud.)

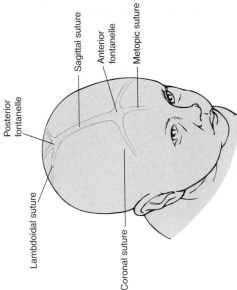

FIGURE 20–11 The infant head.

Posterior fontanelle

Lambdoidal suture

Coronal suture

Sagittal suture

Anterior fontanelle

Metopic suture

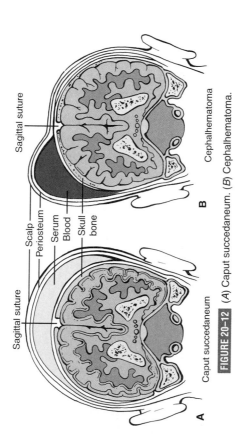

FIGURE 20–12 (A) Caput succedaneum. (B) Cephalhematoma.

PHYSICAL ASSESSMENT (continued)

PROCEDURE	NORMAL FINDINGS	DEVIATIONS FROM NORMAL
• Neck and clavicles	Neck moves freely. Infant attempts to control head when hyperextended, holds head midline position. Clavicles are symmetrical and intact.	• Webbing of neck, abnormal masses, limp. Crepitus when clavicle palpated, along with decreased movement in arm of that side, may indicate fractured clavicle.
• Extremities	Five fingers and toes on each extremity, no webbing, normal palmar creases, bilateral movement with full ROM in arms and legs. Legs have equal length, symmetrical bilateral gluteal/thigh creases, no hip click, normal position of feet.	• Polydactyly, syndactyly, absent digits could indicate genetic abnormality; polydactyly without bone, however, is commonly seen. Positive Ortolani maneuver indicates congenital dislocation of the hip (see Fig. 16–15). Unequal thigh/gluteal creases may indicate unequal leg length or dislocation of the hip.
• Spine	No openings spine flexible and rounded in infants younger than 3 months old (Fig. 20–13).	• Opening in spinal column, pilonidal dimple could indicate spina bifida or other spinal abnormalities.
Assess *GI system.*		
• Mouth	Oral mucosa and lips pink, palate intact; Epstein pearls, retains feedings.	• Cyanosis; white patches on oral mucosa is thrush. Abnormal fusion of lip/palate is seen with cleft lip/palate. Excessive salivation, unable to tolerate feedings may indicate esophageal atresia.

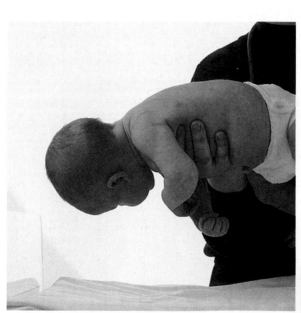

FIGURE 20–13 The spine is rounded in infants under the age of 3 months.

PHYSICAL ASSESSMENT (continued)

PROCEDURE	NORMAL FINDINGS	DEVIATIONS FROM NORMAL
• Anus	• Patent anus, meconium passed within 24–48 hours after birth	• No passage of meconium stool within 24–48 hours after birth could indicate no patency of anus and/or cystic fibrosis.
• Abdomen	• Abdomen shape cylindrical, round, soft; bowel sounds present 30–60 minutes after birth, liver palpable 1–2 cm below costal margin	• Abdomen sunken. Distended abdomen could indicate pyloric stenosis. Hirschsprung disease could also be considered, especially with suprapubic mass palpable.
• Umbilical cord	• Umbilical cord white, drying; three vessels present in cord (two arteries and one vein)	• Abnormal insertion of umbilical cord, discolored cord. Bulge at umbilicus suggests umbilical hernia—may disappear by 1 year of age (Fig. 20–14). Two vessels present in cord could indicate genetic abnormalities; however, is seen in newborns who have no abnormalities.
Assess *genitourinary system.*	Void within first 24 hours after birth	No urinary output beyond 48 hours after birth may indicate kidney problems.
• Male	• Testes descended within scrotal sac, meatus at tip of penis; circumcision site dry, minimal swelling and drainage	• Testes found in inguinal canal, scrotal sac edematous with fluid (hydrocele), meatus positioned above (epispadias) or below (hypospadias) tip of penis; bright red active bleeding at circumcision site

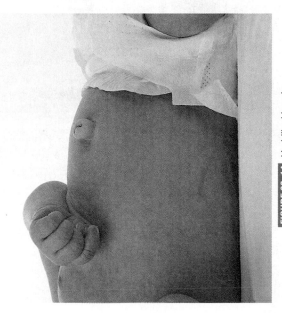

FIGURE 20–14 Umbilical hernia.

PHYSICAL ASSESSMENT (continued)

PROCEDURE	NORMAL FINDINGS	DEVIATIONS FROM NORMAL
• Female	• Labia majora cover labia minora, vaginal discharge	• Edema, tags present
Assess **skin.**	Pink, warm, dry, smooth, soft, good turgor, peeling hands and feet. Nails extend to end of fingers or beyond, well formed. Common variations: Acrocyanosis, harlequin color change, *vernix caseosa* in creases or absent, lanugo sparse, veins rarely visible, milia over nose/chin. Pigmentation: *erythema toxicum*, mongolian spots (Fig. 20–15) common in dark-skinned newborns over dorsal area and buttocks. Stork bites (*nevus flammeus*) (Fig. 20–16)	Minimal adipose tissue indicates fetal wasting; poor turgor, generalized cracking or peeling of skin can be seen in postmature infants. Lacerations, lesions. Yellowish green-stained skin is seen in newborns who have passed meconium in utero secondary to fetal distress. Jaundice within 24 hours after birth is pathologic jaundice caused from blood disorders such as hemolytic disease of the newborn. Cyanosis, generalized edema, pallor, hemangiomas, *nevus vascularis*, café-au-lait spots, skin tags and fibrous tumors may suggest neurofibromatosis.

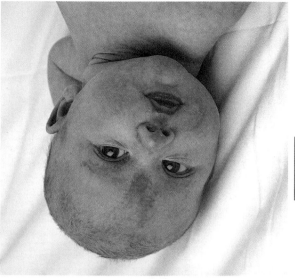

FIGURE 20–16 Stork bites.

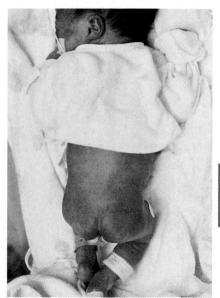

FIGURE 20–15 Mongolian spots.

Possible Collaborative Problems

Elevated bilirubin levels
Infection
   Circumcision
   Nosocomial
   Bacterial

TEACHING TIPS FOR SELECTED NURSING DIAGNOSES

Nursing Diagnosis: Ineffective Breathing Pattern (transient alteration in lung expansion)

☐ Monitor respiratory status every 30 min × 4 until stable, then per protocol. Auscultate breath sounds per protocol. Promote oxygenation and fluid drainage by placing infant on side; use postural drainage with head of bed slightly lower than body. Have suction equipment ready for use.

Nursing Diagnosis: Risk for Suffocation, Sudden Infant Death Syndrome (SIDS)

☐ Healthy infants should be placed on their back when putting them to sleep. Side positioning is an alternative but does carry a slightly higher risk of SIDS [American Academy of Pediatrics, 2000].

Nursing Diagnosis: Ineffective Thermoregulation (cool environment, decrease in body fat)

☐ Assess temperature every 30 min × 4, then per protocol. Maintain temperature at 97.6–99.2°F (−36.4–37.3°C). Keep infant temperature probe attached properly to skin to ensure reading probe accurately. Monitor for signs and symptoms of cold stress. Keep infant warm and dry. Postpone bath until temperature is stable. Apply cap to head and extra blankets to infant if temperature <97.6°F (36.4°C). Teach parents mechanisms of heat loss: radiation, convection, conduction, evaporation. Teach techniques used to prevent cold stress and to maintain or increase infant temperature (eg, dress, cap, blanket wrap, cuddle). Teach parents correct procedure in taking newborn axillary temperature, reading thermometer, interpreting results.

Nursing Diagnosis: Imbalanced Nutrition, less than body requirement

■ Review prenatal history, looking for maternal risk factors such as gestational diabetes. Assess for hypoglycemia, checking blood glucose values at birth and at 1 hour of age or per hospital protocol. Weigh infant on admission and daily. Auscultate bowel sounds every shift. Assess for rooting/sucking behaviors. Initiate breast-bottle-feeding at birth and on demand for breast-feeding and per hospital protocol for bottle-feeding. Record frequency, amount and length of feeding. If regurgitation occurs, note frequency and amount. Monitor newborn stools/voids and record per shift. Observe for feeding problems (refusal to eat, regurgitation, gagging, difficulty swallowing, and difficulty with latching onto breast, etc). Evaluate neonate after feeding for satisfaction of feeding. Observe parents/newborn for feeding problems, encourage questions and problem solving for parents regarding feeding difficulties or concerns.

Nursing Assessment Form Based on Functional Health Patterns

Client Profile

Name _____ Birthdate _____ Sex _____

Ethnic origin _____ Religion _____

Medical diagnoses _____

Present treatment _____

Past treatments _____

Past hospitalizations _____

Allergies _____

Current Medications

Name	Dose	Purpose	Problems

Subjective

HEALTH PERCEPTION–HEALTH MANAGEMENT PATTERN

Reason for seeking health care _____

_____

Health rating	1	2	3
	Poor	Fair	Excellent

Perception of illness _____

Effect of illness on ADLs _____

Use of alcohol _____

tobacco _____

drugs _____

Special health habits _____

Last immunizations _____

Compliance with treatments _____

_____

Objective

Appearance _____

Grooming _____

Posture _____

Expressions _____

Ht _____ Wt _____

P _____ R _____ T _____

(oral, axillary, rectal)

BP sitting R _____ L _____

standing R _____ L _____

Nursing Assessment Form Based on Functional Health Patterns

NUTRITIONAL–METABOLIC PATTERN

Daily Food and Fluid Intake

Breakfast _____

Lunch _____

Supper _____

Snacks _____

Food intolerances _____

Difficulty chewing _____

Dysphagia _____

Sore gums _____

Sore tongue _____

N and V _____

Abdominal pains _____

Antacids _____

Laxatives _____

Skin condition _____

Hair condition _____

Nail condition _____

Ideal wt. _____ Difficulty gaining _____

   losing _____

Cold/heat intolerances _____

Voice changes _____

Difficulty with nervousness _____

Skin: Color _____ Texture _____

Lesions _____ Moisture _____

Temp _____

Turgor _____

Hair: Color _____ Texture _____

Amt _____ Dry _____

Scalp lesions _____

Nails: Color _____

Shape _____ Condition _____

Texture _____ Tenderness _____

Number of teeth _____

Oral Mucosa:

Condition _____

Lesions _____

Gums _____ Tongue _____

ELIMINATION PATTERN

Bowel habits

Frequency _____ Color _____ Pain _____

Consistency _____ Laxatives _____ Umbilicus _____

Enemas _____ Suppositories _____

Ileostomy _____ Colostomy _____

Bladder habits

Frequency _____ Amt _____ Color _____

Pain _____ Hematuria _____

Incontinence _____ Nocturia _____

Retention _____ Infections _____

Catheter _____ Type _____

Abdomen

Contour _____

Lesions _____ Umbilicus _____

Striae _____ Veins _____

Bowel sounds char. _____

Frequency _____

Size of liver dullness _____

Masses palpated _____

Liver palpated _____

Spleen palpated _____

Rectum

Rashes _____

Lesions _____ Tenderness _____

ACTIVITY–EXERCISE PATTERN

Daily Activities

Hygiene _____

Cooking _____

Shopping _____

Housework _____

Yard work _____

Eating times _____

Dyspnea _____ Palpitations _____

Chest pain _____ Stiffness _____

Weakness _____ Aching _____

Leisure activities _____

Exercise routine _____

Occupation _____

Effect of illness on activities _____

_____

Musculoskeletal

Gait _____ Posture _____

Extremity swelling _____

Symmetry _____ ROM _____

Crepitus _____ Tone _____

Strength _____

Respiratory

Thorax shape _____

Symmetry _____ Retractions _____

Tenderness _____

Diaphragmatic level _____

Breath sounds _____

Adventitious sounds _____

Cardiovascular

Jugular venous pressure _____

Pulsations _____ Heaves _____

Lifts _____

PMI _____ S_1 _____ S_2 _____

S_3 _____ S_4 _____ Murmurs _____

Peripheral Vascular Pulses

Carotid R __ L __ Radial R __ L __

Ulnar R __ L __ Brachial R __ L __

Popliteal R __ L __ Femoral R __ L __

Pedal R __ L __ Posterior tibial R __ L __

Bruits R __ L __

SLEEP–REST PATTERN

Sleep time _____ Quality _____
Difficulty falling asleep _____
Difficulty remaining asleep _____
Sleep aids _____
Sleep medications _____

Appearance _____
Yawning _____ Irritability _____
Short attention span _____

SEXUALITY–REPRODUCTION PATTERN

Female Menstruation

Age of onset _____ Last menstrual period _____
Length _____
Problems _____

Gravida _____ Para _____ Abortions _____
Current pregnancy _____
Infertility _____

Breasts

SBE _____ When _____
Shape _____ Symmetry _____
Nipples _____ Discharge _____
Masses _____ Lymph nodes _____

Male Genitalia

Testicular exam _____ When _____
Masses _____ Swelling _____
Texture _____

Nursing Assessment Form Based on Functional Health Patterns

Male–Female

Contraception used _____

Undesirable side effects _____
Problems with sexual activities _____

Effect of illness on sexuality _____

Sexually transmitted diseases _____

Pain _____ Burning _____
Discomfort during intercourse _____

Penile exam

Masses _____ Growths _____
Lesions _____ Discharge _____
Foreskin retraction _____
Urethral opening _____
Lymph nodes _____
Inguinal masses _____

Female Genitalia

Labia _____ Color _____
Swelling _____ Symmetry _____
Urethral opening _____
Discharge _____
Vaginal opening _____
Lesions _____ Discharge _____
Hymen _____ Inflammation _____

SENSORY–PERCEPTUAL PATTERN

Perceptions of: Vision _____ Taste _____
Hearing _____ Sensation _____
Smell _____
Pain _____
Vision aids _____
Hearing aids _____

Visual Acuity: OD _____ OS _____
OU _____ Visual fields _____
EOMs _____
PERRLA _____

Funduscopic Exam: Red reflex _____
Optic disc _____ Macula _____
Arterioles/venules _____

Hearing: Weber _____ Rinne _____
External canal _____
Tympanic membrane _____
Sensations: Superficial _____ Deep pressure _____
2-point discrimination _____
Cranial Nerves
I. Olfactory _____
II. Optic _____
V. Trigeminal _____
III, IV, VI. Oculomotor, trochlear, abducens _____
VII. Facial _____ Acoustic _____

Behavior _____
Speech _____ Vocabulary _____
Mood _____
Thought processes _____
Orientation: Person _____ Place _____
Time _____ Information _____
Attention _____
Vocabulary _____
Abstract reasoning _____
Similarities _____ Judgment _____
Sensory perception and coordination _____

COGNITIVE PATTERN

Understanding of illness _____
Understanding of treatments _____
Ability to express self _____
Ability to recall:
Remote _____
Recent _____
Ability to make decisions _____
Expression of feelings _____

Nursing Assessment Form Based on Functional Health Patterns

ROLE–RELATIONSHIP PATTERN

Role in family _____

Responsibility _____

Work role _____

Social role _____

Level of satisfaction _____

Effect of illness on roles _____

Communication between family members _____

Family visits _____ Length _____

Draw family genogram:

SELF-PERCEPTION–SELF-CONCEPT PATTERN

Identity _____

Perception of abilities _____

Body image _____

COPING–STRESS TOLERANCE PATTERN

Stressors _____

Coping methods _____

Support systems _____

VALUE–BELIEF PATTERN

Values _____

Goals _____

Source of hope/strength _____

Significant religious person _____

Religious practices _____

Relationship with God _____

Presence of religious articles _____

Religious activities _____

Visits from clergy _____

Nursing Assessment Form Based on Functional Health Patterns

Developmental Information—Age 1 Month to 18 Years

AGE	PHYSICAL DEVELOPMENT	LANGUAGE (COGNITIVE) DEVELOPMENT (BASED ON PIAGET)	PSYCHOSOCIAL DEVELOPMENT (BASED ON ERIKSON)	NURSE'S APPROACH TO ASSESSMENT
Overview of birth to 1 year		*Sensorimotor stage of developing.*	*Developmental task: trust vs mistrust.* Learns to trust and to anticipate satisfaction. Sends cues to mother/caretaker. Begins understanding self as separate from others (body image).	Involve caretaker in assessment (eg, allow him or her to hold child in lap for parts of examination).
1–2 months	Lifts chin and chest off bed. Holds extremities in flexion and moves at	Can discriminate between various sensations and prefers certain ones. Follows	Begins to bond with mother during alert periods.	Conserve infant's body heat. Assess while asleep or quiet. Place infant on table or in

	random; weak neck muscles. Activity varies from quiet sleep to drowsiness to alert activity.	moving objects with eyes.		caretaker's arms. Give bottle if awake.
3–4 months	Head and back control developing. Holds rattle. Looks at own hands. Infant reflexes begin to disappear. Able to sit propped. Props self on forearm in prone position. Rolls from side to back and vice versa and from back to abdomen. Takes objects to mouth. Drools with eruption of lower teeth.	Responds to parent. Social smile. Begins to vocalize; coos, babbles. Locates sounds by turning head, looking.	Learns to signal displeasure. Shows excitement with whole body. Begins to discriminate strangers. Squeals.	Speak softly to infant. Use brightly colored toys, bells, rattles to elicit necessary responses and to distract. Assess ears, mouth, nose last. Assess lungs and heart when quiet.

(continued)

Developmental Information—Age 1 Month to 18 Years

AGE	PHYSICAL DEVELOPMENT	LANGUAGE (COGNITIVE) DEVELOPMENT (BASED ON PIAGET)	PSYCHOSOCIAL DEVELOPMENT (BASED ON ERIKSON)	NURSE'S APPROACH TO ASSESSMENT
5–8 months	Begins to develop teeth. Birth weight doubled. Grasps objects. Sits unsupported.	Begins to imitate sounds, two-syllable words ("dada," "mama"). Responds to own name.	Increased fear of strangers. Definite likes/dislikes. Responds to "no."	Place on caretaker's lap (same as above).
9–12 months	Birth weight tripled. Anterior fontanelle nearly closed. Learns to pull in order to stand, creep, and crawl.	Says two-syllable words besides "dada," "mama." Understands simple commands. Imitates animal sounds.	Looks for hidden objects. Unceasing determination to move about. Clings to mother. Shows emotion. Plays peek-a-boo and pat-a-cake.	
1–3 years	Begins to walk and run well. Drinks from cup, feeds self. Develops fine motor control. Climbs. Begins self-	Preoperational stage of development. Has poor time sense. Increasing verbal ability. Formulates sentences of 4 to 5 words by age 3. Talks to self and	Developmental task: autonomy vs shame and doubt. Establishes self-control, decision making, independence (autonomy). Extremely curious	Be flexible. Begin assessment with play period to establish rapport. Be honest. Praise for cooperation. Begin slowly; speak to child. Involve caretaker/

Age	Physical	Cognitive	Psychosocial	Nursing Approach
	toileting. Kneels without support. Steady growth in height/weight. Adult height will be approximately double the height at age 2. Dresses self by age 3.	others. Has misconceptions about cause and effect. Interested in pictures. Fears: • Loss/separation from parents—peak • Dark • Machines/equipment • Intrusive procedures • Bedtime Speaks to dolls and animals. Increasing attention span. Knows own sex by age 3.	and prefers to do things by self. Demonstrates independence through negativism. Very egocentric; believes he or she controls the world. Attempts to please parents. Participates in parallel play; able to share some toys by age 3.	parent in holding on exam table. Let child hold security object. Allow child to play with stethoscope, tongue blade, flashlight before using on child if possible. Assess face, mouth, eyes, ears last. May need to restrain when lying prone. If resistant, save that part of the assessment for later.
4–6 years	Growth slows. Locomotion skills increase and coordination improves. Tricycle/bicycle riding. Throws ball but has difficulty catching. Constantly ac-	Preoperational stage of development continues. Language skills flourish. Generates many questions (eg, How, Why, What?) Simple problem solving. Uses fantasy to understand and problem solve.	*Developmental tasks: initiative vs guilt.* Attempts to establish self like his or her parents, but independent. Explores environment on own initiative. Boasts, brags, has feelings of indestruc-	Establish rapport through talking and play. Introduce self to child. Have parent present but direct conversation to child. Games such as "follow the leader" and "Simon says" can be used to *(continued)*

Developmental Information—Age 1 Month to 18 Years

AGE	PHYSICAL DEVELOPMENT	LANGUAGE (COGNITIVE) DEVELOPMENT (BASED ON PIAGET)	PSYCHOSOCIAL DEVELOPMENT (BASED ON ERIKSON)	NURSE'S APPROACH TO ASSESSMENT
	maximum growth). Secondary sex characteristics. (See Chapter 15, Genitourinary–Reproductive Assessment.)	Understanding of multiple cause-and-effect relationships. May plan for future career. *Fears:* • Mutilation • Disruption of body image • Rejection by peers	group. Early adolescence: outgoing and enthusiastic. Emotions are extreme, with mood swings. Seeking self-identity, sexual identity. Wants privacy and independence. Develops interests not shared with family. Concern with physical self. Explores adult roles.	child. Ask for child's opinions and encourage questions. Allow input into decisions. Be flexible with routines. Explain all procedures/ treatments. Encourage continuance of peer relationships. Listen actively. Identify impact of illness on body image, future, and level of functioning. Correct misconceptions. Involve parent in assessment only if child requests presence.

Recommended Childhood and Adolescent Immunization Schedule—United States, 2003

1. Indicates the recommended ages for routine administration of currently licensed childhood vaccines, as of December 1, 2002, for children through age 18 years. Any dose not given at the recommended age should be given at any subsequent visit when indicated and feasible. ■ Indicates age groups that warrant special effort to administer those vaccines not given previously. Additional vaccines may be licensed and recommended during the year. Licensed combination vaccines may be used whenever any components of the combination are indicated and the vaccine's other components are not contraindicated. Providers should consult the manufacturers' package inserts for detailed recommendations.

2. **Hepatitis B vaccine (HepB).** All infants should receive the first dose of HepB vaccine soon after birth and before hospital discharge; the first dose also may be given by age 2 months if the infant's mother is HBsAg negative. Only monovalent HepB vaccine can be used for the birth dose. Monovalent or combination vaccine containing HepB may be used to complete the series: four doses of vaccine may be administered when a birth dose is given. The second dose should be given at least four weeks after the first dose except for combination vaccines, which cannot be administered before age 6 weeks. The third dose should be given at least 16 weeks after the first dose and at least 8 weeks after the second dose. The last dose in the vaccination series (third or fourth dose) should not be administered before age 6 months. *Infants born to HBsAg-positive mothers* should receive HepB vaccine and 0.5 mL hepatitis B immune globulin (HBIG) within 12 hours of birth at separate sites. The second dose is recommended at age 1–2 months. The last dose in the vaccination series should not be administered before age 6 months. These infants should be tested for HBsAg and anti-HBs at 9 to

Vaccine	Range of recommended ages					Catch-up vaccination					Preadolescent assessment			
	Birth	1 mo	2 mos	4 mos	6 mos	12 mos	15 mos	18 mos	24 mos	4-6 yrs	11-12 yrs	13-18 yrs		
Hepatitis B[2]	Hep B #1 only if mother HBsAg (-)													
		Hep B #2			Hep B #3						Hep B series			
Diphtheria, Tetanus, Pertussis[3]			DTaP	DTaP	DTaP			DTaP		DTaP	Td			
Haemophilus Influenzae Type b[4]			Hib	Hib	Hib	Hib								
Inactivated Polio			IPV	IPV		IPV				IPV				
Measles, Mumps, Rubella[5]						MMR #1				MMR #2		MMR #2		
Varicella[6]						Varicella				Varicella	Varicella			
Pneumococcal[7]			PCV	PCV	PCV	PCV				PCV	PPV			
Hepatitis A[8]										HepA series				
Influenza[9]						Influenza (yearly)								

Vaccines below this line are for selected populations

15 months of age. *Infants born to mothers whose HBsAg status is unknown* should receive the first dose of the HepB vaccine series within 12 hours of birth. Maternal blood should be drawn as soon as possible to determine the mother's HBsAg status; if the HBsAg test is positive, the infant should receive HBIG as soon as possible (no later than age 1 week). The second dose is recommended at age 1 to 2 months. The last dose in the vaccination series should not be administered before age 6 months.

3. **Diphtheria and tetanus toxoids and acellular pertussis vaccine (DTaP).** The fourth dose of DTaP may be administered at age 12 months provided that 6 months have elapsed since the third dose and the child is unlikely to return at age 15 to 18 months. Tetanus and diphtheria toxoids (Td) is recommended at age 11 to 12 years if at least 5 years have elapsed since the last dose of Td-containing vaccine. Subsequent routine Td boosters are recommended every 10 years.

4. **Haemophilus influenzae type b (Hib) conjugate vaccine.** Three Hib conjugate vaccines are licensed for infant use. If PRP-OMP (PedvaxHIB® or ComVax® [Merck]) is administered at age 2 and 4 months, a dose at age 6 months is not required. DTaP/Hib combination products should not be used for primary vaccination in infants at age 2, 4, or 6 months but can be used as boosters following any Hib vaccine.

5. **Measles, mumps, and rubella vaccine (MMR).** The second dose of MMR is recommended routinely at age 4 to 6 years but may be administered during any visit provided that at least 4 weeks have elapsed since the first dose and that both doses are administered beginning at or after age 12 months. Those who have not received the second dose previously should complete the schedule by the visit at age 11 to 12 years.

6. **Varicella vaccine.** Varicella vaccine is recommended at any visit or after age 12 months for susceptible children (ie, those who lack a reliable history of chickenpox). Susceptible persons age ≥13 years should receive 2 doses given at least 4 weeks apart.

7. **Pneumococcal vaccine.** The heptavalant pneumococcal conjugate vaccine (PCV) is recommended for all children aged 2 to 23 months and for certain children aged 24 to 59 months. Pneumococcal polysaccharide vaccine (PPV) is recommended in addition to PCV for certain high-risk groups. See *MMWR* 2000;49(no. RR-9):1–37.

8. **Hepatitis A vaccine.** Hepatitis A vaccine is recommended for children and adolescents in selected states and regions, and for certain high-risk groups. Consult local public health authority and *MMWR* 1999;48(No. RR-12):1–37. Children

and adolescents in these states, regions, and high-risk groups who have not been immunized against hepatitis A can begin the hepatitis A vaccination series during any visit. The two doses in the series should be administered at least 6 months apart.

9. **Influenza vaccine.** Influenza vaccine is recommended annually for children aged ≥6 months with certain risk factors, including but not limited to asthma, cardiac disease, sickle cell disease. HIV, and diabetes, and household members of persons in groups at high risk (see *MMWR* 2002;51[No. RR-3]:1–31), and can be administered to all others wishing to obtain immunity. In addition, healthy children age 6 to 23 months are encouraged to receive influenza vaccine if feasible because children in this age group are at substantially increased risk for influenza-related hospitalizations. Children aged ≤12 years should receive vaccine in a dosage appropriate for their age (0.25 mL if 6 to 35 months or 0.5 mL if ≥3 years). Children aged ≤8 years who are receiving influenza vaccine for the first time should receive two doses separated by at least 4 weeks.

CATCH-UP SCHEDULE FOR CHILDREN AGE 4 MONTHS TO 6 YEARS

Dose one (minimum age)	Minimum Interval between doses			
	Dose one to dose two	Dose two to dose three	Dose three to dose four	Dose four to dose five
DTaP[1] (6 wks)	4 wks	4 wks	6 mos	6 mos[1]
IPV[2] (6 wks)	4 wks	4 wks	4 wks[2]	
HepB[3] (birth)	4 wks	8 wks (and 16 wks after first dose)		
MMR[4] (12 mos)	4 wks[4]			
Varicella (12 mos)				
Hib[5] (6 wks)	4 wks: if 1st dose given at age <12 mos 8 wks (as final dose): if 1st dose given at age 12–24 mos No further doses needed: if 1st dose given at age ≥15 mos	4 wks[6]: if current age <12 mos 8 wks (as final dose)[6]: if current age ≥12 mos and 2nd dose given at age <15 mos No further doses needed: if previous dose given at age ≥15 mos	8 wks (as final dose): this dose only necessary for children aged 12 mos–5 yrs who received 3 doeses before age 12 mos	
PCV[7] (6 wks)	4 wks: if 1st dose given at age <12 mos and current age <24 mos 8 wks (as final dose): if 1st dose given at age ≥12 mos or current age 24–59 mos No further doses needed: for healthy children if 1st dose given at age ≥24 mos	4 wks[6]: if current age <12 mos 8 wks (as final dose): if current age ≥12 mos No further doses needed: for healthy children if 1st dose given at age ≥24 mos	8 wks (as final dose): this dose only necessary for children aged 12 mos–5 yrs who received 3 doeses before age 12 mos	

1. **Diphtheria and tetanus toxoids and acellular pertussis vaccine (DTaP):** The fifth dose is not necessary if the fourth dose was given after the fourth birthday.
2. **Inactivated Polio (IPV):** For children who received an all-IPV or all OPV series, a fourth dose is not necessary if third dose was given at age ≥4 years. If both OPV and IPV were given as part of a series, a total of 4 doses should be given, regardless of the child's current age.
3. **Hepatitis B vaccine (HepB):** All children and adolescents who have not been vaccinated against hepatitis B should begin the hepatitis B vaccination series during any visit. Providers should make special efforts to immunize children who were born in, or whose parents were born in, areas of the world where hepatitis B virus infection is moderately or highly endemic.
4. **Measles, mumps, and rubella vaccine (MMR):** The second dose of MMR is recommended routinely at age 4–6 years, but may be given earlier if desired.
5. **Haemophilus influenzae type b (Hib):** If current age is <12 months and the first 2 doses were PRP-OMP (PedvaxHIB® or ComVax [Merch]), the third (and final) dose should be given at age 12–15 months and at least 8 weeks after the second dose.
6. **Hib:** If current age ≥12 months and the first 2 doses were PRP-OMP (PedvaxHIB® or ComVax [Merch]), the third (and final) dose should be given at age 12–15 months and at least 8 weeks after the second dose.
7. **Pneumococcal conjugate vaccine (PCV):** Vaccine is not recommended generally for children aged ≥5 years.

CATCH-UP SCHEDULE FOR CHILDREN AGE 7 TO 18 YEARS

		Minimum interval between doses	
	Dose one to dose two	Dose two to dose three	Dose three to booster dose
Td:	4 wks	Td: 6 mos	Td[1]: 6 mos: if 1st dose given at age <12 mos and current age <11 yrs 5 yrs: if 1st dose givben at age ≥12 mos and 3rd dose given at age <7 yrs and current age ≥11 yrs 10 yrs: if 3rd dose given at age ≥7 yrs
IPV[2]:	4 wks	IPV[2]: 4 wks	IPV[2]
HepB:	4 wks	HepB: 8 wks (and 16 wks after 1st dose)	
MMR:	4 wks		
Varicella[3]:	4 wks		

1. Tetanus toxoid: For children aged 7–10 years, the interval between the third and booster dose is determined by the age when the first dose was given. For adolescents aged 11–18 years, the interval is determined by the age when the third dose was given.
2. Inactivated Polio (IPV): Vaccine is not recommended generally for persons aged ≥18 years.
3. Varicella: Give 2-dose series to all susceptible adolescents aged ≥13 years.

Psychosocial Development

YOUNG ADULT DEVELOPMENTAL TASK: INTIMACY VS ISOLATION

Behavior to Assess:

Accepts self: physically, cognitively, and emotionally

Establishes independence from parental home

Expresses love responsibly, emotionally, and sexually

Establishes an intimate bond with another human being

Finds a social friendship group

Becomes involved as part of a community

Establishes a philosophy of living and life

Begins a profession or a life's work that provides a means of contribution

Learns to solve problems of life that accompany independence from parental home

MATURE ADULT DEVELOPMENTAL TASK: GENERATIVITY VS STAGNATION

Behavior to Assess:

Establishes/maintains healthful life patterns

Discovers self as a life-mate for another person

Derives satisfaction from contributing to growth and development of others

Establishes an abiding intimacy

Helps children grow and mature

Maintains a stable home

Finds pleasure in an established work or profession

Takes pride in self and family accomplishments and contributions

Contributes to the community to support its growth and development

Adjusts to physical changes of aging

Develops deeper, sustained friendships

Integrates leisure with work life

Develops a philosophy of life that includes an understanding of mortality

Prepares for eventual retirement

Supports aging parents/relatives

AGING ADULT DEVELOPMENTAL TASK: EGO INTEGRITY VS DESPAIR

Behavior to Assess:

Adjusts to changing physical self

Recognizes changes present as a result of aging, in relationships and activities

Maintains relationships with children, grandchildren, other relatives

Continues interests outside self and home

Completes transition from retirement at work to satisfying alternative activities

Establishes relationships with others his or her own age

Adjusts to deaths of relatives, spouse, and friends

Maintains maximum level of physical functioning through diet, exercise, and personal care

Finds meaning in past life and faces inevitable mortality of self and significant others

Integrates philosophical or religious values into understanding of self to promote comfort

Reviews accomplishments and recognizes meaningful contributions he or she has made to community and relatives

Height–Weight–Head Circumference Charts for Children

Published May 30, 2000 (modified 10/16/00).

SOURCE: Developed by the National Center for Health Statistics in collaboration with the National Center for Chronic Disease Prevention and Health Promotion (2000). http://www.cdc.gov/growthcharts

Birth to 36 months: Girls
Head circumference-for-age and
Weight-forlength percentiles

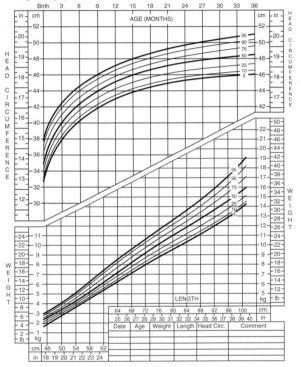

Birth to 36 months: Girls
Length-for-age and Weight-for-age percentiles

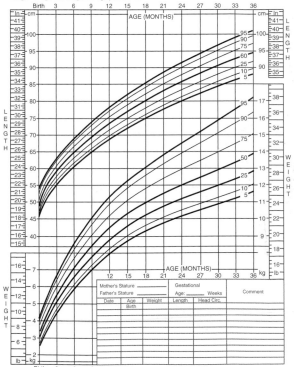

2 to 20 years: Girls
Stature-for-age and Weight-for-age percentiles

Mothers Stature		Fathers Stature		
Date	Age	Weight	Stature	BMI*

* To Calculate BMI: Weight (kg) ÷ Stature (cm) x 10,000
Or Weight (lb) ÷ Stature (in) x 703

AGE (YEARS)

STATURE

WEIGHT

2 to 20 years: Girls
Body mass index-for-age percentiles

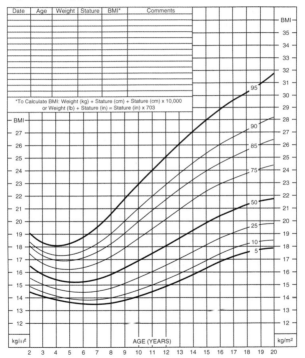

*To Calculate BMI: Weight (kg) + Stature (cm) + Stature (cm) x 10,000
or Weight (lb) + Stature (in) + Stature (in) x 703

AGE (YEARS)

Height–Weight–Head Circumference Charts for Children

2 to 20 years: Boys
Body mass index-for-age percentiles

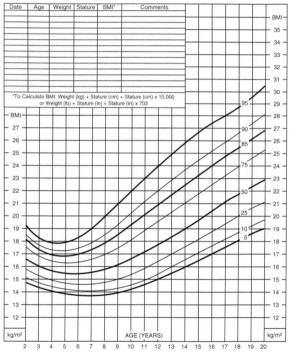

Date	Age	Weight	Stature	BMI*	Comments

*To Calculate BMI: Weight (kg) ÷ Stature (cm) ÷ Stature (cm) x 10,000
or Weight (lb) ÷ Stature (in) ÷ Stature (in) x 703

BMI

AGE (YEARS)

kg/m²

2 to 20 years: Boys
Stature-for-age and Weight-for-age percentiles

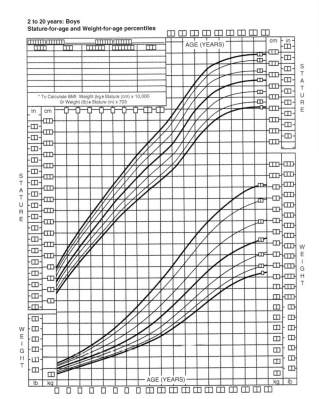

* To Calculate BMI: Weight (kg÷ Stature (cm) x 10,000
Or Weight (lb)÷ Stature (in) x 703

How to Examine Your Own Skin

You can systematically and regularly assess your skin for abnormalities by using the following recommended procedure for skin assessment from the American Cancer Society.

STEP 1

Make sure the room is well lighted, and that you have nearby a full-length mirror, a hand-held mirror, a hand-held blow dryer, and two chairs or stools. Undress completely.

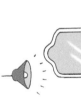

STEP 2

Hold your hands with the palms face up, as shown in the drawing. Look at your palms, fingers, spaces between the fingers, and forearms. Then turn your hands over and examine the backs of your hands, fingers, spaces between the fingers, fingernails, and forearms.

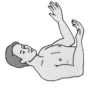

STEP 3

Now position yourself in front of the full-length mirror. Hold up your arms, bent at the elbows, with your palms facing you. In the mirror, look at the backs of your forearms and elbows.

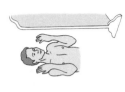

STEP 4

Again, using the full-length mirror, observe the entire front of your body. In turn, look at your face, neck, and arms. Turn your palms to face the mirror and look at your upper arms. Then look at your chest and abdomen, pubic area, thighs, and lower legs.

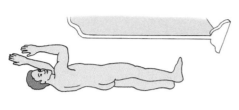

STEP 5

Still standing in front of the mirror, lift your arms over your head with the palms facing each other. Turn so that your right side is facing the mirror and look at the entire side of your body: your hands and arms, underarms, sides of your trunk, thighs, and lower legs. Then turn, and repeat the process with your left side.

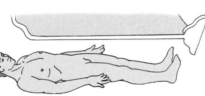

STEP 6

With your back toward the full-length mirror, look at your buttocks and the back of your thighs and lower legs.

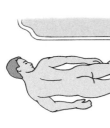

STEP 7

Now pick up the hand-held mirror. With your back still to the full-length mirror, examine the back of your neck, and your back and buttocks. Also examine the backs of your arms in this way. Some areas are hard to see, and you may find it helpful to ask your spouse or a friend to assist you.

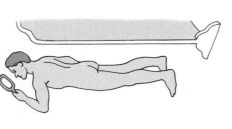

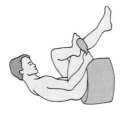

STEP 8

Use the hand-held mirror and the full-length mirror to look at your scalp. Because the scalp is difficult to examine, we suggest you use a hand-held blow dryer, turned to a cool setting, to lift the hair from the scalp. While some people find it easy to hold the mirror in one hand and the dryer in the other while looking in the full-length mirror, many do not. For the scalp examination in particular, then, you might ask your spouse or a friend to assist you.

STEP 9

Sit down and prop one leg up on a chair or stool in front of you as shown. Using the hand-held mirror, examine the inside of the propped-up leg, beginning at the groin area and moving down the leg to your foot. Repeat the procedure for your other leg.

STEP 10

Still sitting, cross one leg over the other. Use the hand-held mirror to examine the top of your foot, the toes, toenails, and spaces between the toes. Then look at the sole or bottom of your foot. Repeat the procedure for the other foot.

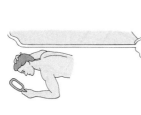

How to Examine Your Own Skin

STEP 5

1. Gently squeeze the nipple and look for a discharge.
2. If you have any discharge during the month—whether or not it is during your BSE—see your doctor.
3. Repeat the examination on your right breast.

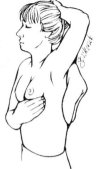

STEP 6

1. Steps 4 and 5 should be repeated lying down.
2. Lie flat on your back with your left arm over your head and a pillow or folded towel under your left shoulder. (This position flattens your breast and makes it easier to check.)
3. Use the same circular motion described above.
4. Repeat on your right breast.

Classification and Management of Blood Pressure for Adults*

BP Classification	SBP* (mm Hg)	DBP* (mm Hg)	Lifestyle Modification	Initial Drug Therapy	
				Without Compelling Indication	With Compelling Indications (See Table 4–3)
Normal	<120	and <80	Encourage		
Prehypertension	120–139	or 80–89	Yes	No antihypertensive drug indicated.	Drug(s) for compelling indications.‡
Stage I Hypertension	140–159	or 90–99	Yes	Thiazide-type diuretics for most. May consider ACEI, ARB, BB, CCB, or combination.	Drug(s) for compelling indications.‡ Other antihypertensive drugs (diuretics, ACEI, ARB, BB, CCB) as needed.

(continued)

CLASSIFICATION AND MANAGEMENT OF BLOOD PRESSURE FOR ADULTS (continued)

BP Classification	SBP* (mm Hg)	DBP* (mm Hg)	Lifestyle Modification	Initial Drug Therapy Without Compelling Indication	Initial Drug Therapy With Compelling Indications (See Table 4–3)
Stage 2 Hypertension	≥160	or ≥100	Yes	Two-drug combination for most† (usually thiazide-type diuretic and ACEI or ARB or BB or CCB).	

DBP, diastolic blood pressure; SBP, systolic blood pressure.
Drug abbreviations: ACEI, angiotensin converting enzyme inhibitor; ARB, angiotensin receptor blocker; BB, beta-blocker; CCB, calcium channel blocker.
*Treatment determined by highest BP category.
†Initial combined therapy should be used cautiously in those at risk for orthostatic hypotension.
‡Treat patients with chronic kidney disease or diabetes to BP goal of <130/80 mm Hg.
From the Seventh Report of the Joint National Committee on Prevention, Detection, Evaluation, and Treatment of High Blood Pressure. (2003). *JAMA, 289*(19), 2560–2572.

Sample Adult Nursing Health History and Physical Assessment

HEALTH HISTORY

A. Client Profile

S.L. is a 72-year-old white female, born on a small farm in southern Missouri. Appears younger than stated age. English speaking, with a German ethnic origin. High school graduate and presently retired from restraint work. Lives in a one-bedroom apartment on first floor. Drives own car. Seeks health care in local community hospital 4 miles from home. Major reason for seeking health care is for routine checkup—has not had one for 8 years. Understands that she has adult-onset diabetes mellitus (type 2), which is controlled with 1800-calorie diet and moderate amount of exercise. Also has "mild rheumatoid arthritic" pains in right hip and finger joints in early mornings; relieved with exercise, warm baths, and ASA.

Treatments/medications:

1. Prescribed: none
2. OTC
   a. ASA gr at H.S. for "arthritis aches." Takes about 2× per month. Denies nausea, abdominal pains or evidence of bleeding while taking.
   b. Mylanta at H.S. for "gas pains."
   c. Dulcolax suppository 3×/week for past 4 years.
   d. Multivitamin 1 qd, for past 4 years.

Past illnesses/hospitalizations:

1. Appendectomy age 18.
2. Left arm fracture age 20.
3. Cholecystectomy age 56, performed for complaint of gas pains after eating fatty foods. Satisfied with care received at local hospital.

Allergies:

Denies food, drug, and environmental allergies.

B. Developmental History

Developmental Level: Integrity vs Despair

Describes childhood as a very happy time for her. Becomes excited and smiles as she relates stories of her childhood on the farm. States she was an average child and ran and played like all the others. Companions were brothers and sisters. Has been married for 55 years. Describes relationship with husband as close and sharing. Owned and operated a restaurant for 30 years with husband and was a waitress at another restaurant after they retired from their own. Lived in a large house until 1988. Currently lives in a one-bedroom apartment. Active in church and society. Volunteers at community functions. She and her husband are active in their church. States she enjoys being retired and lives a "comfortable" life. Does not voice financial concerns. Has begun to write will and distribute personal heirlooms to son and grandchildren. States she is not afraid of death and wishes to have the "business part taken care of" in order to enjoy the rest of her life together with her husband.

C. Health Perception–Health Management Pattern

1. Client's rating of health:
   Scale: 10-best; 1-worst
   5 years ago: 10
   Now: 8

5 years from now: 6

Sees health deterioration as normal aging process and states, "I feel really good when I look at a lot of people my age with all their problems and the medicine they take."

2. Health does not interfere with self-care or other desired activities of daily living. Unaware of signs, symptoms, and Tx of hyperglycemia and hypoglycemia. Denies use of alcohol, tobacco, and drugs.

3. Client seeks health care only in emergencies. Last medical exam September 1996. Keeps active and feels well. Feels lifestyle and faith "keep her going." Does not check own blood sugar or do breast self-exams.

D. Nutritional–Metabolic Pattern

States she is on a "no concentrated sweet" meal pattern as follows: Eats breakfast of whole wheat toast, one boiled egg, orange juice, and decaf. coffee at 7 AM. Eats lunch at noon. Today had tuna, lettuce salad, apple, and milk. Eats light supper around 6 PM. Typical dinner includes small serving broiled meat, green vegetables, piece of fruit, and glass of milk. Tries not to snack but will have fruit if she feels the urge. Drinks two 8-oz glasses of water a day. Drinks decaf. coffee—no tea or colas. Voices no dislikes or food intolerances.

Wears dentures. Last dental exam October 1996. Denies problems with proper fit, eating, chewing, swallowing, sore throat, sore tongue, or colds. Complains of "canker sore" if she eats strawberries. Denies n/v, abdominal pain, or excessive gas. Complains of dyspepsia approx. 2×/month, relieved by Mylanta. Does not associate this with time she takes ASA. Describes skin and scalp as dry. Uses lotions frequently. Denies easy bruising, pruritus, or nonhealing sores. Nails are hard and brittle. Hair is fine and soft.

Current weight: 120 lb; height: 5'4"

Previous weight: 150 lb 10 years ago. Desires to maintain current weight.

Weight fluctuates ± 5 lb/month. Client states, "I've always had to watch what I eat because I gain so easily." Denies intolerance to heat or cold, or voice changes.

J. Cognitive Pattern

Speech clear without slur or stutter. Follows verbal cues. Expresses ideas and feelings clearly and concisely. States she has had a gradual loss of memory over past 5 to 6 years. Believes long-term memory is better than short term. She can recall past weekly events but has trouble recalling dates, times, and places of events. Learns best by writing information down and then reviewing it. Makes major decisions jointly with husband after prayer.

K. Role–Relationship Pattern

Client has been married 55 years. Describes relationship as the best part of her life right now. Only son lives in Minnesota, and they visit one to two times a year. Is very fond of three grandchildren. Expresses desire to visit more often but states, "He has his own life and family now." Communicates once a month by phone. Explains her relationship with other members of the church and community groups as friendly and "familylike." Lives with husband in first-floor apartment. Has casual relationship with apartment neighbors—friendly but distant. Was the oldest of five children. See family genogram.

L. Self-Perception–Self-Concept Pattern

Describes self as a normal person. Talkative, outgoing, and likes to be around people but hates noisy environments. Happy with the person she has become and states, "I can definitely live with myself." States a weakness is that she worries about "little things" more now

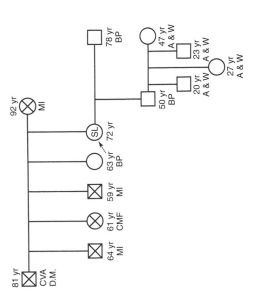

... than she used to and tends to be irritated more easily. Cannot place specific onset of these feelings. Feels good about self-control of diabetes.

M. Coping–Stress Tolerance Pattern

States husband's high blood pressure has never been a source of stress to her. Shares confidences with husband and with a few close friends. Most stressful time in life was losing two brothers and a sister, all in 1994. States with the support of husband and church she handled it "better than most people would have." States she prays and eats when under stress. Cannot identify any major stresses that have occurred in the last year.

N. Value–Belief Pattern

Religious preference is Lutheran. Values relationship with husband, family, and God. Enjoys helping others in the church and community. Believes God is loving, supportive, and forgiving. Places God as first priority in life. States prayer is extremely important to her and practices it daily. States this personalizes her relationship with God. Has been Lutheran all her life and states she and her husband share in church activities together.

PHYSICAL ASSESSMENT

A. General Physical Survey

Ht: 5'4", Wt: 120 lb, Radial pulse: 71, Resp: 16, BP: R arm—120/72, L arm—120/70, Temp: 98.6°F. Client alert and cooperative. Sitting comfortably on table with arms crossed and shoulders slightly slouched forward. Smiling with mild anxiety. Dress is neat and clean. Walks steadily with posture slightly stooped.

B. Skin, Hair, and Nail Assessment

1. *Skin:* Pale pink, warm and dry to touch. Skinfold returns to place after 1 second when lifted over clavicle. Tan "age spots" on posterior hands bilaterally in clusters of four to five and evenly distributed over lower extremities. A 3-cm nodule

with 2-mm macule in center noted in right axilla; indurated, nontender, and nonmobile. No evidence of vascular or purpuric lesions. No edema.

2. *Hair:* Chin length, gray, straight, clean, styled, medium-textured, evenly distributed on head. No scalp lesions or flaking. Fine blond hair evenly distributed over arms bilaterally and sparsely on legs bilaterally. No hair noted on axilla or on chest, back, or face.

3. *Nails:* Fingernails medium length, and thickness, clear. Splinter hemorrhages noted on right thumb near fingertip in midline. No clubbing or Beau lines.

C. Head and Neck Assessment

Head symmetrically rounded, neck nontender with full ROM. Neck symmetrical without masses, scars, pulsations. Lymph nodes nonpalpable. Trachea in midline. Thyroid nonpalpable. Carotid arteries equally strong without bruits. Identifies light and deep touch to various parts of face.

CN V: Identifies light touch and sharp touch to forehead, cheek, and chin. Bilateral corneal reflex intact. Masseter muscles contract equally and bilaterally. Jaw jerk + 1.

CN VII: Identifies sugar and salt on anterior two thirds of tongue. Smiles, frowns, shows teeth, blows cheeks, and raises eyebrows as instructed.

D. Eye Assessment

Eyes 2 cm apart without protrusion. Eyebrows sparse with equal distribution. No scaliness noted. Lids pink without ptosis, edema, or lesions, and freely closeable bilaterally. Sclera white without increased vascularity or lesions noted. Lacrimal apparatus nonedematous. Palpebral and bulbar conjunctiva slightly reddened without lesions noted. Irises uniformly blue. PERRLA, EOMs intact bilaterally. Peripheral vision equal to examiner's.

Visual acuity: With glasses off vision is blurred at 14" away, but can identify number of fingers held up. With glasses on reads newspaper print at 14".

Funduscopic exam: Red reflex present bilaterally. Optic disc round with well-defined margins. Physiologic cup occupies disc. Arterioles smaller than venules. No A-V nicking, no hemorrhages, or exudates noted. Macula not seen. (CNs II, III, IV, VI intact.)

Ear Assessment

Auricle without deformity, lumps, or lesions. Right auricle with tag at top of pinna. Auricles and mastoid processes nontender. Bilateral auditory canals contain moderate amount dark-brown cerumen. Tympanic membrane difficult to view due to wax.

Whisper test: Client identifies one out of two words in four attempts. Weber test: No lateralization of sound to either ear. Rinne test: AC is greater than BC both ears (CN VIII).

F. Nose and Sinuses Assessment

External structure without deformity, asymmetry, or inflammation. Nares patent. Turbinates and middle meatus pale pink, without swelling, exudate, lesions, or bleeding. Nasal septum midline without bleeding, perforation, or deviation. Frontal and maxillary sinuses nontender. Identifies smells of coffee and soap (CN I).

G. Mouth and Pharynx Assessment

Lips moist with peach lipstick. No lesions or ulcerations. Buccal mucosa pink and moist without discoloration or increased pigmentation. No ulcers or nodules. Upper and lower dentures secure. Gums pink and moist without inflammation, bleeding, or discoloration. Hard and soft palates smooth without lesions or masses. Tongue midline when protruded without fasciculations (CN XII intact), lesions, or masses. No lesions, discolorations, or ulcerations on floor of mouth, oral mucosa, or gums. Gag reflex intact, and client identifies sugar and salt on posterior tongue. Uvula in midline and elevates on phonation. (CNs IX and X intact.) Tonsils present without exudate, edema, ulcers, or enlargement.

H. Cardiac Assessment

No pulsations visible. No heaves, lifts, or vibrations. PMI: 5th ICS to LMCL. Clear, brief heart sounds throughout. Physiologic S$_2$. No gallops, murmurs, or rubs. AP = 72/min and regular.

Sample Adult Nursing Health History and Physical Assessment

I. Peripheral Vascular System Assessment

Arms: Equal in size and symmetry bilaterally; pale pink; warm and dry to touch without edema, bruising, or lesions noted. Radial pulses equal in rate and amplitude, and strong. Allen test: Right equal 2-second refill, left equal 2-second refill. Brachial pulses strong, equal, and even. Epitrochlear nodes nonpalpable.

Legs: Legs large in size and bilaterally symmetrical. Skin intact, pale pink; warm and dry to touch without edema, bruising, lesions, or increased vascularity. Superficial inguinal, horizontal, and vertical lymph nodes nonpalpable. Femoral pulses strong and equal without bruits. Popliteal pulse nonpalpable with client supine or prone. Dorsalis pedis and posterior tibial pulses strong and equal. No edema palpable. Homans negative bilaterally. No retrograde filling noted when client stands. Toenails thick and yellowed. Special maneuver for arterial insufficiency: feet regain color after 4 seconds and veins refilled in 5 seconds.

J. Thorax and Lung Assessment

Skin pale pink without scars, pulsations, or lesions. No hair noted. Thorax expands evenly bilaterally without retractions or bulging. Slope of ribs = 40°. No use of auxiliary respiratory muscles and no nasal flaring. Mild kyphosis. Respirations even, unlabored, and regular (16/min). No cough noted. No tenderness, crepitus, or masses. Tactile fremitus decreases below T5 bilaterally posteriorly, and 4th ICS anteriorly bilaterally. Thorax resonance throughout. Diaphragmatic excursion: Left—on inspiration diaphragm descends to T11, and on expiration diaphragm ascends to T9. Right—on inspiration diaphragm descends to T12, and on expiration diaphragm ascends to T9. Vesicular breath sounds heard in all lung fields. No rales, rhonchi, friction rubs, or abnormal whispered pectoriloquy, bronchophony, or egophony noted.

K. Breast Assessment

Breasts moderate in size, round, and symmetrical bilaterally. Skin pale pink with light-brown areola. No dimpling or retraction. Free movement in all positions. Engorged vein noted running across UOQ to areola in right breast. Nipples inverted bilaterally. No discharge expressed. No thickening or tenderness noted. A 2-cm, hard, immobile round mass noted in left breast in LUOQ. Client denies ever noticing this. Nontender to palpation. Lymph nodes nonpalpable. Client does ___ow how to do self breast exam.

L. Abdominal Assessment

Abdomen rounded, symmetrical without masses, lesions, pulsations, or peristalsis noted. Abdomen free of hair, bruising, and increased vasculature. Healed with appendectomy scar. Umbilicus in midline, without herniation, swelling, or discoloration. Bowel sounds low pitched and gurgling at 22/minute × four quads. Aortic, renal, and iliac arteries auscultated without bruit. No venous hums or friction rubs auscultated over liver or spleen. Tympany percussed over all four quads. An 8-cm liver span percussed in RMCL. Area of dullness percussed at 9th ICS in left postaxillary line. No tenderness or masses noted with light and deep palpation in all four quadrants. Liver and spleen nonpalpable.

M. Genitourinary–Reproductive Assessment

No bulging or masses in inguinal area. A 1-cm nodule palpated in right groin. Labia pink with decreased elasticity and vaginal secretions. No bulging of vaginal wall, purulent foul drainage, or lesions. Skene's gland not visible. Anal area pink with small amount of hair. Rectal mucosa bulges with straining.

N. Musculoskeletal Assessment

Posture slightly stooped with mild kyphosis. Gait steady, smooth, and coordinated with even base. Limited ROM of lateral flexion and extension of spine. Paravertebrals equal in size and strength. Shrugs shoulders and moves head to right and left against resistance (CN XI intact); upper extremities and lower extremities have full ROM. Muscles moderately firm bilaterally. No deviations, inflammations, or bony deformities. Small callus on left heel. Moves upper and lower extremities freely against gravity and against resistance. Rheumatoid nodule noted on dorsal surface of left hand.

O. Neurologic Assessment

Mental status: Pleasant and friendly. Appropriately dressed for weather with matching colors and patterns. Clothes neat and clean. Facial expressions symmetrical and correlate with mood and topic discussed. Speech clear and appropriate. Follows through with train of thought. Carefully chooses words to convey feelings and ideas. Oriented to person, place, time, and events. Remains attentive and able to focus on exam during entire interaction. Short-term memory intact, long-term memory before 1992 unclear—especially cannot recall dates and sequencing of events. General information questions answered correctly 100% of the time. Vocabulary suitable to educational level. Explains proverb accurately. Gives semiabstract answers and enjoys joking. Is able to identify similarities 5 seconds after asked. Answers to judgment questions in realistic manner.

Cranial nerves: I–XII intact (integrated throughout exam).

Cerebellar and motor function: Alternates finger to nose with eyes closed; occasionally tends to hit opposite side of nose. Rapidly opposes fingers to thumb bilaterally without difficulty. Alternates pronation and supination of hands rapidly without difficulty. Heel to shin intact bilaterally. Romberg: minimal swaying. Tandem walk: steady. No involuntary movements noted.

Sensory status: Superficial light- and deep-touch sensation intact on arms, legs, neck, chest, and back. Position sense of toes and fingers intact bilaterally. Identifies point localization correctly. Identifies coin placed in hand and number written on palm of hand correctly.

Two-Point Discrimination (in mm)	Right	Left
Fingertips	6	6
Dorsal hand	15	15
Chest	45	49
Forearm	39	35
Back	45	45
Upper arm	40	45

Reflexes	Right	Left
Biceps	2+	2+
Triceps	2+	2+
Patellar	3+	3+
Achilles	2+	2+
Abdominal	1+	1+
Babinski	neg	neg

Motor status: Muscle tone firm at rest, abdominal muscles slightly relaxed. Muscle size adequate for age. No fasciculations or involuntary movements noted. Muscle strength moderately strong and equal bilaterally.

Client's Strengths

- Positive attitude and outlook in life
- Motivation to comply with prescribed diet
- Strong support systems: husband and spiritual beliefs
- No physical limitations

Nursing Diagnoses

- Risk for Ineffective Health Maintenance related to lack of knowledge concerning importance of regular medical checkups, re: lesion in UOQ of left breast not seen by physician, no Pap smear, and no follow-up with diabetes
- Acute right hip pain

- Constipation related to lack of bowel routine and laxative overuse
- Knowledge Deficit: Signs, symptoms, and treatment of hyperglycemia/hypoglycemia
- Knowledge Deficit: Management and causes of constipation
- Knowledge Deficit: self breast exam technique
- Knowledge Deficit: Importance of self-blood glucose monitoring

Collaborative Problems

- Potential complication: Hyperglycemia, hypoglycemia
- Potential complication: Hypertension

Assessment of Family Functional Health Patterns

The nurse obtains data about the family's functional health patterns by interviewing the family as a group or by interviewing one or two family members who are reliable historians and seem knowledgeable about their family's health patterns. If data reveal a particular problem identified with an individual family member, the nurse can then focus attention on obtaining more data from that individual.

I. FAMILY PROFILE

The purpose of the family profile is to obtain biographical family data (age, sex, and current health status of each family member). A genogram may be used to illustrate this information.

II. HEALTH PERCEPTION–HEALTH MANAGEMENT PATTERN

Subjective Data

- Describe your family's general health during the past few years.
- Has your family been able to participate in its usual activities (work, school, sports)?
- Describe what your family does to try to stay healthy (diet, exercise, etc).
- From whom does your family seek health care? When?
- Describe how your family members check their health status (eg, eye exams, dental exams, breast exams, testicular exams, medical checkups).

- Describe any behaviors in your family that are considered unhealthy.
- Who cares for family members who are or who become ill?
- How would you know if a family member were ill?

Objective Data

1. Observe the appearance of family members.
2. Observe the home (hazards and safety devices, storage facilities, cooking facilities).

III. NUTRITIONAL–METABOLIC PATTERN

Subjective Data

- Describe typical breakfast, lunch, supper, and snacks that you eat as a family.
- What type of drinks do you usually have during the day and at night?
- How would you describe your family's appetite in general?
- How often does your family seek dental care? Are there any dental problems in your family?
- Does anyone in your family have skin rashes or problems with sores healing? Explain.
- Who usually prepares the family meals? Who shops for groceries?

Objective Data

1. Observe kitchen appliances, availability of food, and types of foods kept in the home, if possible.
2. Observe preparation of a family meal, if possible.
3. Observe family members for obvious signs of malnutrition or obesity.

IV. ELIMINATION PATTERN

Subjective Data

- How often do family members have bowel movements? Urinate?
- Are laxatives used in your family? Explain.
- Are there problems with disposing of waste or garbage?
- Describe any recycling you do.
- Does your family have pets (indoor or outdoor)? How are their wastes disposed?
- Do you have problems with insects in your home? Explain.

Objective Data

1. Observe bathroom facilities.
2. Inspect home for insects.
3. Observe garbage and waste disposal.

V. ACTIVITY–EXERCISE PATTERN

Subjective Data

- Describe how your family exercises. Frequency?
- How does your family relax?
- What does your family do for enjoyment?
- Describe a typical day of activities in your family (work, school, play, games, meals, hobbies, house cleaning, yard work, cooking, exercise).

Objective Data

1. Observe the pace of family activities.
2. Observe any exercise equipment kept in home.

VI. SLEEP–REST PATTERN

Subjective Data

- When does your family generally go to bed and awaken? Do family members go to bed and arise at different times? Explain.
- Does your family seem to get enough time to sleep? To rest and relax?
- Do any family members work at night? How does this affect other family members?

Objective Data

1. Observe sleeping areas.
2. Observe temperament and energy level of family members.

VII. SENSORY–PERCEPTUAL PATTERN

Subjective Data

- Are there any hearing or visual problems that affect your family members?
- Are there any deficits in a family member's ability to taste and smell that affect how food is prepared for the family?
- Does pain seem to be a family problem? Explain. How is this managed?
- What is the usual form of pain relief used by family members?

Assessment of Family Functional Health Patterns

Objective Data

1. Observe any visual or hearing aids used by family members.
2. Observe medications kept on hand to relieve pain.

VIII. COGNITIVE PATTERN

Subjective Data

- Who makes the major family decisions? How?
- Describe the highest educational level of all family members.
- Does your family understand any illnesses and treatments that affect any of your family members?
- How does your family enjoy learning (eg, reading, watching television, attending classes)?
- Are there any problems with memory in the family? Explain.

Objective Data

1. Observe language spoken by all family members.
2. Observe use of words (vocabulary level), and ability to grasp ideas and express self.
3. Are family decisions present or future oriented? Observe family decision-making strategies.
4. Observe school attended by children.

IX. SELF-PERCEPTION–SELF-CONCEPT PATTERN

Subjective Data

- Describe the general mood of your family (eg, sad, happy, eager, depressed, anxious, relaxed).
- Do you consider yourselves to be a close family? How do you spend time together? Is this time satisfying?

- Do family members share any common goals? Explain.
- What does the family enjoy doing most together?
- How does your family deal with disagreements?
- How do your family members express their affection, feelings, and/or concerns? Are they allowed to do so freely? Explain.
- Does your family seem to discuss problems that affect individual members?
- How does your family deal with change?

Objective Data

1. Observe family discussions.
2. Observe mood and temperament of family.
3. Observe how family members deal with conflict.
4. How do family members show concern and consideration for each other's needs and desires?

X. ROLE–RELATIONSHIP PATTERN

Subjective Data

- Describe how your family members support each other, show affection, and express concerns.
- Describe any problems with relationships between family members.
- Describe your family resources (financial, community support systems, family support systems).
- How active is your family in your neighborhood and/or community?
- Explain family responsibilities for various household chores (washing, cooking, driving, lawn maintenance, etc).
- Explain how discipline is used in your family. How are family members rewarded? Describe any aggression and/or violence that occurs in your family.

Objective Data

1. Observe family interaction patterns (verbal and nonverbal).
2. Explore which family members take responsibility for managing and leading family activities.
3. Observe living space and ownership of rooms by family members.

XI. SEXUALITY–REPRODUCTIVE PATTERN

Subjective Data

If appropriate: Are sexual partners within home satisfied with sexual relationship and activities? Describe any problems.

- Are contraceptives used?
- Is family planning used? How?
- Are parents comfortable answering questions and explaining topics related to sexuality to their children?

XII. COPING–STRESS TOLERANCE PATTERN

Subjective Data

- What major changes have occurred in your family during the past year (eg, divorce, marriage, family members leaving home, new members coming into home, death, illness, births, accidents, change in finances and/or occupation)?
- How does your family *cope* with major stressors (eg, exercise, discussion, prayer, drugs, alcohol, violence)?
- Who in the family copes best with stressors?
- Who has the most difficult time coping with stress?
- Who outside the family (eg, friends, church, support groups) seems to help your family most during difficult times?

Objective Data

1. Observe effect and pace of family interactions.

XIII. VALUE–BELIEF PATTERN

Subjective Data

- What does your family consider to be most important in life?
- What does your family want from life?
- What rules does your family hold most important?
- Is religion important in the family? What religion are family members? What religious practices are important to the family? Is a relationship with God important to the family?
- What does your family look forward to in the future?
- From where do the family's hope and strength come?

Objective Data

1. Observe family rituals and/or traditions.
2. Observe pictures and other articles (religious or other) in home.
3. Listen to general topics discussed in home by family members.
4. Observe the type of television programs viewed by family members and the type of music to which family members listen.

Nursing Diagnoses (Wellness, Risk, and Actual) Grouped According to Functional Health Patterns

1. HEALTH PERCEPTION–HEALTH MANAGEMENT PATTERN

Wellness Diagnoses

Health-Seeking Behaviors
Effective Therapeutic Regimen Management

Risk Diagnoses

Risk for Injury
Risk for Suffocation
Risk for Poisoning
Risk for Trauma
Risk for Perioperative Positioning Injury
Risk for Altered Development
Risk for Altered Growth

Actual Diagnoses

Energy Field Disturbance
Delayed Growth and Development
Ineffective Health Maintenance
Ineffective Therapeutic Regimen: Management Individual
Ineffective Therapeutic Regimen Management: Family
Ineffective Therapeutic Regimen Management: Community
Noncompliance

2. NUTRITIONAL–METABOLIC PATTERN

Wellness Diagnoses

Effective Breast-feeding
Readiness for Enhanced Nutritional Metabolic Pattern
Readiness Enhanced Skin Integrity

Risk Diagnoses

Risk for Imbalanced Body Temperature
  Hypothermia
  Hyperthermia
Risk for Infection
Risk for Imbalanced Nutrition: More than body requirements
Risk for Imbalanced Nutrition: Less than body requirements
Risk for Aspiration
Risk for Imbalanced Fluid Volume
Risk for Constipation
Risk for Delayed Surgical Recovery
Risk for Impaired Skin Integrity

Actual Diagnoses

Decreased Adaptive Capacity: Intracranial
Ineffective Thermoregulation
Fluid Volume Deficit
Fluid Volume Excess
Imbalanced Nutrition: Less Than Body Requirements
Imbalanced Nutrition: More Than Body Requirements
Ineffective Breast-feeding
Interrupted Breast-feeding
Ineffective Infant Feeding Pattern
Impaired Swallowing
Ineffective Protection
Impaired Tissue Integrity
Altered Oral Mucous Membrane
Impaired Skin Integrity
Altered Dentition

3. ELIMINATION PATTERN

Wellness Diagnoses

Readiness for Enhanced Bowel
  Elimination Pattern
Readiness for Enhanced Urinary
  Elimination Pattern

Risk Diagnoses

Risk for constipation
Risk for Impaired Urinary Elimination

Actual Diagnoses

Altered Bowel Elimination
  Constipation
  Perceived Constipation
  Diarrhea
  Bowel Incontinence
Altered Urinary Elimination
  Urinary Retention
  Total Incontinence
  Functional Urinary Incontinence
  Reflex Urinary Incontinence
  Urge Incontinence
  Stress Incontinence

Decreased Adaptive Capacity: Intracranial
Diversional Activity Deficit
Impaired Home Maintenance
Impaired Physical Mobility
Dysfunctional Ventilatory Weaning Response
Impaired Spontaneous Ventilation
Self-Care Deficit: (specify type: Feeding,
Bathing/Hygiene, Dressing/Grooming, Toileting)
Ineffective Tissue Perfusion: (specify type: Cerebral
Cardiopulmonary, Renal, Gastrointestinal,
Peripheral)
Disorganized Infant Behavior
Impaired Walking
Impaired Wheelchair Mobility
Impaired Transfer Ability
Impaired Bed Mobility

5. SEXUALITY–REPRODUCTIVE PATTERN

Wellness Diagnosis

Readiness for Enhanced Sexuality Patterns

Risk Diagnoses

Risk for Ineffective Sexuality Pattern
Risk for Falls

4. ACTIVITY–EXERCISE PATTERN

Wellness Diagnoses

Readiness for Enhanced:
  Cardiac Output
  Diversional Activity Pattern
  Activity–Exercise Pattern
  Home Maintenance Management
  Self-care Activities
  Tissue Perfusion
  Breathing Pattern
  Organized Infant Behavior

Risk Diagnoses

Risk for Disuse Syndrome
Risk for Perioperative Positioning Injury
Risk for Disorganized Infant Behavior
Risk for Peripheral Neurovascular Dysfunction
Risk for Altered Respiratory Function

Actual Diagnoses

Impaired Gas Exchanged
Activity Intolerance
Ineffective Airway Clearance
Ineffective Breathing Pattern
Decreased Cardiac Output

Nursing Diagnoses (Wellness, Risk, and Actual)
Grouped According to Functional Health Patterns

Actual Diagnoses

Sexual Dysfunction
Ineffective Sexuality Patterns

6. SLEEP–REST PATTERN

Wellness Diagnosis

Readiness for Enhanced Sleep

Risk Diagnoses

Risk for Disturbed Sleep Pattern
Risk for Sleep Deprivation

Actual Diagnoses

Sleep Pattern Disturbance
Sleep Deprivation

7. SENSORY–PERCEPTUAL PATTERN

Wellness Diagnosis

Readiness for Enhanced Comfort Level

Risk Diagnoses

Risk for Pain (acute, chronic)
Risk for Aspiration

Actual Diagnoses

Acute Pain
Chronic Pain
Dysreflexia
Disturbed Sensory–Perception (specify Visual
  Auditory, Kinesthetic, Gustatory, Tactile,
  Olfactory)
Unilateral Neglect

8. COGNITIVE PATTERN

Wellness Diagnosis

Readiness for Enhanced Cognition

Risk Diagnosis

Risk for Disturbed Thought Processes

Actual Diagnoses

Acute Confusion
Chronic Confusion
Decisional Conflict (Specify)
Impaired Environmental Interpretation Syndrome
Knowledge Deficit (Specify)
Disturbed Thought Processes
Impaired Memory

9. ROLE–RELATIONSHIP PATTERN

Wellness Diagnoses

Readiness for Enhanced
  Relationships
  Parenting
  Role Performance
  Communication
  Social Interaction
  Caregiver Role
  Grieving

Risk Diagnoses

Risk for Dysfunctional Grieving
Risk for Loneliness
Risk for Impaired Parent/Infant/Child Attachment

Actual Diagnoses

Impaired Verbal Communication
Dysfunctional Family Processes
Dysfunctional Family Processes: Alcoholism
Interrupted Family Processes
Anticipatory Grieving
Dysfunctional Grieving
Impaired Parenting
Parental Role Conflict

Ineffective Role Performance
Impaired Social Interaction
Social Isolation
Caregiver Role Strain

10. SELF-PERCEPTION–SELF-CONCEPT PATTERN

Wellness Diagnoses

Readiness for Enhanced Self-Perception
Readiness for Enhanced Self-Concept

Risk Diagnoses

Risk for Hopelessness
Risk for Body Image Disturbance
Risk for Situational Low Self-Esteem

Actual Diagnoses

Anxiety
Fatigue
Fear
Hopelessness
Powerlessness
Disturbed Personal Identity
Disturbed Body Image

Nursing Diagnoses (Wellness, Risk, and Actual)
Grouped According to Functional Health Patterns

Potential Complication: Muscular/Skeletal

PC: Joint dislocation
PC: Pathologic fractures

Potential Complication: Respiratory

PC: Hypoxemia
PC: Atelectasis/pneumonia
PC: Tracheobronchial constriction
PC: Pneumothorax

Potential Complication: Reproductive

PC: Fetal distress
PC: Postpartum hemorrhage
PC: Pregnancy-associated hypertension
PC: Prenatal bleeding
PC: Preterm labor

Potential Complication: Medication Therapy Adverse Effects

PC: Adrenocorticosteroid therapy adverse effects
PC: Antianxiety therapy adverse effects
PC: Antiarrhythmic therapy adverse effects
PC: Anticoagulant therapy adverse effects
PC: Anticonvulsant therapy adverse effects
PC: Antidepressant therapy adverse effects
PC: Antihypertensive therapy adverse effects
PC: Beta-adrenergic blocker therapy adverse effects
PC: Calcium channel blocker therapy adverse effects
PC: Angiotensin-converting enzyme therapy adverse effects
PC: Antineoplastic therapy adverse effects
PC: Antipsychotic therapy adverse effects

(Carpenito, L. J. (2004). *Nursing diagnosis: Application to clinical practice* (10th ed.). Philadelphia: Lippincott Williams & Wilkins.)
*Frequently used collaborative problems are represented on this list. Other situations not listed here could qualify as collaborative problems.

References and Bibliography

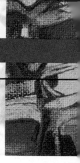

Allal, A., Nicoucar, K., Mach, N., & Dulguerov, P. (2003). Quality of life in patients with oropharynx carcinomas: Assessment after accelerated radiotherapy with or without chemotherapy versus radical surgery and postoperative radiotherapy. *Head & Neck, 25*(10), 833–841.

American Academy of Ophthalmology (1991). *Eye care for the elderly.* San Francisco. www.aao.org

American Academy of Ophthalmology (1997). Policy statement: Breast feeding and the use of human milk. *Pediatrics, 100*(6), 1035–1039. San Francisco: Author.

American Academy of Ophthalmology (2000). *Comprehensive adult medical eye evaluation, preferred practice patterns.* San Francisco. www.aao.org

American Academy of Ophthalmology (2000). Policy statement: Frequency of ocular examinations. San Francisco: Author.

American Academy of Ophthalmology (2001). Policy statement: Vision screening for infants and children. San Francisco: Author.

American Academy of Pediatrics (1997). Policy statement: Breast feeding and the use of human milk. *Pediatrics, 100*(6), 1035–1039.

American Academy of Pediatrics (2000). Task force on infant sleep position and sudden infant death syndrome. *Pediatrics, 105*(3), 650–656.

American Cancer Society (2003). *Cancer facts and figures.* Atlanta: Author.

American Dental Association (2001). *Taking care of teeth and gums.* Chicago: Author.

American Dental Association (2001). *Gum disease: Are you at risk.* Chicago: Author.

American Dental Association (2002). *Your child's teeth.* Chicago: Author.

American Heart Association (2000). *Dietary guidelines for healthy American adults.* AHA Scientific Position. Retrieved March 11, 2004, from http://www.americanheart.org

American Heart Association (2004). *Tips for exercise success: Getting started on an exercise program.* Retrieved March 16, 2004, from http://www.americanheart.org

Andrews, M., & Boyle, J. (2002). *Transcultural concepts in nursing care* (2nd ed.). Philadelphia: Lippincott Williams & Wilkins.

Apgar, V., et al. (1958). Evaluation of the newborn infant: Second report. *Journal of the American Medical Association, 168.*

Atbasogcaronlu, E., Ozguven, H., & Olmez, S. (2003). Dissociation between inattentiveness during mental status testing and social inattentiveness in the scale for the assessment of negative symptoms attention subscale. *Psychopathology, 36*(5), 263–268.

Ballard, J. L. et al. (1991). The new Ballard scale. *Journal of Pediatrics, 119,* 417–423.

Bickley, L. S. (2003). *Bates' guide to physical examination and history taking* (8th ed.). Philadelphia: Lippincott Williams & Wilkins.

Bowles, K., Cater, J. (2003). Screening for risk of rehospitalization from home care: Use of the outcomes assessment information set and the probability of readmission instrument. *Research in Nursing & Health, 26*(2), 118–128.

Campinha-Bacote, J. (2003). *The process of cultural competence in the delivery of healthcare services* (4th ed.). Cincinnati, OH: Transcultural C.A.R.E. Associates.

Carpenito, L. J. (2004) *Nursing diagnosis: Application to clinical practice* (10th ed). Philadelphia: Lippincott Williams & Wilkins.

Criddle, L., Bonnono, C., Fisher, S. (2003). Standardizing stroke assessment using the National Institute of Health stroke scale. *Journal of Emergency Nursing, 29*(6), 541–548.

Daniel, W. A., Jr. (1985). Growth at adolescence clinical correlations. *Seminars in Adolescent Medicine, 1*(1), 15–24.

Dennis, C. (2003). The breastfeeding self-efficacy scale: Psychometric assessment of the short form. *Journal of Obstetric, Gynecologic and Neonatal Nursing, 32*(6), 734–744.

DePaula, T., Lagana, K., & González-Ramirez, L. (1996). Mexican Americans. In Lipton, J., Dribble, S., & Minarik, P., (Eds.). *Culture and nursing care: A pocket guide*. San Francisco: UCSF Press.

Dion, L., Malouin, F., McFayden, B., Richards, C. (2003). Assessing mobility and locomotor coordination after stroke with the rise-to-walk task. *Neurorehabilitation & Neural Repair, 17*(2), 83–92.

Dudek, S. G. (1997). *Nutrition handbook for nursing practice* (3rd ed.). Philadelphia: Lippincott-Raven Publishers.

Erikson, E. (1963). *Childhood and society* (2nd ed.). New York: W. W. Norton.

Ferraro, M., Demaio, J., Krol, J., Trudell, C., Rannekliev, K., & Edelstein, L. (2002). Assessing the motor status score: A scale for the evaluation of upper limb motor outcomes in patients with stroke. *Neurorehabilitation & Neural Repair, 16*(3), 283–289.

Gallagher, L. P., & Kreidler, M. C. (1987). *Nursing and health: Maximizing human potential throughout the life cycle.* Norwalk, CT: Appleton & Lange.

Giger, J., & Davidhizar, R. (2003). *Transcultural nursing: Assessment and intervention.* St. Louis: Mosby.

Gillum, K. (1996). Epidemiology of hypertension in African American women. *American Heart Journal, 13,* 385–395.

Gordon, M. (2002). *Manual of nursing diagnosis* (10th ed.). St. Louis: Mosby-Year Book.

Houston, A., & Cowley, S. (2002). An empowerment approach to needs assessment in health visiting practice. *Journal of Clinical Nursing,* *11*(5), 640–650.

Howard, G., Howard, V. J., Kapholi, C., Oli, M. K., & Huston, S. (2001). Decline in U.S. stroke mortality: An analysis of temporal patterns of sex, race, and geographic region. *Stroke, 32*(10), 2213–2220.

Jacobson, N., Gift, A., & Jacox, A. (1990). Advances in physical assessment. *Nursing Clinics of North America, 25*(4), 743–833.

Kelley, J., Avant, K., & Frisch, N. (1995). A trifocal model of nursing diagnosis: Wellness reinforced. *Nursing Diagnosis, 6*(3), 123–128.

Leininger, M. & McFarland, M. (2002). *Transcultural nursing: Concepts, theories, research and practice.* New York: McGraw-Hill.

Lipson, J., Dibble, S., & Minarik, C. (1996). *Culture and nursing care: A pocket guide.* San Francisco: UCSF Nursing Press.

Manuszak, M., & Ross, Joyce. (2003). Identification and management of vascular risk: beyond low density lipoprotein cholesterol. *Official Journal of the American Association of the Occupational Health Nurse, 51*(12), 521–234.

Marshall, W. A., & Tanner, J. M. (1969). Summary of sequence of sexual development: Boys/girls. *Archives of Disease in Childhood, 44,* 291.

Matucci-Cerinic, M., D'Angelo, S., Denton, C., Vlachoyiannopoulos, P., & Silver, R. (2003). Assessment of lung involvement. *Clinical and Experimental Rheumatology, 21*(3), S19.

Messager, S., Hann, C., Goddard, P., Dettmar, P., & Maillard, J. (2003). Assessment of skin viability: Is it necessary to use different methodologies. *Skin Research and Technology, 9*(4), 321–330.

Metropolitan Life Insurance Company (2000). Height and weight table. *Statistical Bulletin.*

Miller, B. (2002). Breast cancer risk assessment in patients seen in a gynecological oncology clinic. *International Journal of Gynecological Cancer, 12*(4), 389–393.

Murray, R. B., & Zentner, J. P. (1993). *Nursing assessment and health promotion strategies through the life span* (5th ed.). Norwalk, CT: Appleton & Lange.

National Institutes of Health (2003). National high blood pressure education program: The 7th report of the Joint National Committee on Prevention, Detection, Evaluation and Treatment of High Blood Pressure. Bethesda, MD.

Nettina, S. (2001). *The Lippincott manual of nursing practice* (7th ed.). Philadelphia: Lippincott Williams & Wilkins.

Nogami, A. (2002). Idiopathic left ventricle tachycardia: assessment and treatment. *Cardiac Electrophysiology Review, 6*(2), 448–457.

North American Nursing Diagnosis Association. *Nursing diagnoses: Definitions and classification (2003–2004).* Philadelphia: Author.

Olaleye, D., Perkins, B., & Bril, V. (2002). Evaluation of three screening tests and a risk assessment model for diagnosis of peripheral neuropathy in the diabetes clinic. *Journal of the Peripheral Nervous System, 7*(2), 137.

Overfield, T. (1995). *Biological variation in health and illness: Race, age, and sex differences*. Menlo Park, CA: Addison-Wesley.

Pablo, A., Izaga, M., & Alday, L. (2003). Assessment of nutritional status on hospital admission nutritional scores. *European Journal of Clinical Nutrition, 57*(7), 824–831.

Palou, A., Serra, F., & Pico, C. (2003). General aspects on the assessment of functional foods in the European union. *European Journal of Clinical Nutrition, 57*(S1), S12–S17.

Peterson, A., Hryshko-Mullen, A., & Cortex, Y., (2003). Assessment and diagnosis of nicotine dependence in mental health settings. *American Journal on Addictions, 12*(3), 192–197.

Piaget, J. (1967). *Six psychological studies:* New York: Vintage Books.

Pillitteri, A. (2003). *Maternal and child health nursing: Care of the childbearing and childrearing family* (4th ed.). Philadelphia: Lippincott Williams & Wilkins.

Ponzer, S., Skoog, A., & Bergstrom, G. (2003). The short musculoskeletal function assessment questionnaire (SMFA). *Acta Orthopaedica Scandinavica, 74*(6), 756–763.

Purnell, Larry, & Paulanka, B. (2003). *Transcultural health care: A culturally competent approach* (2nd ed.). Philadelphia: F. A. Davis.

Rice, E. M. (1989). Geriatric assessment. *Advancing Clinical Care* (May–June), 8–15.

Sanchez-Muniz, F., Carbajal, A., Rodenas, S., Mendez, M., Raposo, R., & Ruiz, T. (2003). Nutritional assessment, health markers and lipoprotein profile in postmenopausal women belonging to a closed community. *European Journal of Clinical Nutrition, 57*(S1), S26–530.

Schiffman, R., Walt, J., Jacobson, G., Doyle, J., Lebovics, G., & Sumner, W. (2003). Utility assessment among patients with dry eye disease. *Ophthalmology, 110*(7), 1412–1420.

Schmermund, A., Mohlenkamp, S., Stang, A., Gronemeyer, D., Seibel, R., & Hirch, H. (2002). Assessment of clinically silent atherosclerotic disease and established and novel risk factors for predicting myocardial infarction and cardiac death in healthy middle-aged subjects. *American Heart Journal, 144*(2), 212–218.

Schwartz, J., & Vinson, R. (2003). Self-assessment examination of the American academy of dermatology-sparse, brittle hair in a young girl. *Journal of the American Academy of Dermatology, 49*(5), 971.

Shimada, M., Hayat, J., Meguro, K., OO, T., Jafri, S., & Yamadori, A. (2003). Correlation between functional assessment staging and "basic age" by the Binet scale supports the retrogenesis model of Alzheimer's disease: A preliminary study. *Psychogeriatrics, 3*(2). 82–87.

Spector, R. E. (2003). *Cultural diversity in health and illness* (6th ed.). Upper Saddle River, NJ: Prentice-Hall.

Symon, A., MacDonald, A., Ruta, D., (2002). Postnatal Quality of life assessment; introducing the mother-generated index. *Birth 29*(1), 40–46.

Synder, L., Wallerstedt, D., Lahl, L., Nehrebecky, M., Soballe, P., & Klein, P. (2003). Development of breast cancer education and risk assessment program. *Oncology Nursing Forum, 30*(5), 803–811.

Takata, G., Chan, L., Morphew, T., Mangione-Smith, R., Morton, S., & Shekelle, P. (2003). Evidence of assessment of the accuracy of methods of diagnosing middle ear effusion in children with otitis media with effusion. *Pediatrics, 11*(2), 1379–1388.

Tanner, J. M. (1962). *Growth at adolescence* (2nd ed.). Oxford: Blackwell Scientific Publications.

U.S. Department of Agriculture, U.S. Department of Health and Human Services (2000). *Nutrition and your health: Dietary guidelines for Americans* (5th ed.). Washington, DC: Author.

Index

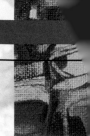

Page numbers followed by the letter "*b*" indicate material in a box; page numbers followed by the letter "*f*" indicate a figure; page numbers followed by the letter "*t*" indicate a table.

A

Abdomen
quadrants of, 269, 270*f*, 271*t*
vascular structures of, 273, 274*f*
viscera of, 269, 272*f*, 273, 274*f*
Abdominal assessment, 269–295
auscultation, 278–279
for bowel sounds, 278–279
for vascular sounds, 279, 280*f*
collaborative problems, 294
equipment for, 273, 275
focus questions for, 275
in geriatric clients, 293
inspection of
abdomen, 277–278
emesis, 278
skin, 276
stools, 278
umbilicus, 277
during labor, 458–461
in newborns, 504
palpation, 284–291
for acute cholecystitis, 291
for appendicitis, 291
for ascites, 288, 290*f*
for asterixes, 291
for kidneys, 288
for liver, 286, 287*b*
of quadrants, 285–286
for spleen, 286, 287*b*
in pediatric clients, 292–293, 295
percussion of, 279, 281–284
liver, 281, 282*f*
quadrants, 281
sequences for, 282*f*
spleen, 281, 283*f*, 284
postpartum, 473–475
risk factors in, 275
teaching tips for, 294–295

Abducens nerve, 375*t*, 395
Abilities, perception of, 30
Abstract reasoning, 383–384
Abuse
child, 480
sexual, 24
Accommodation, eye, 134
Achilles reflex, 417
Acne, 76, 81
Acoustic nerve, 375*t*, 399
Acquired immunodeficiency syndrome (AIDS), 308
Acrochordons, 78
Activities of daily living
assistance with, 371
guideline questions for, 21
and impaired vision, 149
Activity-exercise pattern, 8*b*, 21–22
Adolescents. *See also* Pediatric clients
acne in, 81
breast development in, 267
nutritional assessment in, 440
tobacco use by, 95
tongue piercings in, 95
Adventitious breath sounds, 189, 190*f*, 191
Age, during pregnancy, 445
Age spots, 78
Aging. *See* Geriatric clients
AIDS (acquired immunodeficiency syndrome), 308
Air conduction to bone conduction, 164
Air pollution, 196
Airway clearance, 196–197
Allen test, 227, 231, 234*f*–235*f*
Allergies
patient history of, 15
teaching tips for, 196, 197

Alopecia, 70, 78
Alveolar sacs, 176f, 177
Alveoli, 176f, 177
American Cancer Society
  on breast health, 268
  on nutrition, 294–295
Anemia, iron deficiency, 73
Angiomas, 69f, 78
Angle of Louis, 170, 171f
Angry clients, 11
Anisocoria, 130f, 132
Ankle
  inspection of, 359
  range of motion, 359, 360t, 363f
Ankle clonus reflex, 420
Anterior axillary line (AAL), 172,
    173f, 203, 204f
Anteroposterior (AP) diameter, 193,
    194
Anthropometric measurements,
    427–435
  body mass index, 429, 434t
  height, 427, 428t
  ideal body weight, 427, 429
  mid-arm circumference, 430, 431f
  mid-arm muscle area, 435
  mid-arm muscle circumference,
    432, 435
  triceps skinfold thickness, 432,
    433f
  waist-to-hip ratio, 430
  weight, 427, 428t
Anus
  anatomy of, 318f
  in newborns, 504
  palpation of, 319, 320f
Anxious clients, 11
Aorta, 198, 199f
  abdominal, 273, 274f
  auscultation of, 248, 249f
Aortic area, palpation of, 205, 206f
Aortic valve, 200
Apgar score assessment, 483, 484t
Apical impulse
  in geriatric clients, 218
  inspection and palpation of, 202,
    207f
  location of, 199f, 202, 207f
Apical pulse, 50
  in newborns, 483, 484t, 485
  in pediatric patients, 56
Apnea, 52t

Appearance of client, 379–381
Appendicitis, 291
Arcus senilis, 146
Areolae, 256, 258
Arm recoil, 491
Arms
  arteries of, 223, 224f
  circulation to, 227–228, 231–235
  palpation of, 358
Arterial insufficiency
  impaired skin integrity in, 250
  leg ulcers in, 245t, 246t, 247f
  testing for, 243
  vs. venous insufficiency, 245t
Arterial ulcers, 245t, 246t, 247f
Arteries
  auscultation of, 248, 249f
  of cardiac system, 198, 199f
  in geriatric patients, 59
  palpation of, 228, 229f
  in peripheral vascular system, 223,
    224f
  retinal, 141
Arterioles, retinal, 125
Ascites, 288, 290f
Aspiration, risk of, 295
Assessment techniques. See Physical
    assessment
Asterixes, 291
Asthma, 197
Asymmetrical tonic neck reflex, 422
Atria, 198, 199f
Atrial gallop, 213
Atrioventricular (AV) valves, 198,
    199f, 200
Atrophy, skin, 68f
Auditory canal, 156, 158–159, 166
Auditory function assessment,
    163–165
  gross hearing ability, 163
  Rinne test, 164
  Romberg test for equilibrium, 165
  Weber test, 163, 164f
Auscultation, 36, 42. See also specific
    assessments
Axillary temperature, 48

B

Babinski reflex, 419
Balance
  Romberg test for, 165

tandem walk test for, 410, 411*f*
Barlow maneuver, 366, 367*f*
Barrel chest, 178, 179*f*
Bartholin's glands, 301
Beau's lines, 72
Behavior
 general assessment of, 46
 during labor, 468
 postpartum, 470–471
 during pregnancy, 446
Beliefs of client. *See* Value-belief
  pattern
Biceps reflex, 414, 415*f*
Bicuspid valve, 199*f*, 200
Biographical data of client, 14
Biot's respiration, 181*t*
Birth control
 guideline questions for, 23
 teaching tips for, 335
Bladder
 general assessment of, 20
 location of, 273, 274*f*
 postpartum assessment of,
  477–478
Blepharitis, 129*f*, 131
Blood pressure (BP)
 in adults, 51, 53*t*
 in geriatric patients, 59
 during labor, 467
 and nutrition, 426
 in pediatric patients, 57, 59
 in peripheral vascular assessment,
  228, 251
 postpartum, 470
 in pregnancy, 446
Body build, 46
Body fat, 425
Body image, 30
Body mass index (BMI), 429, 434*t*
Bones. *See also* Musculoskeletal
  assessment
 decalcification of, 371
 in skeletal system, 338, 339*f*
Bowel habits, 20
Bowel sounds, 278–279
Brachial artery, 223, 224*f*, 228
Brachioradialis reflex, 414, 415*f*
Bradycardia, 50, 208
Bradypnea, 52*t*, 180*t*
Brain, 372, 373*f*. *See also* Neurologic
  assessment
Brainstem, 372, 373*f*

Breast
 anatomy of, 252, 254*f*
 development of, 324*f*–328*f*
 landmarks of, 253*f*
 lymph nodes of, 255*f*
 quadrants of, 253*f*
 self-examination of, 268
Breast assessment, 252–268
 areolae, 256, 258
 collaborative problems, 267
 cultural variations in, 267
 equipment for, 256
 focus questions for, 256
 in geriatric clients, 267
 inspection in, 256–260
 lymph nodes, 265
 in males, 265, 266*f*
 in newborns, 493
 nipples, 256, 258, 263
 palpation in, 261–265
 "peau d'orange" appearance, 258,
  259*f*, 260
 in pediatric clients, 265, 267
 positioning for, 257*f*
 postpartum, 471–473
 in pregnancy, 450, 451*f*
 retracted breast tissue, 258, 259*f*
 risk factors in, 256
 teaching tips for, 268
Breast cancer, 256, 267
Breastbone, 170, 171*f*
Breastfeeding
 and breast assessment, 472, 473
 ineffective, 481
 interrupted, 481
 and nutrition, 295
Breath sounds, 188–190
 adventitious, 189, 190*f*, 191
 bronchial, 188
 bronchovesicular, 188, 189*f*
 in geriatric clients, 194
 vesicular, 189, 190*f*
Breathing patterns, ineffective, 196
Bronchi, large-stem, 199*f*
Bronchial breath sounds, 188
Bronchioles, 176*f*, 177
Bronchophony, 192
Bronchospasm, 196–197
Bronchovesicular breath sounds,
  188, 189*f*
Brudzinski sign, 420
Bruits, 230, 248, 279

Buccal mucosa, 102–103
Bullae, 67f

C

Calcium supplements, 371
Caloric requirements, 436, 438t
Cancer
    breast, 256, 267
    cervical, 297
    colorectal, 275, 317
    endometrial, 336
    lung, 177
    oral, 95, 100, 114
    skin, 66
Caput succedaneum, 499, 501f
Cardiac assessment, 198–222
    anatomy in, 198, 199f, 200
    auscultation in, 206f, 208–210, 211,
        213
    chest landmarks in, 204f
    collaborative problems in, 219
    cultural variations in, 218
    equipment for, 200
    focus questions for, 202
    in geriatric clients, 218
    heart murmurs in, 212t
    heart sounds in, 200, 201f, 208,
        209f, 214f
    inspection in, 202–203, 204f
    in newborns, 498
    palpation in, 205, 206f, 207f
    in pediatric clients, 214–215, 216f,
        217
    percussion in, 208
    in pregnancy, 449
    risk factors in, 202
    teaching tips for, 219–222
Carotid artery, 228, 229f, 230
Cataracts, 132, 139f
    in geriatric clients, 146
    risk factors for, 127
Central nervous system (CNS), 372,
    373f
Cephalhematoma, 499, 501f
Cerebellar assessment, 406–411
    in geriatric clients, 410
    techniques for, 406–410, 411f
Cerebellum, 372, 373f
Cerebrovascular accident, 378, 391
Cerebrum, 372
Cerumen, 156, 158f, 168

Cervical cancer, 297
Cervical lymph nodes
    anatomy of, 85f
    palpation of, 88, 90–91
Cervix, palpation of, 301, 302, 304,
    463
Chalazion, 127, 128f
Cherry angioma, 69f, 78
Chest. See also Cardiac assessment;
        Thoracic and lung assessment
    landmarks of, 204f
    pain in, 202
    palpation of, 206f
    in pediatric clients, 215, 216f
Chest circumference, of newborns,
    487
Cheyne-Stokes respirations, 52t, 181t
Chicken pox, 76
Child abuse, 480
Chloasma, 448
Cholecystitis, acute, 291
Clavicles, 170, 171f, 502
Clicks, heart, 211
Clients
    age variations in, 11
    cultural variations in, 12
    emotional variations in, 11–12
    non-English-speaking, 12
    profile of, 14–15
Clinical trials, 54t
Clubbing, nail, 73
Cognitive pattern, 8b–9b, 27–28
    in neurological assessment,
        383–384
Collaborative problems
    in abdominal assessment, 294
    in breast assessment, 267
    in cardiac assessment, 219
    defined, 1
    in ear assessment, 168
    examples of, 5t
    in eye assessment, 147
    format and criteria of, 6t
    in genitourinary-reproductive as-
        sessment, 334
    in head and neck assessment, 94
    during labor, 468
    mental status assessment in, 391
    in mouth and oropharynx assess-
        ment, 113
    in musculoskeletal assessment,
        370

in newborn assessment, 508
in nutritional assessment, 442
in peripheral vascular assessment, 250
in physical surveys, 59
in postpartum maternal assessment, 479
in prenatal fetal assessment, 456
in reflex assessment, 422
in sensory nerve assessment, 404
in skin, hair and nail assessment, 79
in thoracic and lung assessment, 195
treatment for, 2
vs. nursing diagnoses, 4, 5*t*, 6*t*
Collarbones, 170, 171*f*, 502
Colon
anatomy of, 273
cancer of, 275, 317
examinations of, 335–336
Coma, 379, 385, 386*t*
Communication
and age variations, 11
client's ability for, 27
cultural variations in, 12
and emotional variations, 11–12
with non-English speaking clients, 12
questions to use, 10
statements to use, 10–11
styles to avoid, 11
Conchae, 96
Congestive heart failure, 221
Conjunctiva, 124*f*, 131
Conjunctivitis, 129*f*, 131
Consciousness assessment, 378–379
Glasgow Coma Scale for, 385, 386*t*
Constipation, 294–295
Contraception
guideline questions for, 23
teaching tips for, 335
Contractions, 459–460, 469
Coordination, assessment of, 384, 407
Coping methods
guideline questions for, 31
for new infant in family, 480
for stress reduction, 394
Coping-stress tolerance pattern, 9*b*, 31–32

Cornea
anatomy of, 122, 124*f*
inspection of, 131
in pediatric clients, 144
reflex to light, 136
Corneal reflex, 396
Coronary heart disease, risk for, 202
Cortical and discriminatory sensation, 403, 404, 405*f*
Costal angle, 171*f*, 172
Cotton-wool patches, 141–142, 143*f*
Cough reflex, 421
Cover-uncover eye test, 136–137
Crackles, 189, 190*f*, 191
Cranial nerves (CN)
abducens, 375*t*, 395
acoustic, 375*t*, 399
assessment of, 395–402
collaborative problems with, 402
facial, 375*t*, 397, 399
in geriatric clients, 402
glossopharyngeal, 376*t*, 399
hypoglossal, 376*t*, 400
oculomotor, 375*t*, 395
olfactory, 375*t*, 395
optic, 375*t*, 395
spinal accessory, 376*t*, 400, 401*f*
teaching tips for, 402
trigeminal, 375*t*, 396–397, 398*f*
trochlear, 375*t*, 395
type and function of, 374, 375*t*–376*t*
vagus, 376*t*, 400, 401*f*
Cranium, 82, 83*f*
Crawling reflex, 422
Cricoid cartilage, 82, 83*f*
Critical thinking skills, 394
Crust, skin, 68*f*
Cullen sign, 277
Cultural variations
in breast assessment, 267
in cardiac assessment, 218
in communication, 12
in ear assessment, 168
in eye assessment, 147
in genitourinary-reproductive assessment, 323
in mental status assessment, 391
in mouth assessment, 113
in musculoskeletal assessment, 369
in nutritional assessment, 441–442

Cultural variations (*continued*)
  in peripheral vascular disease, 248
  in physical assessment, 59
  in prenatal fetal assessment, 456
  in skin, hair and nail assessment,
    78–79
  in thoracic and lung assessment,
    195
Cushing syndrome, 70, 87
Cyanosis, 64, 65, 79
Cysts, 67*f*

D

Dance reflex, 422
Decision-making, by client, 27
Deep tendon reflexes
  Achilles reflex, 417
  biceps reflex, 414, 415*f*
  brachioradialis reflex, 414, 415*f*
  patellar reflex, 416
  technique for eliciting, 412–417
  triceps reflex, 414, 415*f*
Deep veins, 225, 226*f*
Depressed clients, 12
Dermatomes, 374, 377*f*
Developmental history, 15–16
Deviated septum, 118*f*
Diabetes mellitus, eye examinations
    in, 148*t*, 150
Diagnoses
  medical, 5*t*
  nursing
    categories of, 1, 3*t*
    defined, 1
    examples of, 5*t*
    functional health patterns in, 7
    guidelines for obtaining, 9–12
    treatment for, 1–2
    vs. collaborative problems, 4, 6*t*
  risk, 1, 3*t*
  wellness, 1, 3*t*
Diaper rash, 80–81
Diaphragmatic excursions, 184, 187*f*
Diarrhea, in children, 295
Diastolic pause space, 209*f*, 211
Diencephalon, 372, 373*f*
Diet. *See also* Nutrition
  assessment of
    caloric requirements, 436
    food pyramids, 439*f*
    speedy checklist for, 437*b*

  USDA guidelines in, 438*t*
  guideline questions for, 18
  and heart disease, 220
  and stress, 394
  teaching tips for, 294, 442–443
Dilation of cervix, 463
Discriminatory sensation, 403, 404,
    405*f*
Dorsalis pedis artery, 223, 224*f*
Dorsalis pedis pulse, 240, 241*f*
Dress, client's, 46, 59, 380
Drugs. *See* Medications
Dying, discussing, 12

E

Ear
  anatomy of, 151, 152*f*
  foreign objects in, 169
Ear assessment
  of auditory canal, 156, 158–159
  of auditory function, 163–165
  collaborative problems in, 168
  cultural variations in, 168
  equipment for, 153
  of external ear, 153, 154*f*, 155–156
  focus questions for, 153
  in geriatric clients, 168, 169
  of mastoid process, 156
  in newborns, 493, 498
  in pediatric clients, 165–166, 167*f*,
    169
  risk factors in, 153
  teaching tips for, 168–169
  of tympanic membrane, 159–163
Eardrum. *See* Tympanic membrane
Ecchymosis, 69*f*
Ectropion, 127, 128*f*, 146
Edema, 66
Egophony, 192
Elbow
  inspection of, 353
  palpation of, 358
  range of motion, 353, 354*t*, 356*f*
Elderly. *See* Geriatric clients
Elimination pattern, 8*b*, 19–21
Emesis, color of, 278
Endometrial cancer, 336
Energy level, and nutrition, 425
Entropion, 127, 128*f*, 146
Equilibrium, testing, 165
Erb's point, 205, 206*f*, 215

Erythema
  of breasts, 261
  of skin, 65
Esotropia, 137
Exercise
  assessment focus for, 8*b*
  excessive, 370
  general assessment of, 21
  guideline questions for, 21
  and heart disease, 219, 221–222
  nursing diagnoses for, 22
  during pregnancy, 457
  and skin integrity, 79
  weight-bearing, 370
Exotropia, 137
Extension reflex, 421
Extraocular movements, 135
Extraocular muscles, 122, 124*f*
Extremities
  during labor, 467, 468
  lower
    musculoskeletal assessment,
      359–364
    in pediatric clients, 364–365,
      366, 367*f*
    peripheral vascular assessment,
      236, 238–248
    range of motion, 359, 360*t*,
      361*f*–363*f*
    in newborns, 502
    postpartum assessment of,
      476–477
  upper
    musculoskeletal assessment,
      353–358
    peripheral vascular assessment,
      231, 232*f*–235*f*
    range of motion, 353, 354*t*,
      355*f*–357*f*
Exudates, 141–142, 143*f*
Eye
  external structures of, 122, 123*f*,
    124*f*
  infections of, 149
  internal structures of, 122, 124*f*
Eye assessment, 122–150
  collaborative problems in, 147
  cultural variations in, 147
  equipment for, 125
  of external eye, 127–132
    conjunctiva, 131
    cornea, 131

eyelids and lashes, 127–131
iris, 132
lacrimal apparatus, 132
lens, 132
pupil, 132
sclera, 131
  focus questions for, 125
  frequency of, 147, 148*t*, 150
  functional testing
    abnormal eye movement,
      136–137
    accommodation, 134
    extraocular movements, 135
    peripheral vision, 134
    response to light, 136, 146*f*
    visual acuity, 133
  in geriatric clients, 146, 147, 148*t*,
    149–150
  in newborns, 499
  and nutrition, 426
  ophthalmic examination, 138–143
    of macula, 142
    of optic disc, 140–141
    of red reflex, 139
    of retinal background, 141–142,
      143*f*
    of retinal vessels, 141
  in pediatric clients, 144–145, 149
  risk factors in, 127
  teaching tips for, 147, 149–150
Eyelids and lashes
  anatomy of, 122, 123*f*
  deviations from normal, 127–131
  inspection of, 127, 131
  in pediatric clients, 145

F
Face
  anatomy of, 82, 83*f*
  inspection of, 87–88
  during labor, 467
  in mental status assessment, 380
  postpartum assessment of, 476
  sensory function of, 397, 398*f*, 399
Facial nerve, 375*t*, 397, 399
Failure to thrive, 423
Family
  coping with new infant, 480
  genograms, 29
  roles and responsibilities in, 28
Fat, body, 425

Fear, during labor, 469
Feelings, assessment of, 381
Feet. *See* Foot
Female genitalia, 298*f*
Female genitourinary-reproductive
    assessment, 296–307
    Bartholin's glands, 301
    bimanual examination, 303–307
    equipment for, 296
    focus questions for, 297
    in geriatric clients, 334
    internal genitalia, 301–302
    labia, 299
    in newborns, 494, 506
    risk factors in, 297
    sexual maturity ratings, 324*f*–328*f*
    Skene's glands, 298*f*, 300
    urinary meatus, 299
    vaginal orifice, 299–300, 301
    vaginal wall, 300
Female sexuality, 23–24
Femoral artery, 223, 224*f*
    auscultation of, 248, 249*f*
Femoral pulses, 238, 239*f*
Femoral vein, 225, 226*f*
Fetal heart rate (FHR), 455, 460–461
Fetus. *See also* Prenatal fetal
    assessment
    palpation of, 463–464
    position and station of, 464, 465*f*,
        466*f*
Fibroadenomas, 261, 263, 264*f*
Fibrocystic disease, 263, 264*f*
Fingers
    inspection of, 353
    palpation of, 358
    range of motion, 353, 354*t*, 357*f*
Finger-to-nose test, 407
Flossing, 113, 114
Fluid intake, guideline questions, 18
Fluid volume deficit, 295, 469
Fluid wave test, 288, 290*f*
Fontanelles
    inspection and palpation of, 92,
        93*f*, 499, 500*f*, 501*f*
    risks of injury to, 95
Food pyramids, 436, 439*f*
Foot
    inspection of, 359
    of newborns, 493
Fovea centralis, 125, 126*f*
Friction rubs, 279, 280*f*

Functional health patterns. *See also*
    specific health patterns
    overview of, 7, 13–14
    subjective and objective assess-
        ments in, 8*b*–9*b*
Fundus
    measuring height of, 452, 453*f*, 454*f*
    postpartum, 474, 475*f*

G

Gag reflex, 399, 400*f*
Gait
    assessment of, 46, 343, 380
    in geriatric clients, 59, 371
    in pediatric clients, 366
Gallbladder, 272*f*, 273
Gas exchange, impaired, 196, 197
Gastrointestinal system. *See also*
    Abdominal assessment
    in newborns, 502, 504
    in pregnancy, 450
GDS-5/15 Geriatric Depression Scale,
    391, 392*b*–393*b*
Genitalia
    female, 298f
    male, 309*f*, 329*f*–333*f*
    in newborns, 494, 504
Genitourinary-reproductive assess-
    ment, 296–337
    collaborative problems in, 334
    cultural variations in, 323
    in females, 296–307
        Bartholin's glands, 301
        bimanual examination, 303–307
        equipment for, 296
        focus questions for, 297
        internal genitalia, 301–302
        labia, 299
        in pregnancy, 450
        risk factors in, 297
        sexual maturity ratings,
          324*f*–328*f*
        Skene's glands, 298*f*, 300
        urinary meatus, 299
        vaginal orifice, 299–300, 301
        vaginal wall, 300
    in geriatric clients, 323, 334
    in males, 308–322
        equipment for, 308
        focus questions for, 308
        glans, 310

inguinal area, 313–316
penis, 310, 311
rectum, 316–319
risk factors in, 308
scrotum, 310, 313
sexual maturity ratings,
   329f–333f
testis, 311, 312b, 313
in newborns, 504, 506
in pediatric clients, 323, 324f–333f,
   337
teaching tips for, 334–337
Genograms, 29
Geriatric clients
abdominal assessment in, 293
bone decalcification in, 371
breast assessment in, 267
cardiac assessment in, 218
cerebellar assessment in, 410
cranial nerves assessment in, 402
decreased tear production in, 149
ear assessment in, 168, 169
eye assessment in, 146, 147, 148f,
   149–150
gait in, 371
genitourinary-reproductive assessment in, 323, 334
hair variations in, 78
head and neck assessment in, 94
hearing impairment in, 169
imbalanced body temperature in,
   61
imbalanced nutrition in, 115
impaired gas exchange in, 197
impaired mobility in, 371
impaired vision in, 149
incontinence in, 337
injuries in, 371
interviewing, 11
mental status assessment in, 391,
   392b–393b
mouth assessment in, 111
musculoskeletal assessment in,
   369, 371
nail assessment in, 78, 81
nose and sinus assessment in, 120
nutritional assessment in, 440–441
peripheral vascular assessment in,
   248
physical assessment in, 44, 59
postural hypotension in, 61
promoting sleep in, 371
prostate hypertrophy in, 337
reflex assessment in, 422
sensory nerve assessment in, 404
skin assessment in, 78, 81
thoracic and lung assessment in,
   194, 197
Geriatric Depression Scale, 391,
   392b–393b
Gestational age of newborn, 487–497
determining score rating, 494,
   495f–497f
neuromuscular maturity, 487–493
New Ballard Scale, 487, 488f, 489f
physical maturity, 489f, 493–494
Gingiva. See Gums
Glans, 310
Glasgow Coma Scale (GCS), 385,
   386t
Glaucoma, 127, 148t
Glossopharyngeal nerve, 376t, 399
Goals of client, 32
Goniometer, 341
Gordon, Marjory, 7
Graphesthesia, 404
Grasp reflex, 421
Great vessels, 198, 199f
Grey Turner sign, 276
Gums (gingiva)
anatomy of, 96, 97f
inspection and palpation of,
   103–104
and nutrition, 426
in periodontal disease, 114
receding (periodontitis), 103
Gynecomastia, 265, 266f

H

Hair, pubic
female, 324f–328f
male, 329f–333f
Hair assessment
anatomy in, 62
cultural variations in, 79
focus questions for, 64
in geriatric clients, 78
inspection and palpation of, 70
and nutrition, 18, 425
in pediatric clients, 75, 77
Hand
creases in, 76, 77f
inspection of, 353

Hand (*continued*)
   palpation of, 358
   range of motion, 353, 354*t*, 357*f*
   sensitivity of, 36*t*
Head and neck assessment, 82–95
   anatomy in, 82, 83*f*, 84*f*, 85*f*
   cervical lymph nodes, 88, 90–91
   equipment for, 82
   face, 87–88
   focus questions for, 86
   in geriatric clients, 94
   musculoskeletal function, 349
   neck, 88
   in newborns, 499, 500*f*, 501*f*, 502
   in pediatric clients, 92–94
   in pregnancy, 449
   risk factors in, 86
   scalp, 86–87
   teaching tips for, 95
   thyroid, 88, 89*f*, 90
   trachea, 88, 90
Head circumference, 58, 487, 496*f*
Head injury, 86, 95
Health perception-health management pattern, 8*b*, 16–17
Hearing devices, protective, 168
Hearing loss, 153, 168–169. *See also* Ear assessment
Heart. *See also* Cardiac assessment
   anatomy of, 198, 199*f*, 200
   location of apex in, 216*f*
   rate and rhythm of, 208, 217
   size of, in children, 215, 216*f*
Heart disease
   and diet, 220
   and exercise, 219, 221–222
   fear of, 219
   medications for, 220
   risk factors for, 202
   and sexuality, 220
Heart failure, congestive, 221
Heart rate, fetal, 455, 460–461
Heart sounds
   auscultation of, 208, 210*f*, 211, 213
   in geriatric clients, 218
   murmurs, 211, 212*t*, 218
   normal (S₁ and S₂), 209*f*
   in pediatric clients, 215, 217
   production of, 200, 201*f*
   S₃ and S₄, 213, 214*f*
Heel-to-shin test, 408, 409*f*

Height
   of adults, 45, 51
   anthropometric measurement, 427
   cultural variations in, 59
   of newborns (length), 485
   of pediatric clients, 57
Hematomas, 69*f*
Hemorrhages
   retinal, 142, 143*f*
   splinter, 71, 72*f*
Hepatic coma, 291
Hepatitis B virus (HBV), 275
Hernia, 316
   inguinal, 315*f*
   umbilical, 505*f*
Hips
   congenital dysplasia, 366
   inspection of, 359
   palpation of, 364
   posterior, 348
   range of motion, 359, 360*t*, 361*f*
Hirsutism, 70
HIV (human immunodeficiency virus), 308
Homans sign, 242, 477
Hordeolum (stye), 128*f*, 131
Hospitalizations, patient history of, 15
Human immunodeficiency virus (HIV), 308
Hydrocephalus, 92
Hygiene, 380
Hyoid bone, 82
Hypertension
   classification of, 53*t*
   and peripheral vascular disease, 251
   teaching tips for, 60, 251
Hyperthermia, 47
Hyperventilation, 52*t*, 180*t*, 196
Hypoglossal nerve, 376*t*, 400
Hypotension, postural, 61
Hypothermia, 47, 61
Hypoventilation, 52*t*, 181*t*

I

Ideal body weight (IBW), 427, 429
Identity, perception of, 30
Iliac arteries, 248, 249*f*
Iliac crest, 348

Illness
  patient history of, 15
  patient perception of, 16
  and sexuality, 24
Immunity, passive, 60
Impetigo, 76
Impotence, 336
Incontinence, 337
Indoor Air Quality Hotline, 195
Infants. *See also* Newborn physical
      assessment; Pediatric clients
  aspiration in, 295
  attachment to, 480
  care for, 480
  ear assessment in, 166, 167*f*
  feeding, 481
  growth and development in,
      480
  head assessment in, 92, 93*f*
  liver in, 292
  location of heart apex in, 216*f*
  mouth care for, 115
  musculoskeletal assessment in,
      364–365, 366, 367*f*
  nutrition for, 295, 440, 457, 509
  percussion in, 194
  reflexes in, 421–422
  spleen in, 292
  stranger anxiety in, 394
  thoracic and lung assessment in,
      193–194
Inferior vena cava, 198, 199*f*
Inguinal area, 314*f*
  inspection of, 313
  palpation of, 315–316
Injuries
  due to excessive exercise, 370
  to ears, 169
  to fontanelles, 95
  in geriatric clients, 371
  head, 86, 95
  to nasal cavity, 121
  to neck, 95
  in pediatric clients, 115, 169,
      370–371
  sports, 341
  to teeth, 115
Inspections, 35
Intercostal landmarks, 185*f*–186*f*
Intercostal spaces (ICS), 198,
      202–203
Interviews, nursing

  communication techniques for,
      10–12
  phases of, 9–10
Intestines, 272*f*, 273
Intrapartum maternal assessment,
      457–469
  abdominal assessment, 458–461
  behavioral assessment, 468
  collaborative problems in, 468
  equipment for, 458
  focus questions for, 458
  perineal assessment, 461–466
  peripheral vascular assessment,
      467–468
  teaching tips for, 469
Iris, 122, 123*f*
  in children, 145
  inspection of, 132
Iron deficiency anemia, 73

J

Jaundice, 65, 75
Joints, 338. *See also* Musculoskeletal
      assessment
  chronic pain in, 370
  synovial, 338, 340*f*
Jugular venous pressure, 236, 237*f*

K

Kegel exercises, 337
Keloid, 68*f*
Kernig sign, 420
Kidneys
  location of, 273, 274*f*
  palpation of, 288, 289*f*, 293
  in pediatric patients, 293
Kinesthesia, 404, 405*f*
Knees
  inspection of, 359
  range of motion, 359, 360*t*, 362*f*
Kussmaul respirations, 52*t*, 180*t*
Kyphosis, 194, 344, 345*f*

L

Labia, 298*f*, 299
Labor. *See* Intrapartum maternal
      assessment
Lacrimal apparatus, 122, 123*f*
  in children, 145
  inspection and palpation of, 132

Lacrimal gland, 122, 123f
Lanugo, 493
Large intestine, 272f, 273
Laryngopharynx, 96, 99f
Laxatives, 294
Legs
  arterial insufficiency, 243, 245t,
    246t, 247f
  arteries of, 223, 224f
  bowlegged, 365
  inspection and palpation of, 236,
    238–248
  knock-knees, 365
  postpartum, 476–477
  ulcers of, 245t, 246t, 247f
  veins of, 225, 226f
  venous insufficiency, 244, 245t,
    246t, 247f
Leisure activities, 21
Length, of newborns, 485, 495f
Lens of eye, 124f, 125, 132
Lesions, skin, 66
  primary, 66, 67f
  secondary, 66, 68f
  vascular, 66, 69f
Lethargy, 378
Leukoplakia, 102, 107
Lice, 70
Lichenification, 68f
Light, response to, 136, 146f
Linea nigra, 448
Lips, 101, 426
Liver
  location of, 269, 272f
  normal span, 281, 282f
  palpation of, 286, 287b, 292
  in pediatric patients, 292
  percussion of, 281, 282f
Liver spots, 78
Lordosis, 344, 345f
Lower extremities
  musculoskeletal assessment of,
    359–364
  in pediatric clients, 364–366, 367f
  peripheral vascular assessment
    of, 236, 238–248
  range of motion, 359, 360t,
    361f–363f
Lumbar spines, 344, 346f–347f
Lung assessment, 170–197
  anatomy in, 172, 174f–176f
  auscultation in, 184, 188–192

collaborative problems in, 195
cultural variations in, 195
equipment for, 177
focus questions for, 177
in geriatric patients, 194, 197
inspection in, 178
in newborns, 485
palpation in, 178, 182, 183f
in pediatric patients, 193–194,
  196–197
percussion in, 184, 185f–187f
risk factors in, 177
teaching tips for, 195–197
Lung cancer, 177
Lungs, 172, 174f–176f
Lymph nodes
  anatomy of, 82, 85f
  axillary, 252, 255f, 265
  cervical, 88, 90–91
  in pediatric clients, 94
Lymphatic enlargement, 86

M

Macula, 125, 126f, 142
Macules, 67f
Male genitalia, 309f
  development of, 329f–333f
  in newborns, 494, 504
Male sexuality, 23–24
Males
  breast variations in, 265, 266f
  genitourinary-reproductive assess-
    ment in, 308–322
    equipment for, 308
    focus questions for, 308
    geriatric variations in, 334
    glans, 310
    inguinal area, 313–316
    penis, 310, 311
    rectum, 316–319
    risk factors in, 308
    scrotum, 310, 313
    sexual maturity ratings,
      329f–333f
    testis, 311, 312b, 313
Malnutrition, 70, 427, 430, 432, 435
Manipulative clients, 11
Manubrium, 170, 171f
Mastoid process, 154f, 156
Maternal physical assessment,
  444–481

intrapartum maternal, 457–469
postpartum maternal, 469–481
prenatal fetal, 452–457
prenatal maternal, 445–451
Measles, 76
Mediastinum, 172, 176f, 198
Medical diagnoses, 5t
Medical systems models, 7
Medications
  cardiac, 220
  compelling indications for, 54t
  compliance with, 17
  for hypertension, 53t
  nasal, 120
  patient history of, 14–15
Memory, 27, 383, 394
Menopause, 335
Menstrual history, 23
Mental status assessment, 378–394
  appearance, 379–381
  cognitive abilities, 383–384
  collaborative problems, 391
  cultural variations in, 391
  in geriatric clients, 391, 392b–393b
  Geriatric Depression Scale, 391,
    392b–393b
  Glasgow Coma Scale, 385, 386t
  level of consciousness, 378–379
  Mini-Mental State Examination,
    385, 387b–390b
  mood, 381–382
  movement, 379–381
  in pediatric clients, 385, 391
  perceptions, 382–383
  teaching tips for, 394
  thought processes, 382–383
Metabolism, 18. See also Nutritional-
    metabolic pattern
Microcephaly, 92
Mid-arm circumference (MAC), 430,
    431f
Mid-arm muscle area (MAMA), 435
Mid-arm muscle circumference
    (MAMC), 432, 435
Midaxillary line, 172, 173f
Midclavicular lines (MCL), 172, 173f,
    198, 203, 204f
Midsternal line (MSL), 172, 173f, 203,
    204f
Mini-Mental State Examination, 385,
    387b–390b
Miosis, 130f, 132

Mitral area, palpation of, 205, 206f
Mitral valve, 199f, 200
Mobility, in geriatric clients, 371
Mongolian spots, 65, 75, 78, 506, 507f
Mood, assessing, 46, 381
Moro reflex, 421
Motor function
  assessment of, 406
  in mental assessment, 380
  of trigeminal nerve, 397, 398f
Mouth
  anatomy of, 96–99
  cancer of, 95, 100, 114
Mouth assessment, 100–115
  buccal mucosa, 102–103
  collaborative problems in, 113
  cultural variations in, 113
  equipment for, 100
  focus questions for, 100
  in geriatric clients, 111
  gums, 103–104
  hard and soft palate, 107–108
  lips, 101
  oropharynx, 109–110
  in pediatric clients, 98f, 111, 112f
  risk factors for, 100
  teaching tips for, 113–115
  teeth, 104
  tongue, 105–107
Movement of client, 379–381
Murmurs
  classification of, 212t
  defined, 211
  in geriatric clients, 218
  in pediatric patients, 215
Murphy sign, 291
Muscles, 338, 339f. See also
    Musculoskeletal assessment
  chronic pain in, 370
  and nutritional assessment, 425
Musculoskeletal assessment, 338–371
  collaborative problems in, 370
  cultural variations in, 369
  equipment for, 338
  focus questions for, 341, 364
  gait, 343
  in geriatric clients, 369, 371
  head, 349
  hips, 348, 359, 360t, 361f
  lower extremities, 359–364
  muscle strength, 341, 342t, 400,
    401f

Musculoskeletal assessment
(*continued*)
neck, 349–352
in newborns, 483, 484*t*, 499
paravertebral muscles, 344, 348
in pediatric clients, 364–368,
370–371
in pregnancy, 450
risk factors in, 341
scapula, 348
shoulder, 348, 353, 354*t*, 355*f*
spine, 343–348
stance, 343
teaching tips for, 370–371
temporomandibular joint (TMJ),
349, 352
thorax, 349
upper extremities, 353–358
Mydriasis, 130*f*, 132
Myopia, 133

N

Nails
anatomy of, 62, 63*f*
Beau's lines in, 72
clubbing of, 73
focus questions for assessment,
64
in geriatric clients, 78
inspection and palpation of, 71–74
and nail polish use, 80
and nutrition, 425
in nutritional-metabolic pattern, 18
oncolysis, 74
paronychia, 74
in pediatric clients, 75
splinter hemorrhages in, 71, 72*f*
spoon, 73
thickened, 80
NANDA (North American Nursing
Diagnoses Association), 1
Nasal cavity
anatomy of, 99*f*
injuries to, 121
Nasal speculum, 116
Nasolacrimal duct, 122, 123*f*
Nasolacrimal sac, 122, 123*f*
Nasopharynx, 96, 99*f*
National Eye Care Project, 150
Neck
anatomy of, 82, 83*f*, 84*f*

circulation to, 227–230
injuries to, 95
inspection of, 88
lymph nodes of, 85*f*
muscles and landmarks of, 84*f*
musculoskeletal assessment of,
349–352
in newborns, 502
in pediatric clients, 94
range of motion, 88, 349,
350*f*–351*f*
Neck righting reflex, 422
Nerves
cranial, 374, 375*t*–376*t*, 395–402
sensory, 402–406
spinal, 373*f*, 374, 377*f*
Nervous system
central, 372, 373*f*
peripheral, 373*f*, 374
Neurologic assessment, 372–423
cerebellar assessment, 406–411
of cranial nerves, 395–402
equipment for, 374
focus questions for, 374, 378
of mental status, 378–394
motor assessment, 406
in newborns, 498
in pregnancy, 450
reflex assessment, 412–423
risk factors in, 378
of sensory nerves, 402–406
Neuromuscular maturity of newborns, 487–493
arm recoil, 491
New Ballard Scale for, 487, 488*f*,
489*f*
popliteal angle, 491
posture, 487
Scarf sign, 491, 492*f*
square window sign, 490
Neurovascular dysfunction, 251
Nevus flammeus, 506, 507*f*
New Ballard Scale, 487, 488*f*, 489*f*
Newborn physical assessment,
482–509
Apgar score, 483, 484*t*
collaborative problems, 508
equipment for, 482
focus questions for, 482
gestational age, 487–497
physical examination, 498–507
teaching tips for, 508–509

vital signs and measurements, 485, 486f, 487
Nipples, 256, 258, 263
Nodules, 67f
Non-English speaking clients, 12
North American Nursing Diagnoses Association (NANDA), 1
Nose and sinus assessment, 116–121
  equipment for, 116
  external nose, 117, 119
  focus questions for, 116
  in geriatric clients, 120
  internal nose, 117, 118
  sinuses, 119–120
  teaching tips for, 120–121
  techniques for, 116–120
Nosebleeds, 121
Nursing diagnoses
  categories of, 1, 3t
  collaborative problems vs., 4, 6t
  criteria and format for, 6t
  defined, 1
  examples of, 5t
  functional health patterns in, 7
  guidelines for obtaining, 9–12
  treatment for, 1–2
Nursing health history
  client profile in, 14–15
  definition and purpose of, 1–7
  developmental history in, 15–16
  functional health patterns in
    activity-exercise, 8b, 21–22
    cognitive-perceptual, 8b–9b, 27–28
    coping-stress tolerance, 9b, 31–32
    elimination, 8b, 19–21
    health perception-health management, 8b, 16–17
    nutritional-metabolic, 8b, 17–19
    overview of, 7, 8b–9b, 13–14
    role-relationship, 9b, 28–30
    self perception-self concept, 9b, 30–31
    sexuality-reproductive, 8b, 22–24
    sleep-rest, 8b, 24–25
    value-belief, 9b, 32–33
  guidelines for obtaining, 9–12
Nursing interviews
  communication techniques for, 10–12
  phases of, 9–10
Nursing models, 7
Nutritional assessment, 424–443. *See also* Diet
  anthropometric measurements, 427–435
  collaborative problems, 442
  cultural variations in, 441–442
  dietary assessment, 436, 437b, 438t, 439f
  equipment for, 424
  focus questions for, 424
  general inspection, 425–426
  in geriatric clients, 440–441
  for infants, 457, 509
  in pediatric clients, 295, 436, 440
  during pregnancy, 456–457
  teaching tips for, 294, 442–443
Nutritional-metabolic pattern, 8b, 17–19

O

Obesity, and body mass index, 434t
Objective data, 1, 2t
Obstetric history, 23
Obturator sign, 291
Occupational activities, 21
Ocular fundus, 126f
Oculomotor nerve, 375t, 395
Olfactory nerve, 375t, 395
Onycholysis, 74
Ophthalmic examination, 138–143
  of macula, 142
  of optic disc, 140–141
  of red reflex, 139
  of retinal background, 141–142, 143f
  of retinal vessels, 141
Ophthalmoscope, 138
Optic disc
  anatomy of, 125, 126f
  inspection of, 140–141
Optic nerve, 375t, 395
Oral cancer, 95, 100, 114
Oral cavity. *See* Mouth
Oral temperature, 47, 55
Organs, visceral, 269, 272f, 273, 274f. *See also specific organs*
Oropharynx
  anatomy of, 96, 99f
  inspection of, 109–110

Ortolani maneuver, 366, 367*f*
Osteoporosis, 341
Otitis media, 159, 161*f*
Otoscope, 157*f*
Otoscopic exam
    in adults, 159, 160
    in children, 166, 167*f*
Ovaries, 273, 305

P

Pain
    assessment of, 26
    chest, 202
    chronic, 370
    from labor contractions, 469
Palate, 107–108
Pallor, 65, 79
Palpation, 36, 37*t*–38*t*. *See also spe-
        cific assessments*
Palpebral slant, 144
Pancreas, 269, 272*f*, 274*f*
Pap smears, 335–336
Papilledema, 140
Papules, 67*f*
Paravertebral muscles, 344, 348
Parenting skills, teaching tips for,
        457, 480
Parietal pleura, 172, 176*f*
Paronychia, 74
Patches, skin, 67*f*
Patellar reflex, 416
Pathological reflexes, 419–420
    ankle clonus, 420
    Brudzinski sign, 420
    Kernig sign, 420
    plantar reflex, 419, 421
Pediatric clients. *See also* Infants;
        Newborn physical assessment
    abdominal assessment in, 292–293
    acne in, 81
    asthma in, 197
    blood pressure in, 57, 59
    breast assessment in, 265, 267,
        324*f*–328*f*
    bronchospasm in, 196–197
    cardiac assessment in
        chest wall, 215, 216*f*
        heart rates by age, 217*t*
        heart size, 215
        heart sounds, 213, 215, 217
        location of heart apex, 216*f*

peripheral pulses, 215
    coping with stress in, 394
    developmental level of, 55
    diaper rash in, 80–81
    ear assessment in, 165–166, 167*f*,
        169
    eye assessment in, 144–145, 149
    fluid volume deficits in, 295
    fontanelles in, 92, 93*f*, 95, 499, 500*f*,
        501*f*
    genitourinary-reproductive assess-
        ment of, 323
    head and neck assessment in,
        92–94
    head circumference of, 58, 487,
        496*f*
    height of, 57
    imbalanced body temperature in,
        61
    impaired dentition in, 115
    injuries in, 115, 121, 370–371
    interviewing, 11
    mental status assessment in, 385,
        391
    mouth assessment in, 111
    musculoskeletal assessment in,
        364–368, 370–371
    nutritional assessment in, 295, 436,
        440, 443, 457
    passive immunity in, 60
    physical assessment in, 55–58
    piercings in, 95
    pulse in, 56, 483, 484*t*, 485
    reflex assessment in, 421–422
    respirations in, 57, 193
    risk of aspiration in, 295
    sexual education for, 337
    skin assessment in, 75–77
    teaching tips for, 58
    temperature of, 55–56, 60
    thoracic and lung assessment in,
        193–194, 196–197
    tobacco use in, 95
    toilet-training in, 337
    weight of, 58
Pelvic examinations, 335–336
Penis
    developmental stages of, 329*f*–333*f*
    inspection of, 310
    palpation of, 311
Perception, client's
    of abilities, 30

assessment of, 382–383
of body image, 30
of health, 16
of identity, 30
of illness, 16
of roles at work, 28
of roles in family, 28
of self-worth, 30
of senses, 26
of sexual activities, 23–24
of social roles, 28
of stress, 31
Percussion. *See also specific*
    assessments
defined, 36
sounds elicited by, 41*t*
technique for, 36
types of, 39*t*–40*t*
Perforator veins, 225, 226*f*
Perianal area, 321
Perineal assessment, 461–466
cervix, 463
fetal position and station, 464,
    465*f*, 466*f*
inspection, 461–462
palpation, 463–466
perineum, 462
postpartum, 478–479
presenting part of fetus, 463–464
Periodontal disease, 114
Periodontitis, 103
Peripheral nervous system, 373*f*, 374
Peripheral neurovascular dysfunc-
    tion, 251
Peripheral tissue perfusion, 251
Peripheral vascular assessment,
    223–251
anatomy in, 223, 224*f*, 225, 226*f*
arms and neck, 227–231, 232*f*–235*f*
arterial insufficiency, 243, 245*t*,
    247*f*, 248
auscultation of arteries, 248, 249*f*
collaborative problems in, 250
competency of valves, 244
cultural variations in, 248
equipment for, 225
focus questions for, 225, 227
in geriatric clients, 248, 250
jugular venous pressure, 236, 237*f*
in labor, 467–468
leg ulcers, 245*t*, 246*t*, 247*f*
lower extremities, 236, 238–248

in pregnancy, 449
risk factors in, 227
teaching tips for, 250–251
venous insufficiency, 244, 245*t*,
    247*f*
Peripheral vision, 134
Petechiae, 65, 69*f*, 79
Pharynx, 96
Phlebitis, deep, 242
Physical assessments, 35–44
basic guidelines for, 42–43
general surveys, 45–61
of geriatric clients, 44
of pediatric clients, 43–44
skills for, 35–42
    auscultation, 36, 42
    inspection, 35
    palpation, 36, 37*t*–38*t*
    percussion, 36, 39*t*–41*t*
Physical development, 46, 55
Physical maturity of newborns,
    493–494
Physiologic cup, 125, 126*f*, 141
Piercings, 75, 79, 95
Pinna, 151, 155
in children, 165, 167*f*
Plantar reflex, 419, 421
Pleura, 172, 176*f*
Pleural space, 172, 176*f*
Point of maximum impulse (PMI),
    202, 205
Pollution, 196
Polyps, 161*f*
Popliteal angle, 491
Popliteal artery, 223, 224*f*
Popliteal pulse, 240
Popliteal vein, 225, 226*f*
Position sense, 404, 405*f*
Posterior axillary line, 172, 173*f*
Posterior iliac crest, 348
Posterior tibial pulse, 240, 241*f*
Postpartum maternal assessment,
    469–481
of abdomen, 473–475
of behavior, 470–471
of bladder, 477–478
of blood pressure, 470
of breasts, 471–473
collaborative problems, 479
of extremities, 476–477
of face, 476
focus questions for, 470

Postpartum maternal assessment
(*continued*)
of perineum, 478–479
of pulse, 470
teaching tips for, 479–481
of temperature, 470
of weight, 470
Postural hypotension, 61
Posture
in geriatric patients, 59
in mental status assessment, 379
in newborns, 487
and nutrition, 425
Precordium, 198, 199*f*
Pregnancy. *See* Maternal physical assessment; Prenatal assessments
Pregnancy pigmentation, 448
Prehypertension, 53*t*
Prenatal fetal assessment, 452–457
collaborative problems, 456
cultural variations in, 456
equipment for, 452
of fetal heart rate, 455
focus questions for, 452
fundal height, 452, 453*f*, 454*f*
inspection, 452
palpation, 452
teaching tips for, 456–457
Prenatal maternal assessment,
445–451
equipment for, 445
focus questions for, 445
review of systems in, 445–451
behavior in, 446
blood pressure in, 446
breasts in, 450, 451*f*
cardiovascular system in, 449
gastrointestinal system in, 450
genitourinary-reproductive system in, 450
guideline questions for, 23
head and neck in, 449
maternal age, 445
musculoskeletal system in, 450
neurologic system in, 450
peripheral vascular system in, 449
pulse in, 446
respiratory system in, 450
skin color in, 448
weight gain during, 446, 447*f*

teaching tips for, 456–457
Presbycusis, 153, 168
Presbyopia, 133, 146
Prostate
hypertrophy of, 337
palpation of, 321, 322*f*
Psoas sign, 291
Psoriasis, 71, 72
Ptosis, 129f, 131, 146
Pubic hair growth
female, 324*f*–328*f*
male, 329*f*–333*f*
Pulmonary artery, 198, 199*f*
Pulmonary veins, 198, 199*f*
Pulmonic area, palpation of, 205, 206*f*
Pulmonic valve, 199*f*, 200
Pulse
apical, 50, 56, 210
dorsalis pedis, 240, 241*f*
femoral, 238, 239*f*
in newborns, 483, 484*t*, 485
and nutrition, 426
in pediatric clients, 56, 215
popliteal, 240
posterior tibial pulse, 240, 241*f*
postpartum, 470
in pregnancy, 446
radial, 48, 49*f*, 50, 231, 232*f*
taking, teaching tips for, 220
ulnar, 231, 233*f*
Pulse deficit, 50, 210
Pupils, 122, 123*f*
inspection of, 132
reaction to light, 136, 146
Purpura, senile, 78
Pustules, 67*f*

R

Radial artery, 223, 224*f*
Radial pulse
in adults, 48, 49*f*, 50
palpation for, 231, 232*f*
Range of motion (ROM)
of ankles, 359, 360*t*, 363*f*
of elbow, 353, 354*t*, 356*f*
of fingers, 353, 354*t*, 357*f*
of hips, 359, 360*t*, 361*f*
of knees, 359, 360*t*, 362*f*
measuring, 341
of neck, 88, 349, 350*f*–351*f*

of shoulder, 353, 354t, 355f
of spine, 344, 346f–347f
of toes, 359, 360t, 363f
of wrist, 353, 354t, 356f
Rash, diaper, 80–81
Reasoning, abstract, 383–384
Rebound tenderness, 291
Rectal temperature, 47, 56
Rectovaginal examination, 306, 307f
Rectum, assessment of, 316–322
    anus, 318f, 319, 320f
    equipment for, 316
    focus questions for, 317
    palpation, 319
    perianal area, 321
    prostate, 321, 322f
    risk factors in, 317
    sacrococcygeal area, 321
    teaching tips for, 335–336
Red reflex, 139
Reflex assessment, 412–423
    collaborative problems, 422
    deep tendon reflexes, 412–417
    in geriatric clients, 422
    in newborns, 483, 484t
    nutrition in, 426
    pathologic reflexes, 419–420
    in pediatric clients, 421–422
    superficial reflexes, 414, 418
    teaching tips for, 423
Religious beliefs, 32–33
Renal arteries, 248, 249f
Reproduction. See Sexuality-
    reproduction pattern
Respirations
    in adults, 51, 52t
    in children, 57, 193
    in elderly, 194
    in newborns, 483, 484t, 485
    patterns of, 178, 180t–181t
Respiratory disease, 177
Respiratory system. See Lung
    assessment
Response to light, 136, 146
Responsibilities, perception of, 28
Rest pattern. See Sleep-rest pattern
Retina
    anatomy of, 124f, 125
    hemorrhage of, 142, 143f
    inspection of, 141–142
    retinal vessels, 124f, 125, 141
    onchi, 194

Ribs, 171f, 172, 194
Rinne test, 164
Risk diagnoses, 1, 3t
Role-relationship pattern, 9b, 28–30
ROM. See Range of motion
Romberg test, 165, 408
Rooting reflex, 421

S

Sacrococcygeal area, 321
Saliva, 96
Salivary glands, 96, 98f
Scales, skin, 68f
Scalp, 71, 86–87
Scapula, 348
Scapular lines, 172, 173f
Scarf sign, 491, 492f
Sclera, 122, 123f, 131
Scoliosis, 344, 345f, 368
Scrotum, 310, 313
Seborrheic keratosis, 78
Seizures, 423, 477
Self-perception/self-concept pattern,
    9b, 30–31
Self-worth, 30
Semilunar valves, 200
Senile keratosis, 78
Senile lentigines, 78
Senile ptosis, 146
Senile purpura, 78
Sensations
    decreased, 406
    testing for, 403–404, 405f
Sensitive issues, communication
    about, 12
Sensory function
    of facial nerve, 397
    of trigeminal nerve, 396
Sensory nerve assessment, 402–406
    collaborative problems in, 404
    cortical and discriminatory sensa-
        tion, 403–404, 405f
    in geriatric clients, 404
    primary sensations, 403
    teaching tips for, 406
Sensory perception, 384, 402
Sensory-perceptual pattern, 8b–9b,
    26–27
Septum, 118
Sexual abuse, 24

Sexual dysfunction, 336
Sexual education, 337
Sexual maturity ratings
  female, 324f–328f
  male, 329f–333f
Sexual organs. *See* Female genitalia;
  Male genitalia
Sexuality
  discussing with clients, 12
  and heart disease, 220
Sexuality-reproduction pattern, 8b,
  22–24
Sexually transmitted diseases (STDs),
  24, 335
Shoulder
  inspection of, 353
  palpation of, 348
  range of motion, 353, 354t, 355f
SIDS (Sudden Infant Death
  Syndrome), 508
Simian creases, 76, 77f
Sinus assessment
  equipment for, 116
  focus questions for, 116
  palpation of, 119
  percussion of, 120
Skeleton, 338, 339f. *See also*
  Musculoskeletal assessment
Skene's glands, 298f, 300
Skin assessment
  of abdomen, 276
  anatomy in, 62, 63f
  in arterial and venous insuffi-
    ciency, 250
  collaborative problems, 79
  cultural variations in, 79
  equipment for, 62, 64
  focus questions for, 64
  in geriatric clients, 78, 81
  inspection and palpation, 64–66
  in newborns, 483, 484t, 493, 506,
    507f
  and nutritional status, 18, 425
  in pediatric clients, 75–77, 80–81
  in pregnancy, 448
  primary lesions, 67f
  risk factors in, 64
  secondary lesions, 68f
  teaching tips for, 79–81
  vascular lesions, 69f
Skin cancer, 66
Skin lesions, 66
  primary, 66, 67f
  secondary, 66, 68f
  vascular, 66, 69f
Skull, 82, 83f
  of infants, 92, 93f
Sleep
  aids for, 25
  in geriatric clients, 371
  postpartum, 479
Sleep-rest pattern, 8b, 24–25
Smoking, 196, 220
Snaps, heart, 213
Social roles, 28
Speech, assessment of, 381
Spider angioma, 69f
Spider nevi, 448
Spider veins, 69f
Spinal accessory nerve, 376t, 400,
  401f
Spinal assessment, 343–348
  in newborns, 502, 503f
  normal and abnormal curves, 345f,
    368
  palpation, 344
  in pediatric clients, 368
  range of motion, 349, 350f–351f
Spinal cord, 372, 373f
Spinal nerves, 373f, 374, 377f
Spiritual beliefs, 32–33
Spirituality, discussing, 12
Spleen
  location of, 272f, 273
  palpation of, 286, 287b, 292
  in pediatric patients, 292
  percussion of, 281, 283f, 284
Splinter hemorrhages, 71, 72f
Spoon nails, 73
Sports injuries, 341
Square window sign, 490
Stance, assessment of, 343
Standard Precautions, 35
Startle reflex, 421
Stereogenesis, 404
Sternal angle, 170, 171f
Sternal notch, 203, 204f
Sternocleidomastoid muscle, 400,
  401f
Sternomastoid, 82, 83f
Sternum, 170, 171f, 194
Stethoscopes, 42
Stomach, 272f, 273
Stools, color of, 278

Stork bites, 506, 507f
Strabismus, 137
Stress tolerance, 31–32
    assessment focus for, 9b
    teaching tips for, 394
Striae gravidarum, 448
Stroke, 378, 391
Stupor, 379
Stye (hordeolum), 128f, 131
Subjective data, 1, 2t
Sudden Infant Death Syndrome
    (SIDS), 508
Sun exposure, 80
Superficial reflexes
    technique for eliciting, 414, 418
    umbilicus reflexes, 418
Superficial veins, 225, 226f
Superior vena cava, 198, 199f
Support systems, 31
Suprasternal notch, 170, 171f
Susto, 12
Synovial joints, 338, 340f
Systolic pause space, 209f, 211

T

Tachycardia, 50, 208
Tachypnea, 52t, 180t
Tandem walk, 410, 411f
Tattoos, 75
Teaching tips
    for abdomen, 294–295
    for breast self-examinations, 268
    for cardiac function, 219–222
    for cranial nerves, 402
    for ears, 168–169
    for eyes, 147–150
    for general physical health,
        60–61
    for genitourinary-reproductive sys-
        tem, 334–337
    for hair, 80
    for head and neck, 95
    for labor, 469
    for mental status, 394
    for musculoskeletal system,
        370–371
    for nails, 80
    for newborns, 508–509
    for nose and sinus, 120–121
    for nutrition, 115, 442–443
    for oral care, 113–115

    for peripheral vascular disease,
        250–251
    for postpartum assessment,
        479–481
    for prenatal fetal assessment,
        456–457
    for reflexes, 423
    for respiratory function, 195–197
    for sensory nerves, 406
    for skin, 79–81
Tear production, decreased, 149
Teeth
    anatomy of, 96, 97f, 98f
    care for, 113–114
    inspection and palpation of, 104
    and nutrition, 426
    timetable for, 98f, 112f
Temperature
    axillary, 48
    in geriatric patients, 59
    in newborns, 485, 508
    oral, 47, 55
    in pediatric patients, 55–56, 61
    postpartum, 470
    rectal, 47, 56
    teaching tips for, 60
    tympanic, 48, 49f, 56
Temporomandibular joint (TMJ),
    349, 352
Testes
    developmental stages of, 329f–333f
    palpation of, 311, 313
    self-examination of, 312b, 335
Testicular self-examination (TSE),
    312b, 335
Thoracic and lung assessment,
    170–197
    auscultation in, 184, 188–192
    collaborative problems in, 195
    cultural variations in, 195
    equipment for, 177
    focus questions for, 177
    in geriatric patients, 194, 197
    in newborns, 498, 508
    palpation in, 178, 182, 183f
    in pediatric patients, 193–194,
        196–197
    percussion in, 184, 185f–187f
    in pregnancy, 450
    risk factors in, 177
    teaching tips for, 195–197
Thoracic cage, 170, 171f

Thoracic cavity, 172, 177, 195
Thoracic expansion, 182, 183*f*, 194
Thoracic spines, 344, 346*f*–347*f*
Thorax, 170–177
  auscultation of, 184, 188–192
  cross-section of, 179*f*
  imaginary landmarks of, 172, 173*f*
  inspection of, 178
  intercostal landmarks of, 185*f*–186*f*
  lung position in, 172, 174*f*–175*f*
  major respiratory structures in,
    172, 176*f*
  musculoskeletal assessment, 349
  palpation of, 178, 182, 183*f*
  percussion of, 184, 185*f*–187*f*
  thoracic cage in, 170, 171*f*
  thoracic cavity in, 172, 177
Thought processes
  assessment of, 382–383
  disturbed, 394
Throat (pharynx), 96, 99*f*
Thyroid cartilage, 82, 83*f*
Thyroid disease, 86
Thyroid gland
  anatomy of, 82, 83*f*
  palpation of, 88, 89*f*, 90
Tibial pulse, posterior, 240, 241*f*
Tissue perfusion, 251
TMJ (temporomandibular joint), 349,
  352
Tobacco use
  and heart disease, 220
  and impaired gas exchange, 196
  and oral cancer, 95
Toenails, 78, 81
Toes
  inspection of, 359
  range of motion, 359, 360*t*, 363*f*
Toilet-training, 337
Tongue
  anatomy of, 96, 97*f*, 99f
  black hairy, 105
  inspection of, 105–107
  and nutrition, 426
Tonsillitis, 110
Tonsils, 97*f*, 99*f*, 110
Torus palatinus, 108
Trachea
  auscultation of breath sounds
    over, 188
  palpation of, 88, 90

  in respiratory anatomy, 82, 83*f*,
    172, 176*f*, 177
Trapezius muscle, 82, 400, 401*f*
Treatments
  for collaborative problems, 2
  compliance with, 17
  for nursing diagnosis, 1–2
  patient history of, 14–15
Triceps reflex, 414, 415*f*
Triceps skinfold thickness (TSF), 432,
  433*f*
Tricuspid area, palpation of, 205,
  206*f*
Tricuspid valve, 199*f*, 200
Trigeminal nerve, 375*t*, 396–397, 398*f*
Trochlear nerve, 375*t*, 395
Tropia, 137*f*
Tumors, 67*f*. *See also* Cancer
  breast, 261, 264*f*
Tuning fork, 163, 164
Turbinates, 96, 99*f*, 118
Turgor of skin, 66
Two-point discrimination, 403, 405*f*
Tympanic membrane (TM)
  anatomy of, 151, 152*f*
  assessment of, 159–163
  in elderly, 168
  otitis media, 159, 161*f*
  in pediatric clients, 166
  perforated, 162*f*, 163
  polyps in, 161*f*
  scarred, 162*f*, 163
Tympanic temperature
  in adults, 48, 49*f*
  in children, 56

U

Ulcers
  of legs, 245*t*, 246*t*, 247*f*
  skin, 68*f*
Ulnar artery, 223, 224*f*
Ulnar pulse, 231, 233*f*
Umbilical cord, 504, 505*f*
Umbilicus, inspection of, 277
Umbilicus reflexes, 418
Upper extremities
  musculoskeletal assessment of,
    353–358
  peripheral vascular assessment of,
    231, 232*f*–235*f*

range of motion, 353, 354*t*, 355*f*–357*f*
Urinary incontinence, 337
Urinary meatus, 298*f*, 299
Urination, 334
USDA (US Department of Agriculture)
   food pyramids, 436, 439*f*
   guidelines for calorie requirements, 436, 438*t*
Uterus
   involution of, 475*f*
   during labor, 459–460
   palpation of, 304
   pregnant, location of, 273, 274*f*

V

Vaginal assessment
   in genitourinary assessment, 302
   of orifice, 298*f*, 299–300, 301
   of vaginal wall, 300, 303
Vagus nerve, 376*t*, 400, 401*f*
Value-belief pattern, 9*b*, 32–33
Valves
   aortic, 200
   atrioventricular, 198, 199*f*, 200
   bicuspid, 199*f*, 200
   mitral, 199*f*, 200
   pulmonic, 199*f*, 200
   semilunar, 200
   tricuspid, 199*f*, 200
Varicose veins, 244
Vascular assessment. *See* Peripheral vascular assessment
Vascular skin lesions, 66, 69*f*
Vascular sounds, 279, 280*f*
Veins
   abdominal, 276
   in cardiac system, 198, 199*f*
   in peripheral vascular system, 224*f*, 225, 226*f*
   retinal, 141
   spider, 69*f*
   varicose, 244
Vena cava, superior and inferior, 198, 199*f*
Venous insufficiency
   impaired skin integrity in, 250

   leg ulcers in, 245*t*, 246*t*, 247*f*
   and tissue perfusion, 251
   vs. arterial insufficiency, 244, 245*t*
Venous ulcers, 245*t*, 246*t*, 247*f*
Ventricles, 198, 199*f*
Ventricular gallop, 213
Venules, retinal, 125
Vertebra prominens, 171*f*, 172
Vertebral line, 172, 173*f*
Vesicles, 67*f*
Vesicular breath sounds, 189, 190*f*
Visceral organs, 269, 272*f*, 273, 274*f*
Visceral pleura, 172, 176*f*
Vision. *See also* Eye assessment
   acuity tests for, 133, 145
   impaired, 149
   peripheral, 134
Vital signs, 45
Vitamin B_{12} deficiency, 105
Vitiligo, 65
Voice sounds, altered, 192
Vomiting, in children, 295

W

Waist-to-hip ratio, 430
Weber test, 163, 164*f*
Weight
   cultural variations in, 59
   guideline questions on, 18
   ideal body weight, 370, 427, 429
   measurement of, 427, 428*t*
   of newborns, 485, 486*f*, 495*f*
   of pediatric clients, 58
   in physical survey, 45, 51
   postpartum, 470
   in pregnancy, 446, 447*f*
Wellness diagnoses, 1, 3*t*
Wheals, 67*f*
Wheezes, 189, 190*f*, 191, 194
Whispered pectoriloquy, 192
Work
   guideline questions for, 21
   roles and responsibilities in, 28
Wrist
   inspection of, 353
   palpation of, 358
   range of motion, 353, 354*t*, 356*f*